Biomaterials, Medical Devices and Tissue Engineering

Biomaterials, Medical Devices and Tissue Engineering:

An Integrated Approach

Frederick H. Silver PhD

Professor of Pathology
Robert Wood Johnson Medical School
Director, Graduate Program in Biomedical Engineering
Rutgers University
New Jersey, USA

CHAPMAN & HALL
London · Glasgow · New York · Tokyo · Melbourne · Madras

Published by Chapman & Hall, 2–6 Boundary Row, London SE1 8HN, UK

Chapman & Hall, 2–6 Boundary Row, London SE1 8HN, UK

Blackie Academic & Professional, Wester Cleddens Road, Bishopbriggs, Glasgow G64 2NZ, UK

Chapman & Hall Inc., One Penn Plaza, 41st Floor, New York NY10119, USA

Chapman & Hall Japan, Thomson Publishing Japan, Hirakawacho Nemoto Building, 6F 1-7-11 Hirakawa-cho, Chiyoda-ku, Tokyo 102, Japan

Chapman & Hall Australia, Thomas Nelson Australia, 102 Dodds Street, South Melbourne, Victoria 3205, Australia

Chapman & Hall India, R. Seshadri, 32 Second Main Road, CIT East, Madras 600 035, India

First edition 1994

© 1994 Chapman & Hall

Commissioned by Technical Communications (Publishing) Ltd

Typeset in 10 on 12pt Times by Fleetlines Typesetters Limited, Southend-on-Sea, UK

Printed in Great Britain at Clays Ltd, St. Ives plc, Bungay, Suffolk

ISBN 0 412 41260 8

Apart from any fair dealing for the purposes of research or private study, or criticism or review, as permitted under the UK Copyright Designs and Patents Act, 1988, this publication may not be reproduced, stored or transmitted, in any form or by any means, without the prior permission in writing of the publishers, or in the case of reprographic reproduction only in accordance with the terms of the licences issued by the Copyright Licensing Agency in the UK, or in accordance with the terms of licenses issued by the appropriate Reproduction Rights Organization outside the UK. Enquiries concerning reproduction outside the terms stated here should be sent to the publishers at the London address printed on this page.

The publisher makes no representation, express or implied, with regard to the accuracy of the information contained in this book and cannot accept any legal responsibility or liability for any errors or omissions that may be made.

A catalogue record for this book is available from the British Library
Library of Congress Cataloging-in-Publication data
Silver, Frederick H., 1949–
    Biomaterials, medical devices, and tissue engineering : an integrated approach / Frederick H. Silver. – 1st ed.
        p. cm.
    Includes bibliographical references and index.
    ISBN 0–412–41260–8 (alk. paper)
    1. Implants, Artificial–Materials. I. Title.
    [DNLM: 1. Biocompatible Materials. 2. Implants, Artificial.
    3. Biomedical Engineering. QT 34 S587ba 1993]
RD132.S55 1993
617.9'5–dc20
DNLM/DLC
for Library of Congress   93-23542
                                                                          CIP

∞ Printed on permanent acid-free text paper, manufactured in accordance with ANSI/NISO Z39.48-1992 and ANSI/NISO Z39.48-1984 (Permanence of Paper).

Intro & summary

Contents

1	**Scope and markets for medical implants**	**1**
	1.1 Introduction	1
	1.2 Markets for medical implants	2
	1.3 Materials of construction	4
	1.4 Pre-clinical and clinical biocompatibility evaluation	25
	1.5 Biology of transplantation of tissue products matching	29
	1.6 Federal Food and Drug Administration (FDA) regulations	38
	1.7 Summary	44
2	**Wound dressings and skin replacement**	**46**
	2.1 Introduction	46
	2.2 Biochemistry of skin	51
	2.3 Mechanical properties of skin	57
	2.4 Repair of skin	62
	2.5 Incidence of skin wounds	66
	2.6 Wound dressings	73
	2.7 Summary	91
3	**Replacement of skeletal tissues**	**92**
	3.1 Introduction	92
	3.2 Anatomy and physiology of tendons and ligaments	93
	3.3 Biochemistry and biophysics	96
	3.4 Mechanical properties of ligament	100
	3.5 Repair of ligament	103
	3.6 Clinical evaluation of ligament function	105
	3.7 ACL reconstruction using biological and synthetic materials	107
	3.8 Total joint replacement	113
	3.9 Materials used in total knee replacement (TKR)	116
	3.10 Summary	118
4	**Biomaterials used in ophthalmology**	**120**
	4.1 Introduction	120
	4.2 Anatomy of the eye	121
	4.3 Biochemistry of eye structures	123
	4.4 Mechanical properties of ocular tissues	125
	4.5 Corneal wound healing	126
	4.6 Viscoelastic solutions	126
	4.7 Intraocular lenses	143
	4.8 Contact lens materials	145

vi Contents

	4.9	Eye shields	148
	4.10	Other ocular materials	149
	4.11	Summary	151

5 Cardiovascular implants — **153**
- 5.1 Introduction — 153
- 5.2 Physiology and anatomy of vessel wall and heart valve — 153
- 5.3 Anatomy and physiology of blood components — 164
- 5.4 Mechanical properties of aorta and valve — 168
- 5.5 Repair of cardiovascular tissue — 180
- 5.6 Pathophysiology of aortic and valvular diseases — 181
- 5.7 Aorta and heart valve replacements — 183
- 5.8 Cardiac valve replacements — 189
- 5.9 Summary — 192

6 Facial implants — **194**
- 6.1 Introduction — 194
- 6.2 Biochemistry of facial tissues — 199
- 6.3 Mechanical properties of facial tissues — 200
- 6.4 Repair of facial structures — 204
- 6.5 Types of procedures performed in facial plastic surgery — 206
- 6.6 Synthetic implant materials — 213
- 6.7 Solid facial implants — 216
- 6.8 Mesh materials — 219
- 6.9 Summary — 219

7 Dental implants — **220**
- 7.1 Introduction — 220
- 7.2 Impression materials — 221
- 7.3 Denture base resins — 225
- 7.4 Restorative resins — 225
- 7.5 Cements for restorations — 229
- 7.6 Dental porcelains — 231
- 7.7 Base metal alloys for dental castings — 231
- 7.8 Other materials, collagen — 232
- 7.9 Summary — 235

8 Breast implants — **236**
- 8.1 Introduction — 236
- 8.2 Anatomy and physiology of the breast — 237
- 8.3 Psychology of breast augmentation — 239
- 8.4 Types of breast implants — 240
- 8.5 Complications associated with use of breast implants — 243
- 8.6 Complications with poly(urethane)-covered implants — 247

	8.7	Implant placement	248
	8.8	Current concerns	248
	8.9	Summary	249
9	**510 (k) and PMA regulatory filings in the US**		**250**
	9.1	Introduction	250
	9.2	Components of a 510 (k) regulatory filing	252
	9.3	Premarket approval (PMA) application	255

References   **262**

Index   **301**

1.
Scope and Markets For Medical Implants

1.1 Introduction

Medical devices are used routinely in the practice of medicine not only in the United States but throughout the world. The use of polymers, metals, ceramics and composite materials in the formulation of medical devices dates back centuries to the use of plant and animal skins for the amelioration of pathological conditions that resulted from mechanical, chemical or pathogenic trauma to tissues and organs. The word 'device' as defined by the US Federal Drug and Food Administration (FDA) includes any instrument, apparatus, implement, machine, contrivance, implant, *in vitro* reagent, or a combination of these elements that is intended for diagnosis, prevention or treatment of a disease (Phelps and Dormer, 1986). Materials such as synthetic and natural polymers, metals, ceramics, and composites of these materials are by themselves not considered devices and are approved by the FDA when formulated into an end-use device. Prior to 1976, the use of medical devices was unregulated in the US. In 1976, the US Congress enacted the Medical Device Amendments to the Federal Food, Drug, and Cosmetic Act of 1938, which called for the regulation of three classes of devices. Class I devices are those that present little or no risk to the user. Class II devices present some risk and are subject to performance standards while class III devices are the most dangerous and require pre-market approval prior to their widespread distribution. Most of the biomaterials that we will discuss in this book are used in class II and III medical devices and require extensive safety and effectiveness testing prior to commercial sale. The purpose of this book is to review the types of materials that are used to replace or augment tissues and organs of the human body, and to look to the future in predicting the directions for new material development.

In order to properly assess the state-of-the-art in tissue replacement and augmentation, it is first necessary to carefully review the physiology, anatomy, biochemistry and biomechanics of normal tissues as well as the pathophysiological changes that require intervention to restore normal function. In addition, since most medical implants require surgical intervention for installation, it is necessary to be familiar with the repair and regeneration responses that result before it is possible to define the biocompatibility of an implant material.

The biocompatibilty and engineering uses of devices are intimately associated with the chemical and mechanical properties of the materials used in device construction. Therefore, we will briefly review the relationship between chemical and physical structures and mechanical properties of implant materials prior to establishing the utility of each type of material in medical applications. After reviewing this material, it will be easier to understand the types of pre-clinical biocompatibility tests that are required before clinical tests can begin.

1.2 Markets for medical implants

Development of biomaterials used in medical devices has occurred in response to the growing numbers of patients afflicted with traumatic and non-traumatic conditions. As the population grows older, there is an increased need for medical devices to replace damaged or worn tissues.

Many of us are aware of the trauma associated with severe burn injuries that can be a result of thermal, chemical and electrical etiologies. About two million people suffer burns each year and 100 000 (Table 1.1) of these patients require hospitalization (Nicosia and Petro, 1983). In the case of severe burns, the immediate problem is to stabilize the patient's breathing, respiration and cardiac output. Once the patient is stabilized, it is critical to remove dead tissue from the wounds and to apply appropriate wound dressings and bandages. Ultimately, the degree of scarring and disfigurement is related to the area and depth of the burn injury as well as the time it takes to regenerate the epithelial layer of the skin. Active burn dressings that promote skin regeneration facilitate healing and help to minimize long-term adverse cosmetic effects.

A far more pressing problem that results in skin loss, is the formation of bed sores (skin loss due to ulceration) in patients who experience prolonged bed rest or immobilization. This problem is complicated further by a weak heart. Approximately eight million (Table 1.1) people in the US are affected by this condition. Deep skin wounds that remain unhealed for prolonged periods of time result in systemic infection and even death. This problem is severe in 3.7 million diabetic patients primarily because skin wound healing is impaired by this condition. These data indicate the significant need for burn and wound dressings.

Rupture of the anterior cruciate ligament (ACL) occurs during sports activities and results in impaired ability to make fine cutting motions. The anterior cruciate ligament is one of two ligaments that connect the femur to the tibia through the knee joint and limit rotational and translational motion of the tibia with respect to the femur. Rupture of the ACL leads to loss of stability of the knee joint and a loss of athletic ability. Approximately 150 000 people each year suffer traumatic injury to the

Table 1.1 Number of yearly implant procedures in the US*

Type of procedure	Number in million
Bed sores	8.0
Breast prostheses	0.240
Burns	0.100
Corneal grafts	0.0369
Dental implant	0.045
Diabetic skin wounds	3.7
Fixation devices	0.100
Heart valves	0.43
Hip and knee implants	0.245
Intraocular lens	1.2
Skin excision	0.59
Tendon and ligament replacements	0.150
Total hip	0.170
Total knee	0.100
Vascular grafts	0.200
Vascular bypass grafts	0.194

* adapted from Biomedical Business International, Tustin, CA, October 22, 1986, April 7, 1988, May 10, 1988, July 20, 1989, August 17, 1989, December 7, 1989, March 23, 1990.

ACL. Repair to the ACL is normally achieved using either biological or synthetic replacements.

As the average age of our population increases, more and more people suffer from osteoarthritis and rheumatoid arthritis. These two conditions lead to joint disease and the inability to walk effectively without excruciating pain. Approximately 245 000 US citizens each year have a total knee or hip replaced using implants that are composites of metal, polymers and ceramics. Steady growth in the number of joint replacements is expected over the next decade.

Ophthalmologists have aggressively pioneered the use of medical devices including lens implants, viscoelastic solutions for eye surgery, corneal transplants and protective corneal shields. About 1.2 million implants are used each year to replace intraocular lenses that are removed because of decreased transparency.

Debakey in the 1950s pioneered the use of vascular grafts made of synthetic polymers to replace the aorta in patients with pathologic conditions. Since the 1950s biologic and synthetic grafts have been routinely used in the clinic for replacement of the thoracic and abdominal aorta. Only vessel grafts are used for bypassing blocked coronary arteries. Approximately 194 000 cases of coronary artery bypass are reported each year in the

4 Scope and markets for medical implants

US as well as 200 000 cases where a graft is used to replace the aorta. Since coronary artery disease is a major cause of death in the US, vigorous growth of the market for synthetic small diameter vascular prostheses is expected.

Facial implants are becoming widely used by surgeons for reconstructive as well as purely cosmetic reasons. As our society continues to have a heightened awareness of cosmetic surgery, the number of facial cosmetic procedures and the number of implants will increase.

Although the number of cavities and dental procedures conducted in the US each year has been limited by the introduction of fluoridated water and routine prophylactic cleanings, there are still about 45 000 dental implant procedures conducted each year. Far more procedures are conducted that involve filling and crown materials. Biomaterials scientists are continually evaluating new inert high strength composite materials to replace conventional amalgams and other metal containing implants.

Implants are used for cosmetic and reconstructive surgery of the breast. Each year approximately 240 000 surgical procedures are conducted involving breast implants. Recently, concern has been expressed in scientific literature over the problems associated with use of silicone gel filled breast implants.

Only a few of the procedures conducted in the US each year that involve medical implants have been discussed. The wound care market alone totals almost US $1.2 billion a year. Clearly the economic and medical impact of medical devices is very large and underscores the importance of continued research and development to improve the quality of health care. Because of the size and importance of the field, it is not possible in this text to cover all implant applications in detail. Therefore, a few areas of implant usage have been selected that can be covered in detail in a text of several hundred pages.

1.3 Materials of construction

All medical implants are composed of either polymers, metals, ceramics, or composites of these materials. Tissue replacement with synthetics is achieved by selecting the material that has physical properties most similar to those of natural tissue. Table 1.2 lists the physical properties of soft and hard tissues as well as typical ranges observed for polymers, metals, ceramics and composites. For soft tissue applications (skin, tendon, ligament, breast, eye, vascular system, and face) natural and synthetic polymers are used to replace the function of tissues damaged as a result of genetic or acquired diseases as well as traumatic injury. Metals, ceramics and composites are widely used for replacement or reinforcement of bone and dentin. A brief review of the structure and properties of each of these materials is given below.

Soft tissues have strengths and tensile moduli that are normally below 100 MPa and therefore polymers with similar strengths and slightly higher

Table 1.2 Physical properties of tissues and materials used for their replacement

Material	Ultimate strength (MPa)	Modulus (MPa)	Ref.
Soft tissue			
Arterial wall	0.5–1.72	1.0	Silver 1987
Hyaline cartilage	1.3–18	0.4–19	Silver 1987
Skin	2.5–16	6–40	Silver 1987
Tendon/ligament	30–300	65–2500	Silver 1987
Hard tissue (bone)			
Cortical	30–211	16–20 (GPa)	Cowin 1989
Cancellous	51–193	4.6–15 (GPa)	Cowin 1989
Polymers			
Synthetic rubber	10–12	4	Black 1988
Glassy	25–100	1.6–2.6 (GPa)	Black 1988
Crystalline	22–40	0.015–1 (GPa)	Black 1988
Metal alloys			
Steel	480–655	193 (GPa)	Black 1988
Cobalt	655–1400	195 (GPa)	Black 1988
Platinum	152–485	147 (GPa)	Black 1988
Titanium	550–860	100–105 (GPa)	Black 1988
Ceramics			
Oxides	90–380 (GPa)	160–4000 (GPa)	Heimke 1986
Hydroxylapatite	600	19 (GPa)	Heimke 1986
Composites			
Fibres	0.09–4.5 (GPa)	62–577 (GPa)	Black 1988
Matrices	41–106	0.3–3.1	Black 1988

moduli are most frequently used to replace these tissues. In contrast, bone has a slightly higher tensile strength while its modulus is a factor of ten higher than that found for soft tissues. Since polymers do not have moduli above 10 GPa, metal alloys, ceramics and fibre reinforced composites are used to replace bone. Below we consider each classification of materials that are used as replacements for soft and hard tissues.

1.3.1 Polymers

Polymers have physical properties that most closely resemble those of soft tissues and therefore this class of materials is used extensively to replace the function of tissues including skin, tendon, cartilage, vessel wall, lens, and mammary tissue. On a molecular level, tissues are composed of polymers that are organized into unique hierarchical structures. The properties reflect the content and arrangement of the constituent molecules.

Polymer formation and structure

Polymers by definition are molecules that are made up of a unit or units that are repeated many times. These units are covalently connected forming a large molecule commonly referred to as a macromolecule. Synthetic polymers are synthesized by either **addition polymerization** that occurs by growth of a polymer chain using a free radical mechanism or by **condensation polymerization** of two bi- or multi-functional molecules (Figure 1.1). Condensation polymerization yields a by-product in addition to the growing polymer chain.

A number of different physical variations can exist for even a single chemistry of a polymer chain. These variations arise because the polymer chain can be **linear** if the reactants are bifunctional or **branched** if one of the reactants is tri-functional or multi-fuctional (Figure 1.2). If the reactants have an asymmetric carbon, (one that has four different groups bonded to it) and they are able to react in different physical forms with the growing polymer, then the chain can be regular (**isotactic**). If the monomers add in alternating configurations, then it is termed atactic (Figure 1.3). If the chain is composed of random sequences of both physical arrangements then it is termed **syndiotactic**.

The three-dimensional form of a polymer chain is dictated by the ability of the individual units that compose the chain to freely rotate about the backbone. The size of the repeat unit is indirectly proportional to the ability

Figure 1.1. Types of polymerization processes.

Addition	$H_2C=CH_2 + H_2C=CH_2 \longrightarrow$	$-CH_2-CH_2-CH_2-$
Condensation	HOOC-R-COOH + HOOC-R-COOH $\longrightarrow$	-CO-R-CO- + H_2O

Figure 1.2 Types of Polymer Chain Physical Structures.

Bifunctional reactant

    A-B + A-B $\longrightarrow$ -A-B-A-B- linear chain

Trifunctional reactant

    A-B-B + A-B-A $\longrightarrow$ A
                                          B
                                          A   branched chain
                                          |
                                   A-B-B

Monomers that have two functional groups react to form a linear chain. In comparison, if one monomer is trifunctional the chain can be branched.

Figure 1.3 Chain structural differences in polymers formed from monomers with an asymmetric carbon.

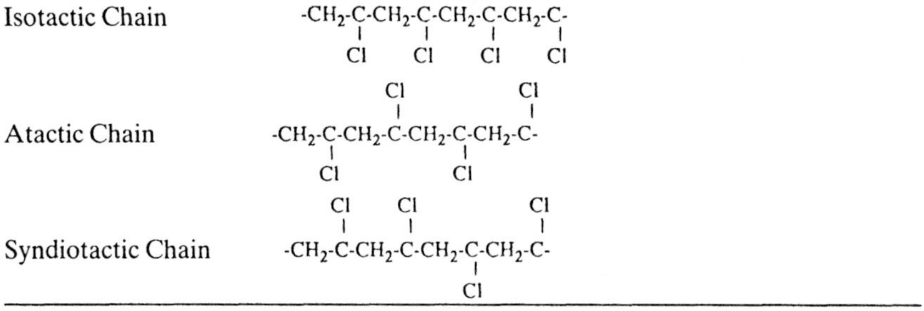

Isotactic Chain	-CH$_2$-C-CH$_2$-C-CH$_2$-C-CH$_2$-C-
	     | | | |
	     Cl Cl Cl Cl

Atactic Chain	Cl Cl
	     | |
	-CH$_2$-C-CH$_2$-C-CH$_2$-C-CH$_2$-C-
	     | |
	     Cl Cl

Syndiotactic Chain	Cl Cl Cl
	     | | |
	-CH$_2$-C-CH$_2$-C-CH$_2$-C-CH$_2$-C-
	                      |
	                      Cl

Isotactic chains have functional groups that are superimposed by chain translation on one side of the backbone (i.e. Cl shown below), while in an atactic chain the functional group alternates. In a syndiotactic chain the functional groups are randomly arranged.

of the backbone of the chain to undergo free rotation. Chains with large bulky side groups, rings that make up part of the backbone, or double bonds that are in the backbone do not undergo free rotation and are therefore stiff (Figure 1.4). The flexibility of a polymer chain is proportional to Boltzmann's constant, k, times the natural log of the number of allowable configurations (*omega*) of the backbone. In thermodynamic terms the entropy, S, is a measure of the chain randomness and is proportional to the chain flexibility.

Mathematically,

$$S = k \ln (omega) \qquad (1.1)$$

The relationship between entropy and the **number of conformations** (*omega*) of a polymer chain are given by equation 1.1. The number of allowable conformations is obtained by comparing the theoretically allowable conformations, found by computer simulation, and those determined from x-ray diffraction on polymer crystals. Silver (1987) goes into further

Figure 1.4 Conditions for limited rotation around a chain backbone.

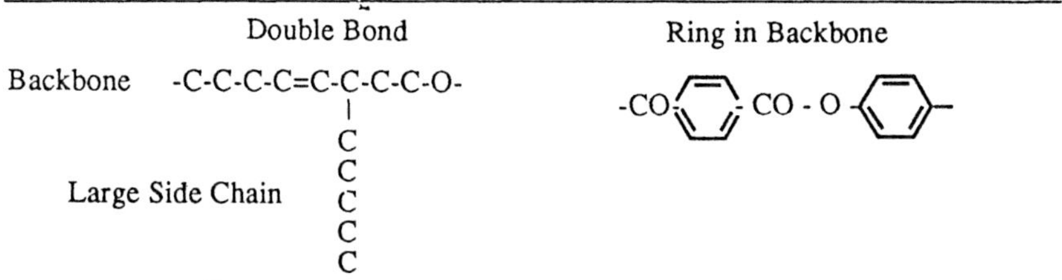

	Double Bond	Ring in Backbone

Backbone	-C-C-C-C=C-C-C-C-O-
	                |
	                C
		-CO-⟨ ⟩-CO-O-⟨ ⟩-

Large Side Chain	C C C C	

Typical backbone sequence showing a double bond, aromatic rings and large side chains all of which limit free rotation about the backbone of the chain.

details as to how conformational maps are made for each chemical unit that is repeated in a polymer chain.

Polymer chains with large bulky side groups are not flexible and form **glasses** without long range order at low temperature. In comparison, flexible chains can pack into **crystals** that stabilize polymers into three-dimensional arrays. At room temperature, polymer chains can be flexible or rigid depending on the bulkiness of the side chains. Polymers with large side chains that are glasses at room temperature become flexible when heated. Addition of thermal energy initiates backbone rotation.

Polymers used in medical devices

Polymeric materials are used in the construction of medical devices that are found in almost every phase of medicine and dentistry. From the construction of blood bags to breast protheses (Table 1.3), polymers have found applications in every specialty area and continue to be the most widely used material in health care. They include **condensation polymers** typically formed from reaction of alcohols and acids to form poly (esters), reaction of acids and amines to form poly(amides) and reaction of acids and a combination of these reactants to form poly(urethanes). **Addition polymers** are formed by free radical polymerization of unsaturated compounds. Polymerization requires initiation by a free radical mechanism, propagation of the chain and free radical termination. Typical addition polymers include poly(ethylene), poly(methyl methacrylate), poly(vinyl chloride), and poly(ethylene terephthalate). The average chain length of these materials is determined by methods described in Table 1.4. Processing of polymers into end-products involves compounding with several other ingredients listed in Table 1.5.

Table 1.3 Typical polymers used in medical devices*

Polymer	Medical device applications
Poly(ethylene)	Hip, tendon/ligament implants and facial implants
Pol(ethylene terephthalate)	Aortic, tendon/ligament and facial implants
Poly(methyl methacrylate)	Intraocular lens, contact lenses and bone cement
Poly(dimethyl siloxane)	Breast, facial and tendon implants
Poly(urethane)	Breast, vascular and skin implants

* adapted based on Batich and DePalma, 1992; Black, 1988; Dardik, 1986; DeVore, 1991; Friedman and Ferkel, 1988; Glasgold and Silver, 1991; and Rovee, 1991

Table 1.4 Molecular weight characterization of polymers*

Method	Molecular weight	Comments
Chromatography	Weight average	Number average can be calculated, shape dependent
Light scattering	Weight average	Angular and concentration dependence
Osmometry	Number average	Affected by counter ions
Ultracentrifugation	Weight average	Number average, can be calculated
Viscometry	Viscosity average	Depends on shape

* Silver, 1987 for additional details

Fabrication of medical devices

The fabrication of polymers into end-use medical devices involves compounding, characterization of the raw polymer, processing into final device form, sterilization and final characterization. Most polymeric materials are synthesized in large batches for general use and are not produced solely for medical applications. These polymers contain additives that enhance the polymerization process (Table 1.5). In addition, a number of additives are used in a process termed compounding, which enhances the mechanical properties and simplifies formation of complex shapes.

Raw polymer must be characterized to validate the chemistry of the backbone as well as that of the surface. This can be accomplished by mass and infrared spectroscopy. Once the chemistry of the repeat unit and surface have been characterized, it is necessary to identify the distribution of chain lengths that make up the sample. This is accomplished by determination of several average molecular weights. The number average molecular weight can be determined by gel permeation chromatography, ultracentrifugation and by measurement of the osmotic pressure. It represents the molecular weight of the average chain and reflects the chain size (Table 1.4). The distribution of chain lengths that make up a polymer cannot be determined from a single molecular weight determination.

Table 1.5 Additives used to process polymers into engineering materials*

Additive	Function
Accelerators	Increase kinetics of crosslinking
Antioxidants	Minimize cracking of device when exposed to oxidants
Crosslinking agent	Prevents viscous flow of final product
Plasticizers	Facilitate flow of polymer into desired shape
Reinforcing agents	Used to improve mechanical properties of polymers

* Black, 1988

To better evaluate the distribution of lengths, the weight average molecular weight is determined from light scattering, or based on calculations made from ultracentrifugation and chromatography data (Table 1.4). The weight average molecular weight is an average calculated using the molecular weight of each chain as the weighing factor. A ratio of the weight average and the number average molecular weights, termed **polydispersity index**, gives a measure of the distribution of chain lengths. If this ratio is one then all the chains are of uniform length. If the ratio is greater than one then a mixture of large and small chains exists. Polymers with polydispersity indices of twenty or greater are processed using conventional moulding techniques more easily than polymers that have lower indices. Some polymers that have very high molecular weights are formed into final shapes by fusing fine powders under heat and pressure because they do not flow evenly using conventional injection and compression moulding equipment.

Placticizers are low molecular weight compounds that enable individual macromolecular chains to exhibit backbone flexibility under applied stresses. Typically, plasticizers are less expense than polymers and are added as extenders to lower the cost of the final product (Table 1.5). However, these low molecular weight additives may leach out of the finished product if it is in contact with biological fluids for long periods of time. Therefore, care must be taken to select the appropriate plasticizer/polymer system.

Fillers, including mould release agents as well as antioxidants are added to polymers to enhance mechanical properties, facilitate processing and prevent product breakdown during storage. However, these agents can leach from the implant and may have deleterious side effects if used in permanent implants.

Polymer processing into a wide variety of shapes occurs by extrusion, moulding, spinning, weaving, knitting and casting techniques (Table 1.6). **Extrusion** is a process by which polymers are heated until they become viscous liquids and then fed using a moving screw through an aperture. If the aperture is an annulus then a tube results. Other shapes are formed by changing the geometry of the aperture. **Moulding** involves either direct placement or injection of the polymer into a mould in association with heat and pressure to allow the polymer to conform to the size and shape of the mould. In some cases the shape is made using air pressure to inflate the polymer. Polymer fibres are formed by either melt or solvent **spinning** techniques. In melt spinning, a polymer is heated until it is a viscous fluid and then is forced through an orifice to form a fibre. The fibre is solidified by cooling and is collected as continuous monofilament. Monofilament is then knitted, woven or formed into fabrics. Solution spinning involves forming a viscous liquid by mixing the polymer with a solvent and pumping it through an orifice at which time it comes into contact with a poor solvent causing

Table 1.6 Processes used to form polymeric devices*

Process	Type of device
Extrusion	Fibre, tube, sheet and other cross-sections
Moulding	Bottles, sheets, connectors, syringes and complex shapes
Spinning	Fibre
Weaving	Fabric (woven and non-wovens)
Knitting	Fabric
Casting	Film, sheet

* Black, 1988, Rodriguez, 1982

coagulation. Solvent **casting** involves solidification of a polymer solution by allowing the solvent to evaporate. Polymeric materials can also be processed using lathes, grinders and shapers in a similar manner to metals.

Crystalline polymers can be heated above their crystalline melting temperatures and processed by one of the above techniques. Upon cooling, crystals reform providing mechanical reinforcement. If the crystals are small then the polymer can be transparent or translucent. If the crystals are larger than about $0.025 \mu m$ then the polymer is translucent or opaque. The chains of crystalline polymers do not always need to be crosslinked together unless the material is constantly loaded for long periods of time. However, the chains of non-crystalline polymers need to be cross-linked into a three-dimensional network because the polymer will behave like a viscous liquid and flow under applied loads. Crosslinking agents may be added to the polymer prior to final processing or the polymer may be end-treated prior to packaging.

Polymer sterilization may be conducted on the final product or it may be accomplished by fabrication in a clean room using liquids that are sterile filtered. Typically, final product end-sterilization is achieved by exposing the material to gamma radiation (2.5 Mrads is a standard dosage), ethylene oxide or formaldehyde. Treatment with ethylene oxide and formaldehyde may lead to adverse biological reactions such as anaphylaxis and immune responses. In some cases an antibiotic coating is impregnated on the device to minimize the risk of infection.

Mechanical properties of polymers
Mechanical properties of polymers are a consequence of the degree of crystallinity and the transition temperature at which they change from a viscoelastic material to a rigid glass. Typical properties for polymers in comparison to natural tissues, metals, ceramics and composites are given in Table 1.2.

1.3.2 Metals

Although polymers are easy to process into a variety of end-use sizes and shapes, their moduli and strengths are much lower than those of bone and dentin. Therefore, hard tissue replacement is achieved using materials with higher values of the modulus and strength. These materials include metals, ceramics and composites.

Metals have a large range of applications including devices for fracture fixation, partial and total joint replacement, surgical instruments, external splints, braces and traction apparatus as well as dental amalgams (Table 1.7). The high modulus and yield point coupled with the ductility of metals makes them suitable for bearing large loads without leading to large deformations and permanent dimensional changes. They can be processed into final parts using a number of conventional techniques and have good resistance to degradation in a biological environment.

Structure of metals

Metals are crystalline materials built up by the repeat of a unit cell containing a specific number of atoms in defined positions. Several types of unit cells which maximize the number of nearest neighbour atomic contacts are frequently observed including: face-centred cubic (FCC), hexagonal-close packed (HCP) and body-centred cubic structures (BCC). Figure 1.5 shows the location of the atoms in the FCC, HCP and BCC structures. These structures are characterized by the distance between nearest neighbours and the distance between two unit cells. This depends on the atoms in the unit cell and the type of unit cell.

Unit cells are formed when metal atoms in a liquid come close enough to form physical bonds through van der Waals attractions. This is followed by sharing of valence electrons. The atoms reach an equilibrium separation distance, that can be computed based on the Lenard-Jones 6-12 potential energy function, and then form **metallic bonds** by sharing secondary or outer

Table 1.7 Medical applications of metals*

Application	Metal
Dental appliances	Cobalt-chromium alloys
Conductive leads	Titanium alloys
Fracture plates	Stainless steel (austenitic), Cobalt-chromium alloys
Heart valves	Cobalt-chromium alloys
Joint components	Cobalt-chromium alloys, titanium alloys
Nails	Cobalt-chromium alloys, titanium alloys
Pacemaker cases	Titanium alloys
Screws	Cobalt-chromium alloys, titanium alloys

* adapted based on Black, 1988

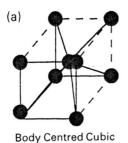
(a) Body Centred Cubic

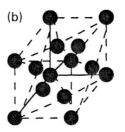
(b) Face Centred Cubic

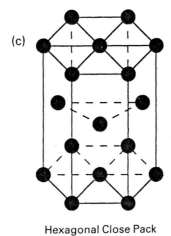
(c) Hexagonal Close Pack

Figure 1.5 Diagram illustrating atomic positions in BCC, FCC and HCP crystal structures: (a) body centred cubic; (b) face-centred cubic; and (c) hexagonal close pack.

electrons. The ability of metals to conduct electricity is a consequence of the rapid electron movement through a metal.

In response to mechanical loading, metal atoms if unimpeded move into positions occupied by other atoms in the crystalline lattice. Deformation is only limited by the imperfections in the lattice. The limits of a perfect crystal lattice are defined by **grain boundaries**. Grain boundaries are the points at which neighbouring crystals come together. Crystal imperfections are concentrated at the interface between neighbouring grains.

Deformation of metals initially results in stretching of the bonds that hold the atoms together. This generates a linear response between stress and strain that is the atomic consequence of Hooke's law. As illustrated by Figure 1.6, *Hooke's law* mathematically describes the linear relationship between stress and strain as well as the reversibility of this relationship. On the atomic level, the reversibility is associated with the reestablishment of the equilibrium interatomic distances. The deformability of a metal can be modified by mixing metal atoms of two or more sizes to form an **alloy**. The addition of carbon to iron based alloys provides resistance to atomic sliding within the crystal lattice. **Work hardening** and control of crystal lattice size are two other mechanisms that limit the deformability of metals. During work hardening, atomic sliding occurs as a result of deformation of the metal which limits further atomic sliding. If the crystal lattice is limited in its size then deformation is also limited.

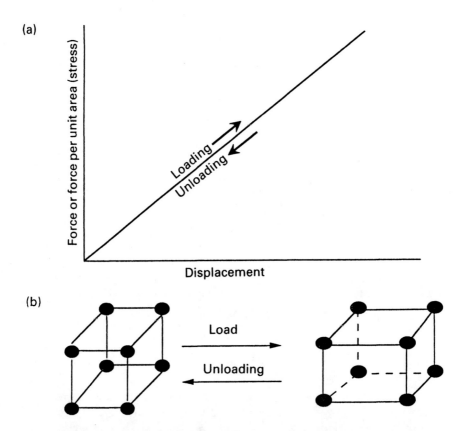

Figure 1.6 Mechanical and atomic aspects of Hooke's law: (a) schematic diagram illustrating the linear relationship between force and stress and displacement for metals; (b) during loading the atomic bond distances are stretched (bottom) while during unloading the atomic distances return to normal which is mathematically represented by the Lenard-Jones 6-12 potential energy function.

Atoms used in the formation of metallic implants include aluminium (Al), cobalt (Co), chromium (Cr), iridium (Ir), iron (Fe), manganese (Mn), molybdenum (Mo), nickel (Ni), niobium (Nb), palladium (Pd), platinum (Pt), tantalum (Ta), titanium (Ti), vanadium (V), tungsten (W), and zirconium (Zr) as tabulated in Table 1.8. The atoms are either alloying elements or elements that make up the base metals. Stainless steels are composed of iron and carbon atoms in the presence of several alloying elements including chromium, nickel, manganese, molybdenum and vanadium. These metals are used for fracture hardware, braces, and surgical instruments (Black, 1988). Cobalt-based alloys include chromium, manganese, tungsten, molybdenum, nickel, niobium, and tantalum and are used for the construction of joint replacement components. Titanium-base alloys include aluminium, vanadium, iron, niobium and zirconium and are used to construct hardware for fracture fixation and joint component replacement. Finally, platinum or precious alloys, include alloying elements such as iridium and palladium are used in construction of electrodes.

Engineering of alloys

Alloy formation begins with extraction of ore which is a compound of metals with oxygen, and other elements. These unwanted elements must be removed before the metals can be melted together, under conditions that prevent side reactions to form the alloys of interest.

Table 1.8 Elements found in metallic implants*

Element	Abbreviation	Atomic number	Weight	Application
Aluminium	Al	13	26.98	alloying element
Cobolt	Co	27	58.93	base element
Chromium	Cr	24	52.0	alloying element
Iridium	Ir	77	192.2	alloying element
Iron	Fe	26	55.85	base element
Manganese	Mn	25	55.94	alloying element
Molybdenum	Mo	42	95.94	alloying element
Nickel	Ni	28	58.71	alloying element
Niobium	Nb	41	92.91	alloying element
Palladium	Pb	46	106.4	alloying element
Platinum	Pt	78	195.1	base element
Tantalum	Ta	73	181.0	alloying element
Titanium	Ti	22	47.90	base element
Tungsten	W	74	183.9	alloying element
Vanadium	V	23	50.94	alloying element
Zirconium	Zr	40	91.22	alloying element

* adapted based on Black, 1988

The formation of alloys occurs by first melting two metals at a temperature above the melting temperature of both metals. Under these conditions the metals form a homogeneous mixture. If these two metals form homogeneous crystalline phases on cooling, then the product is referred to as an **alloy**. This alloy may have different **phases**; each phase has a distinct atomic composition. The grain size of each phase can be increased by heating the alloy to a temperature below the melting temperature of the phase for a predetermined period of time. This process is called **heat treatment** or **annealing**. Once the heat treatment step is completed the alloy is rapidly cooled, a process termed **quenching**. Liquids are normally poured into moulds to be **cast** into ingots or parts for the fabrication of medical devices.

Casting of an alloy into bars, rods and other shapes that are then machined into medical devices is rarely done. Alloys are infrequently cast in temperature resistant dies in which many parts can be manufactured at one time.

Another process more frequently used involves the production of a wax model of the shape that is placed in an inexpensive mould material. The mould is heated to strengthen it and to vapourize the wax. After the part is formed, the mould is broken to remove the part and then it is discarded.

Cast alloys can then be processed in a number of ways depending on the desired mechanical properties of the final product (Table 1.9). **Drawing** is used to pull an ingot into wire or into sheets of metal. A sheet can then be pressed by placing it between a male and female die to form a cuplike structure. Structures can be hardened by **machining** or **forging**. Forging involves heating a metal and then using a series of pairs of dies to change stepwise the shape of the part. If an ingot can be ground to form micron sized particles then the particles can be placed in a mould and heated until the particles fuse. This process is termed powder metallurgy. Two parts with similar composition can be joined by local heating in an inert gaseous environment. This process is termed **welding**. If an additional metallic material is added then the process is termed **brazing**.

Table 1.9 Processing of cast alloys*

Process	Formed product
Brazing	Complex part formed by heating metals in presence of another metallic material
Drawing	Wire and sheet formed from ingot
Forging	Unusual shape formed using dies
Machining	Part of complex geometry
Welding	Combination of parts produced by local heating and fusion

* adapted based on Black, 1988

Mechanical forming of alloys Cast structures are relatively weak because the grain size is large. Grain size can be controlled by the cooling rate used to solidify liquid solutions. Rapid cooling can limit grain size, yielding more desirable mechanical properties; however, there are additional postforming treatments that are also used to improve mechanical properties (Table 1.10).

Thermal treatment, termed **annealing**, is commonly used to improve properties. Metals are worked at temperatures above their yield points which mechanically hardens them and results in a loss of ductility and toughness. Work hardening under large deformations may require additional heating to $\frac{1}{3}-\frac{1}{2}$ of the melting temperature followed by controlled cooling.

During annealing, large grains grow by assimilating metal atoms from small grains. A single grain size provides better mechanical properties than a mixture of grain sizes. **Tempering** is a partial annealing used to toughen brittle strong alloys used as cutting edges. Tempering involves the rapid cooling, **quenching**, of a heated metal surface.

Metals are also **aged** at slightly elevated temperatures to permit the formation of precipitates that limit grain ductility. **Precipitation hardening** by formation of oxides and carbides form very small crystals that act to raise the ultimate tensile strength and yield point without affecting the moduli.

Additional treatments including anodization, carburization, electroplating, grinding, nitriding, passivation, polishing, sand blasting and surface alloying. **Anodization** involves formation of an oxide film on aluminium and titanium-base alloys by placing them in an electrolyte bath and passing a current through the metal rendering it anodic. In **electroplating**, the metal is

Table 1.10 Treatments used to modify mechanical properties of metals*

Treatment	Process and Result
Annealing	Thermal treatment below melting temperature; increases modulus and toughness
Grinding, polishing and sand blasting	Removal of surface impurities to improve surface aesthetics and properties
Precipitation hardening (carburization)	Formation of an oxide layer on heating a metal to elevated temperatures; increases tensile strength
Tempering	Thermal treatment by annealing followed by rapid cooling; increases toughness of brittle alloys
Work hardening	Mechanical conditioning below melting temperature; increases modulus

* adapted based on Black, 1988

rendered cathodic. **Surface alloying** is accomplished by electroplating or by vacuum deposition which is sometimes followed by heat treatment.

Carburization involves reaction of carbon with steel surfaces to produce carbide precipitates. Steel and titanium-base metals can react with ammonia or potassium cyanide to form **nitrides**.

Grinding is a physical process that results in surface layer abrasion and is used to remove surface impurities. **Polishing** is a smoothing process also used to remove surface impurities and improve the aesthetics of the final product.

Sand blasting, involves forcing a high speed stream of particles using air to collide with the surface of a material cleaning the surface.

Passivation, involves acid surface treatment forming oxides and hydroxides. This improves corrosion resistance of orthopaedic implants.

Types of stainless steel alloys used in implants A variety of alloys are used in the production of medical devices including stainless steels, cobalt-base alloys, titanium-base alloys, platinum-base alloys and new materials including refractory metals and nickel-titanium alloys.

Steels were the first modern metallic alloys used in orthopaedics (Black, 1988). The initial corrosion problem, i.e. rusting, of early implants was corrected by addition of carbon, chromium and molybdenum. Carbon is added at low concentrations to initiate carbide formation, while chromium facilitates formation of a stable surface oxide layer and molybdenum controls corrosion. There are four types of stainless steels that are distinguished by the appearance of characteristic phases at room temperature; these types are austenitic, ferritic, martensitic and precipitation hardenable. **Austenitic steel** is characterized by a solid phase termed austenite which is a solid solution of iron with 2% or less of carbon. Superior corrosion resistance has led to its use in implant applications. **Ferritic steel** contains a small amount of nickel, and in the presence of the austenitic phase at high temperature dissociates into iron and carbon on cooling. **Martensitic steel**, is formed by rapidly cooling and heating the austenitic phase. Precipitation hardenable steel has a high enough carbon content to form a carbide precipitate on heating. These steels are hard and tough and find applications as surgical and cutting instruments.

Standards for the composition and mechanical properties of materials, found in the Annual Book of the American Society For Testing Materials, Volume 13.01 (Medical Devices), can be obtained from ASTM at 1916 Race Street, Philadelphia, Pa 19103. Reference to these standards will be made below.

Standard stainless steels are designated by ASTM for sheet and strip (F56, F139), bar and wire for surgical implants (F55, F138). The compositions of these steels are given in Table 1.11. It should be noted that the compositions and properties of F55 are identical to F56 and those of F138 are the same as F139.

Table 1.11 Chemical composition of stainless steel alloys*

Composition, %	F55 %		F138 %		F745 %
Element	Grade 1	Grade 2	Grade 1	Grade 2	
Carbon	0.08 max	0.03 max	0.08 max	0.03 max	0.06 max
Manganese	2.0 max	2.0 max	2.0 max	2.0 max	2.0 max
Phosphorus	0.030 max	0.03 max	0.025 max	0.025 max	0.045 max
Sulphur	0.030 max	0.03 max	0.010 max	0.010 max	0.030 max
Silicon	0.75 max	0.75 max	0.75 max	0.075 max	1.0
Chromium	17 to 19	17 to 19	17 to 19	17 to 19	17 to 19
Nickel	12 to 14	12 to 14	13 to 15.5	13 to 15.5	11 to 14
Molybdenum	2.0 to 3.0	2.0 to 3.0	2.0 to 3.0	2.0 to 3.0	2.0 to 3.0
Nitrogen	0.10 max	0.10 max	0.10 max	0.10 max	
Copper	0.50 max	0.50 max	0.50 max	0.50 max	
Iron	balance	balance	balance	balance	balance

* adapted from ASTM, Vol. 13.01

The difference between these types of stainless steels is the amount of each element added. F55 and F138 are casting alloys with high ductility, and can undergo extensive postcasting mechanical processing. They are the most common stainless steel alloys used in medical device fabrication as wrought materials. F745 is a high strength alloy that is cast and solution annealed for surgical implant applications. Mechanical properties of stainless steels are listed in Table 1.12.

Stainless steels that are treated by annealing have higher ultimate strains, lower ultimate tensile strengths and lower yield points than do cold-worked products. Cold-worked products are work hardened, which increases strength at the expense of ductility.

Table 1.12 Mechanical properties of stainless steels†

Type and condition	UTS* (MPa)	Yield at 2%**	US, %***
F55, F138, annealed	480–515	170–205	40
F55, F138 cold-worked	655–860	310–690	12–28
F745, annealed	480 min	205 min	30 min

* Ultimate tensile strength
**Yield strength at 2% offset in MPa
***Ultimate tensile strain
min = minimum
† adapted based on ASTM, Vol. 13.01

Table 1.13 Chemical compositions of cobalt-base alloys*

Element	F75 %	F90 %	F562 %	F563 %
Manganese	1.00 max	1.0 to 2.0	0.15	1.0 max
Silicon	1.0 max	0.4 max	0.15 max	0.5 max
Chromium	27–30	19–21	19–21	18 to 22
Nickel	1.0 max	9–11	33–37	15 to 25
Molybdenum	5.0 to 7.0	9 to 10.5	3 to 4	
Carbon	0.35 max	0.05 to 0.15	0.025 max	0.05 max
Iron	0.75 max	3.0 max	1.0 max	4 to 6
Phosphorus		0.04 max	0.015 max	
Sulphur		0.03 max	0.01 max	0.01 max
Tungsten		14 to 16		3 to 4
Titanium			1.0 max	0.5 to 3.5
Cobalt	balance	balance	balance	balance

* adapted based on ASTM, Vol. 13.01

Cobalt-base alloys There are at least four compositions of cobalt-base alloys that are designated by ASTM including, F75, F90, F562 and F563. F75 is a cast alloy that is commonly used in many applications. F90 is a wrought alloy that is more suitable for hot rolling. F562 and 563 are less frequently used. Table 1.13 lists the chemical compositions of these alloys.

Cobalt-base alloys have an austenitic phase that is partially converted to a martensitic phase. These phases have similar structures to the crystalline structures found in stainless steels, however, there are compositional differences between these alloys. Mechanical properties of these alloys are tabulated in Table 1.14.

In comparison to stainless steels, cobalt-base alloys exhibit higher moduli and much higher strengths; however, these alloys have lower ductilities. Other aspects of implant design to consider with cobalt-base alloys are the difficulty of machining and the higher cost of cobalt and tungsten elements.

Titanium-base alloys Titanium-base alloys are found in many commercial medical devices. The two alloys that are covered by ASTM specifications are F67 and F136. F67 grade 4 is used for surface coating of orthopaedic implants and is one of four grades specified in ASTM standards. F136 is commonly referred to as Ti6Al4V because it contains on average 6% aluminium and 4% vanadium as described in Table 1.15. There is some concern over the possible biologic side effects due to the addition of vanadium. In addition to Cobalt-Chromium alloys, Ti6A14V is used extensively in the medical device industry.

Table 1.14 Mechanical properties of cobalt-base alloys†

Type and condition	UTS* (MPa)	Yield at 2%**	US, %***
F75, cast	655	450	8
F90, annealed	896	379	30–45 min
F562, solution annealed	793–1000	241–448	50
F562, cold worked	1793 min	1586 min	8
F563, annealed	600	276	50
F563, cold worked & aged	1000–1586	827–1310	12–18

* Ultimate tensile strength
** Yield strength at 2% offset in MPa
*** Ultimate tensile strain
† adapted based on ASTM, Vol. 13.01

Titanium alloys have two major phases, an *alpha* phase that is formed at high temperatures and a *beta* phase referred to as martensitic which occurs at lower temperatures.

Although titanium and its alloys have moduli that are roughly half of those of stainless steel and cobalt-base alloys and lower ductility, they have ultimate tensile strengths that approach those found for these alloys. Mechanical properties of titanium-base alloys are found in Table 1.16.

Platinum-base alloys are used primarily in electrodes for electrical stimulation, because of their relatively high cost. Their corrosion resistance and mechanical properties contribute to their success in these applications. Platinum is used unalloyed or alloyed with rhodium. Ultimate tensile strengths, moduli and strains to failure of 147 MPa, 152–485 MPa and 35%, respectively, are reported for these alloys.

Table 1.15 Elemental composition of titanium-base alloys*

ASTM specification	F67	F136
Element	%	%
Nitrogen	0.05 max	0.05 max
Carbon	0.10 max	0.08 max
Hydrogen	0.15 max	0.012 max
Iron	0.50 max	0.25 max
Oxygen	0.40 max	0.13 max
Aluminium		6.5 max
Vanadium		4.0 max
Titanium	balance	balance

* adapted based on ASTM, Vol. 13.01

Table 1.16 Mechanical properties of titanium-base alloys†

Type and condition	UTS* (MPa)	Yield at 2%**	US, %***
F67	240–550	170–485	15–24 min
F136	860–896	795–827	10 min

* Ultimate tensile strength
***Yield strength at 2% offset in MPa
*** Ultimate tensile strain
† adapted based on ASTM, Vol. 13.01

Ceramics

This classification includes inorganic materials such as SiO_2 or other metal oxides in crystal and glassy phases similar to polymers. Physically, ceramics are stiff, hard, brittle materials that are insoluble in water. Their primary advantages include high strength and modulus. The properties of these materials reflect the types of atomic bonding that exists between atoms as well as the atomic radii (Black, 1988, Park, 1984).

Ceramic materials are held together by ionic and covalent bonds. Ionic bonds are highly directional and require very high energies of dissociation. For this reason, ceramic materials containing ionic bonds, tend to be resistant to chemical and mechanical dissolution. Ceramic materials such as hydroxyapatite, the mineral phase of bone, are being studied because of their stabilities in a number of orthopaedic and dental applications as replacements for bone and dentin.

Carbons are another class of ceramics. They are typically made by heating carbon containing polymer chains to high temperatures in the absence of oxygen. These materials once held high potential for replacement of heart valves, ligaments, and dental implants. Recent evidence suggests that the long term biocompatibility of these materials in some applications is questionable.

Elements such as sodium and chloride are ionized by electron transfer and in the process can make an ionic compound as a result of coulombic attractions. Negatively charged ions have increased atomic radii as a result of addition of an electron while positively charged ions have smaller radii compared to the uncharged atom.

Ceramics can be classified by their structural components as compounds containing metal (M) and nonmetal (N) atoms using the general formula $M_x N_y$ where x and y represent the number of atoms of each species in a unit crystal. In the simplest case the the unit cell has equal numbers of atoms and can be represented by the formula MN largely due to the similar radii of the metal and nonmetal atoms (radius metal/radius nonmetal > 0.732).

The unit cell becomes a simple cubic structure as shown for CsCl in Figure 1.7 when the radii are similar. If the relative radii of the metal and non-metal atoms are quite different, then the face centred cubic (FCC) structure is observed. Examples of ceramics in the FCC structure are NaCl and ZnS. If unequal numbers of metal and non-metal atoms are found in the unit cell then the formula becomes more complicated such as for aluminium oxide which is Al_2O_3. In this ceramic, the O^{-2} ions are in hexagonal close packed structure and the aluminium ions fill $\frac{2}{3}$ of the spaces between the negatively charged ions.

Another group of ceramic materials includes the silicates that form sheet or network structures. These include crystalline forms such as quartz and the glassy form, fused silica.

Piezoelectric ceramics (these materials convert electrical energy into mechanical energy) such as barium titanate are of interest because these types of crystals can elongate or shorten in an electric field due to displacement between the positive and negative charges.

Mechanical properties of ceramics

Ceramics are generally known for their high hardness and hence high modulus values. On the Moh's scale, diamond, which is a carbon base ceramic, has a hardness of ten, alumina nine, quartz eight and hydroxyapatite five. Hydroxyapatite is the ceramic that forms the mineral phase of bone. Values for moduli and compressive strengths of bone are given in Table 1.2 as well as for ceramics in Table 1.17.

Carbons have mechanical properties that depend in part on the organization of the atoms and aggregates of atoms. Graphite is composed of

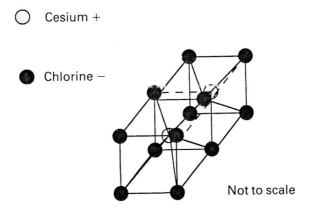

Figure 1.7 Crystal structure of cesium chloride.

Table 1.17 Mechanical properties of some ceramics and carbons*

Ceramic	Modulus of elasticity (GPa)	Compressive strength (MPa)
Al_2O_3 (crystals)	379	345–1034
Sintered Al_2O_3	365	207–345
Silica glass	72	107
Pyrex glass	69	69
Carbons		
Graphite	24	138
Glassy	24	172
Pyrolytic	28	517

* adapted based on Black, 1988

aggregates of crystallites containing parallel layers of carbon atoms in a hexagonal close packed structure. The layers of crystals are held together by carbon to carbon crosslinks. Large numbers of crosslinks are present in pyrolytic carbons giving these materials their high compressive strength. Pyrolytic carbons are formed from a hydrocarbon in a gaseous state by heating the gas to about 1200°C in the absence of oxygen.

Glassy or vitreous carbons are made by heating cross-linked carbon base polymers such as phenol formaldehyde in the absence of oxygen. Although short range crystallinity does exist, a well defined crystal structure is absent. It is the absence of a well defined crystal structure that explains the lower value of the compressive strength of glassy compared to pyrolytic carbons.

Unlike metals, ceramics tend to deform minimally during loading, a result which is a consequence of the electronic charge that prevents atoms from moving large distances. This phenomenon makes ceramics very brittle and these materials tend to fracture at lower strengths when they are tested in tension as compared to compression. The low value of the failure tensile strength is a consequence of stress concentration that occurs around cracks or flaws in the structure. For this reason, ceramics have medical applications that require only limited deformability.

1.3.4 Composites

These materials are made up of two or more types of phases and usually include stiff fibres embedded in a ductile matrix yielding a material with properties that are between those of each phase. For example, carbon fibres are embedded in epoxy or poly(lactic acid) matrix to obtain a material that has a strength and stiffness approaching that of the fibres and a ductility and toughness approaching that of the matrix. Many composite materials are under development for a number of medical applications.

1.4 Pre-clinical and clinical biocompatibility evaluation

The development of materials that are intended for use in medical devices is a complicated process. The complicated part is that exact design criteria have not been established based on sound scientific principles. Another way to state this concept is that many devices have been designed based on a trial-and-error approach. These designs work, for reasons that are not well understood. Many of the currently used materials have been adapted from aviation, marine and automotive engineering since high demands (corrosion resistance, strength and flexibility) are made on materials used in these applications.

The next generation of materials used in medical devices will be designed based on analysis of the properties of normal tissues since a limit has been reached in adapting old materials to new applications. The length of time required to introduce any new material into general clinical practice can vary from several to over ten years depending on the application. Therefore, it is essential to understand the physiology and anatomy of the application to minimize the start up time for any design.

1.4.1 Medical device design

The design process by its very nature is complex and requires the ability to synthesize anatomical and physiological data. In addition, the design should include reasonable benchmarks at each step of development. Initially, the design is directed at mimicking the structure and properties of natural tissue which have been optimized by evolutionary forces over millions of years. The first step in the design is to make a table of physical properties that are displayed by natural tissue. Next, it is necessary to set realistic boundary conditions as to which of these properties are critical to the design and which are less critical. In addition, biocompatibility requirements should be used to rule out materials that do not merit further consideration. Once this has been accomplished, a set of design specifications are determined and the development concepts are initiated. The first question that is asked is, 'what materials possess the properties that meet or come close to the specifications given?'

Once an approach to the design is chosen, a prototype of the design is made and evaluated to determine whether it matches the design specifications. Normally, only a few test specifications are evaluated so that time is not wasted conducting extensive testing if the material does not meet the most important design criteria. If initial evaluation or screening studies show positive results, a complete evaluation of the specifications is normally undertaken. Once a complete specification evaluation is achieved, the design is modified based on analysis of the test results. The design process is cyclic since the results of each step may lead to new hypotheses, which in turn lead to continued testing until the prototype produced performs in a similar manner to the tissue to be replaced.

To facilitate the design, the objectives must be clearly formulated in terms of design specifications and the designer must have a specific hypothesis to evaluate through construction of a prototype. Included in the design at a later stage is consideration of the cost and availability of raw materials, the possibility of mass production of the design, and the pathway for FDA approval. However, in order to prevent stifling novel ideas, the later concepts should not be used to discard new approaches since it may be difficult to judge the future cost of raw materials or processes.

Most novel ideas that are generated by inventors are achieved by free thinking. In this process a designer spends a great deal of time just collecting information about the topic and the subject of the design without really evaluating how this information relates to the problem. After a preset period of free thinking the designer integrates background material and generates a large list of characteristics important to the design. This list is eventually shortened and integrated into a design by one of many processes. There is no formula for creative thinking and therefore each individual will learn under what conditions he thinks best. The most important concept is that the test results should be interpreted without bias. Many medical device designs are studied in animals for decades with limited progress because a designer or scientist is unwilling to carefully interpret experimental results or is infatuated with 'his' design. The success of any design is dependent on the choice of the design specifications and final end-use testing. However, before end-use testing is warranted, a series of laboratory studies directed at evaluating the safety and efficacy of the prototype must be completed.

1.4.2 Safety and efficacy testing

The testing conducted on a biomaterial intended for use in a medical device must address safety and effectiveness criteria as outlined in several recently published texts (Ciarkowski, 1986; Black, 1988). The specific tests required vary with the type of device and application; however, some general testing is usually recommended. Normally, animal testing is conducted to demonstrate that a medical device is safe, and that when implanted in humans that the device will reduce, alleviate or eliminate the possibility of adverse medical reactions or conditions.

According to the ASTM Medical Devices Standards (Annual Book of ASTM Standards, Section 13, Medical Devices, ASTM 1916 Race Street, Philadelphia, Pa, 19103) the types of generic biological test methods for materials and devices depends on the end-use application. Biological reactions that are detrimental to the success of a material in one device application may not be applicable in a different end-use. A list (Table 1.18) of potentially applicable biocompatibility tests that are related to end-use of a material or device is given as a starting point.

A description of some of these tests is given in annual ASTM Medical Device Standards book and in chapters 14–21 of the *Handbook of*

Table 1.18 Biologic tests used to evaluate biocompatibility*

Test	ASTM standard
Cell culture cytotoxicity	F748
Skin irritation	F719
Intramuscular and subcutaneous implantation	F748
Blood compatibility	F748
Hemolysis	F756
Carcinogenesis	F748
Long-term implantation	F748
Mucous membrane irritation	F748
Systemic injection acute toxicity	F750
Intracutaneous injection	F749
Sensitization	F720
Mutagenicity	F748
Pyrogenicity	F748

* ASTM Medical Devices Standards, Section 13

Biomaterials Evaluation that is edited by A.F. von Recum (1986). Additional information on the theory of these tests and the biological systems that are involved are found in chapter 4 of *Biocompatibility* (Silver and Doillon, 1989).

Cell culture cytotoxicity studies evaluate the in vitro toxicity of substrate materials to cultured cells. Tests used include Agar Diffusion, Fluid Medium, Agar Overlay and Flask Dilution. All of these tests measure the toxicity of substrates or extracts of materials on cells. Cell death is measured normally by the inability of cells to incorporate vital dyes.

Skin irritation assay involves applying a patch of the material to be evaluated to an area of rabbit skin that has been shaved and in some cases abraded. After 24 hours of contact, the patch is removed and the skin is graded for redness and swelling.

Short-term intramuscular implantation is designed to evaluate the reaction of tissue to an implant for periods of 7 and 30 days. At the conclusion of the test period, the samples are graded both visually and based on analysis of histological sections. A test described in the United States Pharmacopeia (USP) is widely used.

Short-term subcutaneous implantation involves placement of an implant in a tissue pocket beneath the skin for a period of days to weeks. Normally the implant is placed away from the site of suturing to eliminate the possibility of reaction to the suture material. In some cases the wounds are clipped closed.

Blood compatibility is normally assessed by determination of clotting times and platelet aggregation initiated by a test surface or by blood exposed to a surface. Tests are conducted in vitro, in vivo and ex vivo.

Hemolysis is determined by placing powder, rods or extracts of the material in human or rabbit plasma for about 90 minutes at 37°C. The amount of hemoglobin released into solution is determined by measuring the absorbance at a characteristic wavelength after red blood cells have been removed by centrifugation. Hemolysis of 5% of the red blood cells or less is generally considered acceptable. Hemolysis is also measured in vivo by determining the red cell half-life after implantation of a device.

Carcinogenicity testing involves long term implantation to evaluate the potential for cell transformation and tumour formation.

Long-term implant tests are covered by ASTM specifications F 361 and F 469 for muscle and bone respectively. Implant materials are placed in the muscle as a soft tissue model and in bone as a model of hard tissue. The implantation site is evaluated grossly and histologically for inflammation, giant cell formation and signs of implant movement and tissue necrosis.

Mucous membrane irritation is evaluated by placing the material in close proximity to a mucous membrane. The amount of irritation and inflammation is determined from gross and histological measurements. The hamster cheek pouch is a model that is becoming more frequently used for this test procedure.

Systemic injection (acute toxicity) is designed to determine the biological response to a single intravenous or intraperitoneal injection of extract (50 ml/kg) of a material over a 72 hour time period. Extracts are prepared in saline or other solutions that simulate body fluids. Animals are monitored for immediate signs of toxicity and at specific time intervals.

Intracutaneous injection involves the reaction of an animal to a single intracutaneous injection of a saline or vegetable extract of a material. Rabbits are commonly used and they are studied for signs of redness and swelling at the injection site for periods of 72 hours.

Sensitization assay involves mixing the material or an extract with Freund's complete adjuvant and injection of the material into the animal's subcutaneous tissue during a two week induction period. After two weeks, the animal (normally a guinea pig) is challenged with the material or extract by placing it in contact with the skin near the injection site for 24 hours. The skin is graded for allergic reactions.

Mutagenicity is evaluated using the Ames test. This test employs genetically altered bacteria which are placed in contact with an extract of the material. The bacteria have altered nutritional needs. Mutations that cause reversion back to the 'wild type' phenotype lead to bacteria that will grow only under the original nutritional conditions and not under conditions the mutant grows. This test is used to screen materials for carcinogenic potential.

Pyrogenicity is used for fever producing substances that are either components of gram negative bacterial cell membranes (endotoxins) or are materials of chemical origin. Endotoxins are determined by injection of an extract of material into the rabbit circulatory system and measuring the resulting elevation in body temperature. Another method involves contact of the material with cells that are lysed specifically by endotoxins (Limulus Amebocyte Lysate Test). Chemical pyrogens are determined only by the rabbit test.

1.5 Biology of transplantation of tissue products matching

A number of biomaterials are derived directly from human tissues, without processing to remove cellular materials. These tissues must be matched to avoid rejection. Tissue matching involves matching the gene products of the major histocompatibility complex that is found on chromosome six in the human genome. In order to understand the process of tissue matching, it is first necessary to review a few priniciples of immunobiology.

The **major histocompatibility complex** (MHC), the Ia region, codes for products that are expressed on the surface of cells found throughout the body (Abbas, Lichtman, and Pober, 1991). These products vary between individuals and are used as markers to reflect genetic differences. Proteins derived from these genes turn genes on and off in the MHC that controls graft rejection. Thus, individuals who express the same MHC product molecules accept grafts from one another. The genes that control this response are called the immune response genes.

The immune response genes code for two classes of products that are involved in foreign antigen recognition by **T lymphocytes** (T cells). These products are termed the **class I and class II MHC products** and are found embedded in the cell membrane of host cells (Figure 1.8). **Class I molecules** contain two separate protein chains: a heavy MHC encoded chain with a molecular weight of about 44 000 (*alpha*) and a non-MHC encoded chain with a molecular weight of 12 000 (*beta*) (Table 1.19). The *alpha* **chain** is embedded into the cell membrane and extends out into

Table 1.19 Molecular structure of class I and class II MHC products†

Class	Chain types	Molecular weights	Type of protein
I	heavy (alpha)	44 000	integral*
	light (beta)	12 000	peripheral*
II	heavy (alpha)	33 000	integral*
	heavy (beta)	31 000	integral*

* extends extracellularly
† Abbas, Lichtman and Pober, 1991

30 Scope and markets for medical implants

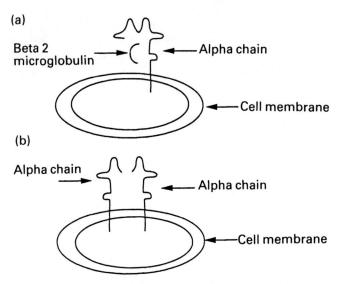

Figure 1.8 Diagram illustrating differences existing between (a) class I and (b) class II cell surface antigens.

the extracellular environment while the *beta* **chain** (also termed *beta*-2 microglobulin) is found physically associated with the extracellular component of the *alpha* chain.

All class II products are composed of two non-covalently linked polypeptide chains that have similar structures. The *alpha* chain (molecular weight of about 33 000) is slightly larger than the *beta* chain (molecular weight of about 31 000) as a result of a greater degree of sugar chain attachment. Both of the chains extend through the membrane into the extracellular matrix. Both class I and class II molecules have peptide binding clefts by which foreign antigens become attached to the cell membrane of host lymphocytes.

The MHC is located on the short arm of **chromosome six.** *Beta*-2 microglobulin is encoded by a gene on **chromosome 15**. Based on studies of serum from humans, the class I and II MHC products on leukocytes (**human leukocyte antigens**, HLAs) are encoded by regions of the MHC termed A, B and C (Figure 1.9). They are referred to as HLA-A, HLA-B and HLA-C genes. Products of these genes are present on donor tissue (white blood cells) and they react with antibodies that are present in the host's blood. In the presence of complement, the recipient's serum lyses donor lymphocytes.

Other regions of the MHC involved in graft rejection were later indentified based on the induction of proliferation of foreign T cells in the **mixed leukocyte reaction** (D and DR regions). Other genes (DQ and DP) were

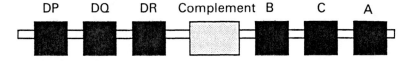

Figure 1.9 Diagram of human MHC loci located on chromosome six.

subsequently located and named for their proximity to R in the alphabet. Specifically, the HLA antigens coded for by the MHC are HLA-A, HLA-B and HLA-C, the class I MHC molecules, and HLA-DQ, HLA-DP and HLA-DR, the class II MHC products.

The human MHC extends about 3500×10^3 base pairs which is equivalent to the length of the entire DNA in a bacteria. The class II genes are closest to the centromere in the order DP, DQ, and DR. Further from the class II region is the complement region which codes for components of the complement system (Figure 1.9). The class I region which codes for the A, B and C HLA antigens is found further down the chromosome.

MHC molecules are found in as many as 40 different varieties for even a single gene product. Both class I and class II products are involved in triggering T-cell responses that cause **rejection of transplanted cells**. Both class I and II products are found embedded within the cell membrane and bind foreign protein antigens to form complexes that are recognized by antigen-specific T-lymphocytes. Antigens that are associated with class I molecules are recognized by **CD8+ cytolytic T-lymphocytes** (CTLs), whereas class II associated antigens are recognized by CD4+ helper T cells (Figure 1.10). Tissue rejection is minimized by matching the HLA antigens of the donor and host.

1.5.1 Types of tissue grafts and rejection processes

Transplantation involves the removal of cells, tissues or organs from one individual and then placing them into another individual. If the graft is returned to the same patient it is termed an **autograft**, while if it is placed in another individual of the same species it is termed an **allograft**. Tissue transferred to another species is termed a **xenograft**. If it is placed in the same anatomic location from which it was derived the transplantation procedure is termed **orthotopic**, while if the location to which it is moved is different from the original anatomic site, it is termed **heterotopic**. If tissue is transplanted from one individual to another unrelated individual there is high probability that the vascular supply to the graft will be destroyed and that it will be **rejected**.

First set rejection occurs seven to ten days after a graft is transferred between unrelated individuals. A subsequent skin graft transplanted from the same

32 Scope and markets for medical implants

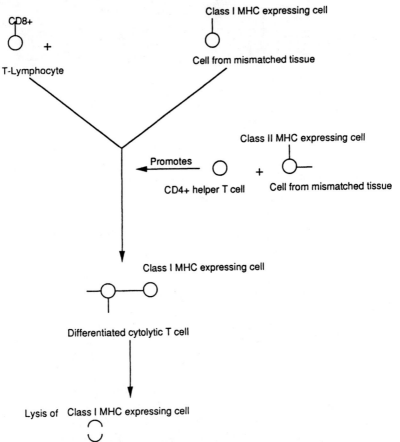

Figure 1.10 Recognition of antigen by T cells.

donor to the same recipient will be rejected in only two to three days by an accelerated mechanism (**second set rejection**). If the second graft is from a third donor unrelated to the first two individuals, then the new graft elicits only a first set rejection.

The immune response to an antigen can be both **cell mediated** and **humoral**. Cell-mediated responses are, in general, more important for graft rejection. Recognition of transplanted cells is determined by inheritance of genes from both parents who have equal potential to be active (co-dominant genes).

The **mixed leukocyte reaction** (MLR) is induced by culturing mononuclear leukocytes from one individual with mononuclear leukocytes from a potential donor. If there are differences in the class I and class II HLA antigens on cells from both the donor and recipient, a large number of the mononuclear cells will proliferate over a period of four to seven days. Cell proliferation denotes cellular incompatibility.

Two types of cell populations are stimulated during the MLR. One type of T-cell expresses the CD8 molecule but not the CD4 molecule and functions as a **cytolytic T lymphocyte** (CTL) by destroying cells that do not bear the appropriate antigens. The molecules on stimulator and target cells recognized by CD8+ CTL are the class I MHC molecules that are coded for by the HLA-A, B and C regions. The full differentiation of CTLs in the MLR requires stimulation by class I molecules as well as help that is provided by CD4+ helper T-cells. CD4+ helper T-cells release **interleukin-2** (IL-2) that stimulates T-cell proliferation. CD4+ helper T-cells are specific for allogenic class II MHC products.

Stimulation of alloreactive T cells in vivo

Allografts that are different from the host at both class I and II loci (CD8+ and CD4+) result in T cell activation and proliferation. CD8+ cells recognize class I MHC products, which are expressed on the surface of all cells in the graft. Differentiation of these cells (CD8+) is largely dependent upon CD4+ T cells being stimulated by allograft class II molecules present on **antigen presenting cells** (APCs) in the allograft.

If the class II containing cells, including the APCs, are removed prior to graft transplantation, the rate of rejection of the graft will proceed more slowly or not at all despite differences in the class I MHC products. Class II MHC products can be eliminated from the graft by several treatments including: prolonged cell culture, treatment with antibodies to class II MHC products plus complement, extensive graft profusion of blood vessels to wash out APCs (Table 1.20). The problem of graft rejection can be ameliorated by removal of passenger leukocytes.

Rejection is stimulated by CD4+ helper cells activated by foreign cells expressing class II MHC products that are different than those of the recipient. The CD4+ cells then stimulate the growth and differentiation of reactive CD8+ cytolytic T cells (Figure 1.10). Stimulation is normally provided by passenger leukocytes that are APCs carried within the vessels of the graft. Elimination of the passenger leukocytes serves to reduce the activation of helper cells and differentiation and growth of CD8 + cells, and thereby decreases the severity of the rejection reaction. However, in

Table 1.20 Processes that limit graft rejection†

Process	Effect
Prolonged cell culture	Loss of class II MHC markers
Treatment with antibodies	Blockage of class II MHC receptors
Extensive graft profusion	Wash out antigen presenting cells

† Abbas, Lichtman and Pober, 1991

humans, the stimulatory effects of endothelial cells activate CD4+ helper cells and can initiate graft rejection.

The mechanism for production of antibodies against foreign MHC products is not clearly understood, but it is believed that B cells specific for antigens are stimulated in a similar manner to any other foreign protein. Both antibody dependent and T cell mediated graft rejection can occur independently by different mechanisms. In the case of T cell mediated rejection, CD4+ T cells can recruit and activate macrophages, initiating graft injury by a **delayed type hypersensitivity** response. CD8+ T cells directly lyse graft endothelial and parenchymal cells. In contrast, antibodies to donor MHC products activate the complement system and injure graft blood vessels.

Mechanism of graft rejection

Both **acute and chronic rejection** are processes that can occur simultaneously and are characterized by the cell types present. **Hyperacute rejection** is characterized by occlusion of vascular channels, by deposition of platelets and fibrin networks and begins within minutes of surgical completion of the suturing of donor and host vessels (Table 1.21). **Blood clotting** and **platelet aggregation** (thrombosis) occurs prior to the development of inflammation and is mediated by pre-existing antibodies that attach to endothelial cells, which subsequently activate complement. Endothelial cells secrete a form of von Willebrand factor which mediates platelet adhesion and aggregation and activates blood clotting. In early experimental transplantation procedures, hyperacute rejection occurred as a result of mismatching of blood types.

Table 1.21 Differences between hyperacute, acute and chronic rejection†

Type of rejection	Characterization
Hyperacute	Occlusion of vascular channels blood clotting and platelet aggregation mediated by circulating antibodies that activate complement
Acute humoral	Mediated by IgG antibodies to endothelial cell antigens and involves complement
Acute cellular	Necrosis of parenchymal cells in presence of lymphocytes and macrophages
Chronic	Deposition of collagen and loss of normal tissue architecture

† Abbas, Lichtman and Pober, 1991

Differences between **ABO blood group antigens** of the donor and recipient limit blood transfusions by causing antibody and complement dependent lysis of red blood cells. The red blood cell has antigens in the form of cell surface macromolecules that differ because of variations in the attached sugar units. All normal individuals synthesize a **core sugar** called the **O antigen**. A single gene encodes three common forms of the enzyme which transfers sugars to this cell surface macromolecule. The O form is devoid of enzymatic activity whereas the **A gene product** transfers a terminal N-acetyl galactosamine and the **B gene product** transfers a terminal galactose moiety (Table 1.22). If the recipient of a blood transfusion receives red blood cells that express a form of an antigen (A or B or a combination) not expressed on red cells of the host then massive red cell lysis will result (Table 1.23). Individuals with AB blood type can tolerate transfusions from all potential blood donors and are universal recipients. In contrast, individuals with OO blood type can tolerate transfusions from only donors with OO blood type and are universal donors (Table 1.23).

Although ABO antigens are also expressed on vascular endothelial cells, hyperacute rejection by anti-ABO antibodies is not a clinical problem because all donors and recipients are matched for these groups. **Hyperacute rejection** is infrequent and is caused by antibodies directed against MHC products or against other antigens expressed on endothelial cells and blood monocytes (E-M antigens).

Table 1.22 Types of blood group antigens and blood types

Antigens	Blood type
OO*	O
AA	A
AO	A
BB	B
BO	B
AB	AB

* A maximum of two types of antigens exist in each individual because two copies of each gene are present.

Table 1.23 Acceptable blood transfusions between unrelated individuals

Recipient blood type	Acceptable donor blood type
O	O
A	A, O
B	B, O
AB	A, B, O

Acute humoral rejection is characterized by death of individual cells of the graft blood vessels with inflammation of the vascular wall (Table 1.21). This process is mediated by **IgG** antibodies to endothelial cell antigens (**E-M or MHC products**) and involves activation of complement. Lymphocytes may contribute by responding to antigens present on vascular endothelial cells or they may produce cytokines that activate inflammatory cells. Both of these processes lead to endothelial cell lysis.

Acute cellular rejection is characterized by necrosis of the parenchymal cells in the presence of lymphocytes and macrophage infiltrates (Table 1.21). Effector mechanisms include **cytolytic lysis, activated macrophage lysis** and natural killer cell lysis. Evidence suggests that recognition and lysis by CD8+ T cells is probably the most important mechanism of acute cellular rejection. **Natural killer (NK) cells** are large lymphocytes found in blood and lymphoid tissues and are derived from bone marrow. They are primitive cytolytic T cells that lack specific cell receptors. They are able to kill target cells without previous exposure to the target; however, the exact mechanism of NK cell lysis is unclear at this time.

Chronic rejection is characterized by deposition of collagenous tissue (fibrosis) with loss of normal organ architecture (Table 1.21). Although the pathogenesis of chronic rejection is unknown, the product is similar to the result of chronic inflammatory diseases and therefore chronic rejection may involve inflammation and subsequent wound healing. One form of rejection is characterized by proliferation of intimal smooth muscle cells in the wall of arteries which are observed in renal and cardiac transplants. This form exhibits morphological changes characteristic of accelerated arteriosclerosis.

Prevention of rejection

If a graft is transplanted into an individual with a normal immune system, some form of rejection results. If rejection is left untreated it will result in organ failure. The two methods that have been used to limit the immune response to a transplant include treatments to the graft and to the host immune system.

Elimination of passenger leukocytes improves the 'take' of rodent transplants but it has not been shown to improve the survival of transplants in humans (Table 1.24). In humans, matching of blood ABO group antigens between donor and recipient eliminates hyperacute rejection. In addition, tissue typing of donors and recipients improves the probability for graft take. Matching of MHC antigens appears sufficient to prevent rejection if three out of four of the A and B antigens are similar (each MHC gene product can have two forms termed **alleles**). In the case of kidney transplantation, in depth matching is possible since kidneys are stored in organ banks prior to transplantation. For heart and liver transplantation, storage of the organ is more difficult and therefore matching is less frequently done.

Suppression of the recipient's immune system is normally required to prevent chronic rejection even if tissue typing is done (Table 1.24).

Plasmapheresis is a process used to suppress a patient's immune response. It is for the removal of blood plasma (containing antibodies to transplant antigens) that is done outside of the body and then the washed cells are returned to the patient. This process is used to treat acute humoral rejection with limited success. Pre-treatment of the recipient with **transfusions** of the donor's blood is sometimes used to induce tolerance to the donor's antigenic molecules.

Immune suppression is more commonly achieved by use of drugs including **corticosteroids, azathiaprine, cyclosporin** and **cyclophosphamide** as well as by **irradiation** of lymphoid tissue. Corticosteroids act by either selective lysis of T cells or by blocking cytokine gene transcription inhibiting inflammation. Azathioprine and cyclophosphamide are metabolic toxins that inhibit growth of lymphocytes. Irradiation of T cells is another method of selective destruction since they are more sensitive than most other cell types to radiation.

Cyclosporin A, a cyclic peptide that is a fungal product, inhibits gene transcription resulting in suppression of cytokine mediated response to foreign cells in the graft.

Clinical organ transplantation

Kidney transplantation has been conducted clinically since the 1950s forming the basis for transplantation of a number of tissues. Selection of donor and recipient matches in renal transplantation is based on blood group matching (ABO), absence of pre-formed antibodies in blood of the recipient to donor cells (E and M antigens) and HLA typing. Matching of three out of the four A and B alleles promotes graft take. The HLA-C allele is not normally matched and is believed to be less important as a target of T cell recognition. Matching of the HLA-DR alleles is important independent

Table 1.24 Methods used to prevent rejection of transplants*

Method	Mode of action
Wash tissue extensively	Eliminate passenger leukocytes
Match MHC antigens AB	Decrease possibility of acute rejection
Match blood type	Prevent hyperacute rejection
Plasmapheresis	Minimize acute humoral rejection
Corticosteroids	Suppress immune system (T-cell lysis)
Azathioprine or Cyclophosphamide	Inhibit lymphocyte growth
Cyclosporin A	Suppress cytokine induced response
Irradiation	Destroy lymphocytes

* Abbas, Lichtman and Pober, 1991

of HLA-A and HLA-B matching. Since the HLA-DQ gene is linked to the DR gene, HLA-DR matching often matches HLA-DQ.

Immunosuppression with corticosteroids, azathioprine and anti-T cell antibodies is sufficient to allow survival of 50–60% of unrelated cadaveric donor grafts at 1 year, compared to a survival rate of 90% with grafts from donors who are related to the recipient. Graft function is normally measured by **plasma creatinine** levels except in the case of cyclosporin immunosuppressed patients, since this drug causes kidney toxicity and impaired function. In this instance, transplant survival is assessed based on histopathological examination of biopsy specimens.

Liver allograft rejection can be evaluated based on bile excretion, since cyclosporin is not as toxic to liver as it is to kidney. In heart transplants, functional impairment usually indicates that rejection may be irreversible. Therefore cardiac allograft biopsies are routinely done as a follow-up procedure by catheterization through the right ventricle via the venous circulation. Biopsies of the intraventicular septum are taken with little risk to the patient for diagnostic purposes. Cardiac transplant rejection is the most common cause of graft failure.

Immunosuppression prevents rejection; however, transplant recipients are susceptible to viral infections and tumour formation that may be fatal. Infections with a **herpes** family of viruses as well as **B cell lymphomas**, squamous cell carcinoma of the skin and **Kaposi's sarcoma** are consequences of this treatment (Table 1.25).

1.6 Federal Food and Drug Administration (FDA) regulations

Prior to 1976 the FDA exercised little authority over production and distribution of medical devices. The Federal Food, Drug and Cosmetic Act of 1938 was chiefly concerned with devices that made fraudulent claims. Many of the devices used were relatively simple and presented little risk to the

Table 1.25 Side effects of immunsuppression*

Medical condition	Effect on immunosuppressed patient
Infection	
Cytomegalovirus	Viral infection leading to death
Malignancies	
B cell lymphoma	Tumours involving lymph nodes and other sites such as G.I., skin, bone or brain
Squamous cell carcinoma	Malignancy of skin epithelial cells
Kaposi's sarcoma	Multiple disseminated skin lesions

* Abbas, Lichtman and Pober, 1991

patient. In 1976 after lengthy hearings, Congress enacted the **Medical Device Amendments** to the **Federal Food, Drug and Cosmetic Act**.

The Medical Device Amendments required that the FDA impose varying regulatory controls over devices by establishing a system of classes with varying requirements based on the relative risk presented. The definition of device that was used included any instrument, apparatus, implement, machine, contrivance, implant, in vitro reagent or other article, including any component, part, or accessory which was recognized in the official National Formulary, the **United States Pharmocopeia**, intended to be used in the diagnosis, treatment, mitigation, cure or prevention of disease in man or animals or, in the case of components used to affect the structure or function of the body of man or animals. An unwritten definition exists suggesting that devices do not have any chemical effect on the body.

There are three classifications of medical devices depending on the amount of risk and invasiveness associated with their use (Table 1.26). **Class I devices** include crutches, bedpans, depressors, adhesive bandages and hospital beds. This class of device requires that the manufacturer notify the FDA prior to marketing the product so that the product meets any existing performance standards set by the FDA (Phelps and Dormer, 1986).

Class II devices present some risk to the patient and include a list of performance standards that must be met before the products can be marketed. These devices include hearing aids, blood pumps, catheters, contact lenses, and electrocardiograph electrodes. **Class III devices** pose a significant risk to the patient and could lead to injury if used incorrectly. They include cardiac pacemakers, intrauterine devices, intraocular lenses and heart valve replacements (Ciarkowski, 1986). All class III devices require pre-market approval involving detailed pre-clinical and clinical studies prior to marketing. All devices introduced after 1976 that are not

Table 1.26 Classification of medical devices*

Class	Types of devices	FDA filing
I	crutches, bedpans, depressors, adhesive bandages, hospital beds	PMN/510 (k)
II	hearing aids, blood pumps, catheters, contact lenses, electrodes, catheters	510 (k)
III	cardiac pacemakers, intrauterine devices, intraocular lenses, heart valves, orthopaedic devices	PMA

PMN = pre-market notification, 510 (k) = substantial equivalence to pre-1976 device, PMA = pre-market approval
* Phelps and Dormer, 1986

40 Scope and markets for medical implants

substantially equivalent to devices on the market before 1976 are automatically classified into class III.

1.6.1 Regulatory pathways for medical devices

The manner by which a medical device can be brought to market depends on a number of factors. Although, in theory, devices that are similar to devices marketed pre-1976 are technically covered by **paragraph 510(k)** of the **1976 Medical Device Amendments**, the interpretation of what is defined as substantially equivalent is not clear and is sometimes only determined after submission of safety and efficacy documents to the FDA (Table 1.27).

In theory all medical devices developed after 1976 are classified under class III and require pre-market approval and therefore involve detailed pre-clinical and clinical testing. However, depending on the claims that are made for the device, many medical devices have been approved as substantially equivalent to pre-1976 devices. The approval of **510(k)** devices is facilitated over the pre-market approval route (Phelps and Dormer, 1986; Black, 1988).

Until 1990, manufacturers of post-1976 devices that are 'substantially equivalent' to pre-1976 devices are required to give the FDA 90 days' notice of their intent to market a device and to demonstrate that the device is substantially equivalent to a pre-1976 device. The FDA was required to respond to the 510(k) submission within 90 days or the product could be marketed. Normally, the FDA requires more than 90 days to respond

Table 1.27 FDA approval for medical devices*

Classification	Requirements	Time for approvals
510 (k)	safety data (animal testing)	months
	sterility and pyrogenicity	months
	cytotoxicity	months
	efficacy (literature)	months
	equivalence to device marketed pre-1976	at least 90 days at FDA
PMA	safety testing (animals)	months
	sterility and pyrogenicity	months
	cytotoxicity	months
	efficacy (animals)	months
	clinical efficacy	years
	PMA filing	at least 180 days at FDA

* Phelps and Dormer, 1986; Black, 1988

and may request information in addition to that which is presented in the application.

In contrast, **pre-market approval (PMA)** requires detailed safety and effectiveness data. In the case of a PMA application, the FDA has 180 days to respond. However, normally additional data is required which extends this period by many months. The data submitted to the FDA include pre-clinical and clinical data related to the safety and efficacy of the device. Biomaterials, per se, are not approved by the FDA. The FDA approves medical devices and therefore a particular material must be shown to be safe and effective in that application.

Both PMAs and 510 (k)s require labelling and manufacturing controls to be clearly spelled out before a device can actually be marketed. In addition, the manufacturer must spell out how the product will be sterilized and validated based on testing done by an independent laboratory.

Medical devices must bear labelling that contains adequate directions for use and list the name and place of business of the manufacturer, packer, or distributor. In addition, the label must give the quantity of the material, product name and detailed instructions on how the product should be used by the physician who must prescribe the medical device. Finally, the product insert must describe all inappropriate uses of the device that may bring about adverse reactions.

Each manufacturer must establish in order to get regulatory approval that the medical device is manufactured in accordance with **good manufacturing practices** (GMP). To do this, manufacturers or distributors must register their production facilities with the FDA and be inspected for compliance with GMP regulations. Notification of the intent to ship devices in inter-state commerce must be made 90 days prior to the initial shipment of devices and be updated semi-annually indicating all the types of devices that have been shipped.

1.6.2 Good manufacturing practices

GMP regulations are designed to establish that the manufacturer has control over process variables critical to the performance of the product as well as routine practices to maintain the performance of personnel and equipment (Phelps and Dormer, 1986). GMPs require written procedures for evaluation and sterilization of the final product as well as for maintenance of records for the manufacture and shipment of each batch of product.

Medical device reporting (MDR) regulations require maufacturers and importers of medical devices to report to the FDA any deaths or serious injuries that may have been caused by a marketed device. These regulations require a telephone call to the FDA within 5 days of initial receipt of information that a device caused or contributed to a death or serious injury. Recurring malfunctions that are likely to cause or contribute to death or serious injury must be reported within 15 working days.

1.6.3 Selection of preclinical testing

Whether a device is submitted for 510(k) or PMA approval, it is important to establish its safety and effectiveness so that a maufacturer will not spend unnecessary time and money on a device which is likely to have little medical value. Therefore a broad spectrum of studies should be undertaken to establish without prejudice that the device is safe and effective. The FDA does not publish a specific list of tests that are required for a regulatory submission. Instead they place the burden on the manufacturer to provide substantial evidence that the device is both safe and effective.

Selection of biological tests therefore is not a standardized practice and involves selection of one or more tests listed in Table 1.18. At the very minimum, the FDA will look for acceptable levels of cytotoxicity, mutagenicity, carcinogenicity and pyrogenicity. In addition, results of intramuscular or subcutaneous implantation are also advised. Finally, an implantation is recommended in the end-use application to establish safety and effectiveness. Prior to conducting any of these studies the product sterilization procedure must be validated so that all cell culture and animal tests can be conducted on the final product.

1.6.4 Clinical trials on medical devices

All class III medical devices require that the effectiveness of the device be established prior to marketing (Table 1.26). Therefore, clinical trials on the device must be submitted as part of the final approval process. The goal of the clinical study is to provide evidence, in a blinded study if possible, that the product performs a certain therapeutic function based on a comparison with a control device. It is the clinical data that forms the basis for the product claims that are approved by the FDA for use on the package and in the package insert.

In 1980, the FDA published guidelines detailing the provisions under which devices would be granted exemptions for purposes of investigating safety and effectiveness of class III devices (Hurley, 1986). **The investigational device exemption** (IDE) regulations apply to all medical devices except nonhuman research, custom devices, veterinary devices, diagnostic devices and investigations of currently approved indications of a device. The later case covers the testing of pre-amendment devices and testing combinations of approved devices.

Custom devices are exempted from IDE regulatory filings as are clinical investigations for the advancement of science that do not determine the safety and effectiveness of a device for commercial distribution. Diagnostic devices are exempted if the device is labelled for research purposes only, testing does not require invasive sampling that presents risk to the subject, and the device is not used for diagnostic purposes without confirmation by another approved test.

The IDE regulatory filing required to do clinical trials on non-exempted devices depends on the subclassification of the intended use and the degree of risk to the subject. Significant risk studies involve an investigational device that presents a potential for serious risk to the health, safety or welfare of a subject and its use to support or sustain human life. An application must be submitted to the FDA before any clinical studies can be initiated for devices that pose a significant risk to the subjects.

Devices which pose no significant risk to the subjects do not require FDA regulatory approval before clinical studies can proceed. Their application is considered approved if it has been approved as a non-significant risk study by a **Hospital Internal Review Board** that has evaluated the proposed investigation. The sponsor must also comply with appropriate requirements for labelling, monitoring, reporting and recording the results of the investigation.

1.6.5 The Safe Medical Device Act of 1990

On 28 November, 1990, the US Congress passed a bill entitled 'The Safe Medical Devices Act of 1990' (Table 1.28). The act requires that all user facilities (hospitals, ambulatory surgical facilities, nursing homes and out-

Table 1.28 Provisions of the safe medical device act of 1990*

Provision	Significance
Device injury	All user facilities must report all injuries or deaths resulting from use of a device to the FDA and manufacturer within 10 days
Semi-annual reports	All user facilities must submit report to FDA concerning device related deaths
Distributor reports	All distributors must report adverse reactions or deaths to FDA annually and to manufacturers
Tracking system	Manufacturers of life-sustaining or supporting devices must establish a tracking system
Device performance	FDA will establish device performance standards one year after fourth original PMA
Equivalence	Substantial equivalence is defined as when the intended use of both the pending device and propose device is the same and both devices have the same technological characteristics

* Bruck and Silver, 1991

patient facilities) report to device manufacturers and the FDA within ten working days any device which has caused injury or contributed to the death of a patient. The bill also requires that user facilities submit semi-annually a report of all device related deaths and serious injuries to the FDA. The manufacturer is also required to report any cases of adverse reactions to the FDA separately. Medical device reporting requirements are extended to distributors of medical devices. Distributors of medical devices who submit annual reports to the FDA must also submit reports to the manufacturer. Manufacturers or distributors of permanently implantable, life-sustaining or life-supporting medical devices whose failure have serious adverse health consequences, are required to establish a medical device tracking system.

Another provision of the law states that one year from the date of the fourth original PMA of a kind (same end-use), the FDA will be allowed to use the manufacturer's pre-clinical, animal and clinical information included in regulatory submissions to establish **performance standards** for approval of similar devices. Data on PMAs becomes available on 15 November, 1992 regardless of whether or not the FDA announces its availability sooner in the **Federal register**. Such data will become available one year after the FDA has issued an approval letter to the sponsor.

The bill also clarifies the definition of **substantial equivalence**. Substantial equivalence occurs when the use of both the pending device and the proposed device is the same, both devices have the same technological characteristics, and if the devices have the same technological characteristics and the sponsor includes information demonstrating that it is as safe and effective as one that is legally marketed. In no case can substantial equivalence be argued for a device removed from the market by the FDA because of misbranding or adulteration. Class III medical devices whose manufacturers claim substantial equivalence to pre-1976 devices must include in their application under section 510(k) a summary of and citation to all adverse safety and effectiveness data.

The FDA must review the status of pre-1976 Device Amendments class III devices prior to 1 December, 1995 to determine whether or not each class III device should be reclassified into class I or class II, or whether it should remain in class III.

1.7 Summary

The design and testing of medical devices is an interdisciplinary effort involving scientists, engineers and physicians. Not only must the choice of materials for a device be carefully considered, but also a design should be planned in detail.

Typically, the initial design criteria are based on the physiology and properties of the host tissue to be replaced. Materials including polymers, metals, ceramics, and composites with the appropriate physical properties are then selected and must meet the general 'biocompatibility' requirements. Prototypes are built and tested to include biocompatibility evaluations based on ASTM standard procedures. The device is validated for sterility and freedom from pyrogens before it can be tested on animals or humans.

Medical devices are classified as class I, II or III depending on their invasiveness. Class I devices can be marketed by submitting notification to the FDA. Class II and III devices require either that they show equivalence to a device marketed prior to 1976 or that they receive pre-marketing approval. The time from device conception to FDA approval can range from months (class I device) to in excess of ten years (class III device). Therefore, much planning is necessary to pick the best regulatory approach.

2.

Wound Dressings and Skin Replacement

2.1 Introduction

Wounds to the skin are encountered every day. Minor skin wounds cause some pain, but these wounds will heal by themselves in time. Even though many minor wounds heal effectively without scarring in the absence of treatment, they heal more rapidly if they are kept clean and moist. Devices such as Band-Aids are used to assist in wound healing. For deeper wounds, a variety of wound dressings have been developed including cell cultured artificial skin. These materials are intended to promote healing of skin damaged or removed as a result of skin grafting, ulceration, burns, cancer excision or mechanical trauma.

Synthetic materials in the form of dressings are used primarily for treatment of superficial wounds. These devices prevent moisture and heat loss from the skin and bacterial infiltration from the environment. Artificial skin is used not only to limit entrance of foreign matter into the skin and prevent mass and heat transfer out of the skin, but to provide a continuous cellular layer over the skin. The objective of the use of any implant material is to restore the normal skin structure and physiology. Therefore, it is essential to understand the structure and properties of normal skin before designing a dressing or artificial skin.

2.1.1 Anatomy and physiology of skin

Human skin is a functional organ that covers about two m^2 of surface area. Skin tissue is involved in regulation of body temperature, repair of wounds, immunity from disease, removal of waste and synthesis of growth factors, vitamins, and other important molecules (Geesin and Berg, 1991) (Table 2.1). It also protects the internal organs from mechanical and electrical injury as well as providing shape to the various parts of the body. These physiological functions are maintained as it continually undergoes development and remodelling. Continual loss and replacement of the epithelial cells that are found on the skin surface is just one of the dynamic processes that occur within skin.

The skin is divided into two anatomically distinct regions, the **epidermis** and the **dermis** (Wasserman and Dunn, 1991) (Table 2.2). The outer layer of

Table 2.1 Physiological functions of skin*

Function	Unit conferring function
Immunity from disease	Langerhans and other cells
Protects against mechanical and electrical injury	Collagen and elastic fibres and keratin filaments
Provides shape to various parts of the body	Collagen fibres
Regulation of body temperature	Sweat glands
Repair of wounds	Inflammatory and connective tissue cells
Removal of waste	Tissue macrophages
Synthesis of growth factors, vitamins, etc	Cells

* adapted from Geesin and Berg, 1991

Table 2.2 Anatomical regions of skin*

Region	Function
Epidermis	Protects and insulates skin externally
Stratum basal	Layer of cuboidal single cells that differentiate as they move upward in the skin
Stratum spinosum	Layer several cells thick that shows flattened cell morphology
Stratum granulosum	Transition layer between living and dead cells
Stratum corneum	Uppermost layer of dead cells containing keratin
Stratum lucidum	Translucent lower cellular layer of stratum corneum
Stratum disjunctum	Upper layer of stratum corneum where sloughing of dead cells occurs
Dermis	Provides support for epidermis
Papillary layer	Upper dermal layer containing thin collagen and elastic fibres
Reticular layer	Lower dermal layer containing thick collagen and elastic fibres
Functional units	Dermis contains hair follicles, sebacious and sweat glands, nerves and vessels

* adapted from Wasserman and Dunn, 1991

skin, the epidermis, varies in thickness depending on the location. It is thickest on the palms of the hands and on the soles of the feet where mechanical loads applied to the skin are highest. The epidermis is composed of four cellular layers including the **stratum basal, stratum spinosum, stratum granulosum,** and **stratum corneum**. It is variable in thickness and contains undulations termed **rete pegs**.

The growth of the upper most portion of skin starts at the interface between the dermis and epidermis in the cell layer termed **stratum basal**. This layer is a single cell thick and is composed of cuboidal or low columnar epithelium. It serves as a reservoir of potential cells and is responsible for maintaining the progeny of cells that differentiate in the upper layers of the epidermis. In effect, cells that are formed at the epidermis–dermis interface migrate upward in the skin and take on specific functions until they die and are sloughed off at the air–skin interface (Figure 2.1). Because of their ability to synthesize keratin (a highly insoluble protein) these cells have been termed keratinocytes. Cells adhere to each other by specializations termed hemidesmosomes. Beneath this cell layer is a thin collagenous film termed the **basement membrane** which is the line of demarcation between the epidermis and dermis.

Immediately above the basal cell layer is the **stratum spinosum**, a layer that is several cells thick. It is in this layer that cells show a transition from cuboidal cells to flattened squamous cells near the surface. The uppermost cells of this layer contain sterols and glycolipids creating a lipidous barrier that establishes a seal preventing excessive water loss.

The **stratum granulosum** is a transition layer between the epidermal cells (below) and the dead squamous cells (above). These cells are characterized by the presence of dense granules. These granules are released into the extracellular space near the top of this layer.

The uppermost layer of the epidermis is the **stratum corneum**, which consists of non-viable cells that contain mostly keratin filaments and remnants of cellular material. Cell nuclei are absent as well as junctions between the cells. Cells in contact with the air are observed to slough off. Within the stratum corneum the following two subdivisions are found. The **stratum lucidum** is a translucent layer of tightly packed cells that is in contact with the granulosum. The **stratum disjunctum** is the location where cellular sloughing occurs.

Cells found within the epidermis include keratinocytes, Merkel cells, dendritic cells, melanocytes, Langerhans cells, Schwann cells, mast cells and macrophages (Table 2.3). These cells are involved in protein production, sensory transmission, protection against radiation damage, immune system activation, and inflammatory responses. It is important to note that failure to repair each of these cell types leads to impaired physiologic function.

The **dermis** is a bi-layer material consisting of the **papillary layer** which is in direct contact with the epidermis and the **reticular dermis** which is found

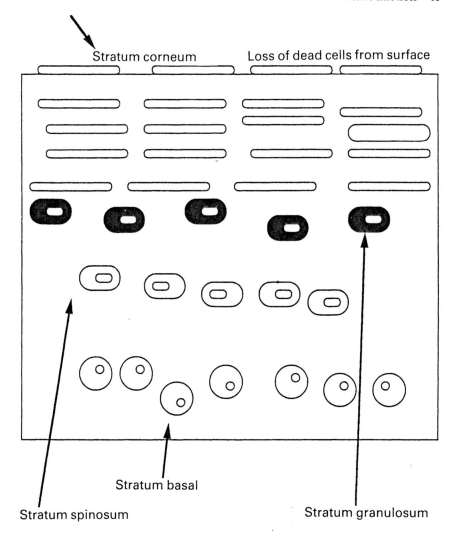

Figure 2.1 Diagram illustrating skin loss by attrition.

below. In the papillary dermis abundant numbers of fibroblasts and other cell types are found as well as wavy fibres consisting of types I and III collagens. In addition, oxytalan fibres, which are similar in composition to elastic fibres, are found in this layer. The reticular layer contains larger diameter collagen and elastic fibres and thicker fibre bundles (compared to the papillary layer). The dermis and epidermis are connected via type VII collagen and oxytalan that extend from the basement membrane into

Table 2.3 Cells found in the epidermis*

Cell type	Function
Dendritic cells	Involved in sensory processes
Langerhans cells	Involved in immune responses
Merkel cells	Involved in sensory processes
Macrophage	Involved in phagocytosis
Mast cells	Involved in inflammation
Melanocytes	Produce melanin and protect against radiation damage
Keratinocytes	Produce keratins, tough fibrous proteins
Schwann cells	Insulate nerve cells

* Wasserman and Dunn, 1991

the dermis. Collagen fibril diameters range from 60–100 nm while fibre diameters range from 10–40 μm.

Dermis contains a variety of functional units including hair follicles, sebacious glands, sweat glands, nerves and vessels (Table 2.4). In addition, it is in close proximity to adipose tissue, veins and arteries and muscle that are immediately below.

Hair follicles originate below the dermis and pass through the dermis and epidermis. They are supported by elastin and collagen fibres and are raised and lowered by a network of smooth muscle, called arrector pili. Sebacious glands are associated with hair follicles except on the palms of the hands and soles of the feet. They secrete a waxy fluid through a duct and onto the epidermal surface.

Sweat glands in the skin are primarily involved in secreting a watery fluid directly onto the epidermis, thereby dissipating heat and maintaining normal body temperature. They are lined by epithelium that are contiguous with the cells that are at the tissue–environment interface.

Nerve endings located in the epidermis and dermis provide sensation of touch, pain and temperature. Free nerve endings are found in the epidermis and around hair follicles.

Blood vessels in and below the dermis, provide nutrition as well as assist in pressure and thermal regulation. A series of blood vessels termed rete cutaneum, supplies blood to the lower portion of the hair follicles and sweat glands. Branches from these vessels feed the sub-capillary plexus which is the blood vessel layer located between the papillary and reticular dermis.

Table 2.4 Functional units found in dermis*

Unit	Function
Blood vessels	Provide nutrition, and assist in pressure and thermal regulation
Hair follicles	Epithelial lined shafts in which hair is formed and directed upward
Nerve endings	Provide sensation of touch, pain and temperature
Sebacious glands	Associated with hair follicles and secrete waxy substance
Sweat glands	Epithelial lined tubes that secrete watery fluid to dissipate heat

* Wasserman and Dunn, 1991

Capillaries derived from these vessels feed the epidermis, and sebacious and sweat glands. Lymphatic vessels are dense in the papillary layer but are not associated with hair, sweat and sebacious glands.

Glandular structures and blood vessels in the skin are often damaged as a result of severe burns and skin ulcers. Although the connective tissue components can be repaired during wound healing, the glandular structures and normal vascular patterns are not easily regenerated. Wound dressings and artificial skin that regenerate these structures are desirable, since in their absence the patient may survive but suffer cosmetic scarring as well as physiologic limitations including problems with thermal regulation.

2.2 Biochemistry of skin

Skin is a multi-component composite of cells and macromolecules (Geesin and Berg, 1991). The major component of the epidermis is the keratinocyte, which forms overlapping structures held together by desmosomes which provide cell-to-cell adhesion. The dermis is composed largely of extracellular matrix components including collagen, elastin, fibrillin, hyaluronic acid and proteoglycans. Collagen fibres give shape to the skin as well as prevent premature mechanical failure. Elastin fibres composed of fibrillin and elastin, are believed to be responsible for recovery of skin after removal of a mechanical load.

The fibroblast is the cell type which is most prevalent in skin and is responsible for synthesizing and depositing collagen fibres in continuous networks that form the structural scaffold. This cell type is also responsible for recognition, removal and turnover of proteins that are damaged or are being recycled.

2.2.1 Intracellular components

Keratinocytes produce a protective cytoskeleton composed of a class of proteins termed keratins. These keratins differ depending on the state of differentiation of keratinocytes observed as the cells move toward the air-skin interface (Table 2.5). The four cellular layers of the epidermis represent different levels of differentiation and therefore have different sets of keratin molecules. **Intermediate filaments** are composed of a number of double helical keratin molecules. The molecules are products of different genes.

Production of keratin fibres is assisted by another protein termed **filaggrin**, a filament aggregating protein. In the lower layers of the epidermis this protein is synthesized in a precursor form termed **profilaggrin**. Profilaggrin is processed in the intermediate layers to form several filaggrin molecules. Filaggrin is reduced to amino acids as cells migrate toward the surface of the epidermis.

Keratinocytes develop a rigid structure within the cytoplasm as they migrate towards the air-skin interface. This structure is formed by cross-linking several proteins together via lysine derived chemical bonds.

2.2.2 Extracellular components

Lipid components of skin result in its hydrophobicity. Lipids in skin provide for water retention, and stratum corneum cohesion. They consist of

Table 2.5 Non-connective tissue proteins and lipids in skin*

Protein	Function
Keratin	Forms insoluble structural component found in intermediate filaments in epidermis
Filaggrin	Filament aggregating protein
Phosphatidylcholine	Lipids in lower layers of skin
Phosphatidylethanolamine	Lipids in lower layers of skin
Sphinomyelin	Lipids in lower layers of skin
Cholesterol sulphate	Lipids in upper layers of skin
Ceramide	Lipids in upper layers of skin
Fatty acids	Lipids in upper layers of skin

* Geesin and Berg, 1991

phosphatidylcholine, phosphatidylethanolamine and **sphingomyelin** in the lower layers and **cholesterol sulphate, ceramide** and **fatty acids** in the upper layer (Table 2.5).

Pigmentation of the skin is achieved by cells located above the basal layer, termed melanocytes. These cells secrete vacuoles, termed melanosomes, containing the pigment, melanin, and introduce them into keratinocytes. The number, size and distribution of melanocytes dictates the resulting skin color. Melanocytes in the epidermis are believed to protect proliferative cells from damage by radiation that penetrates the skin surface.

Epidermis and dermis are separated by a membrane, termed basement membrane, which provides a barrier between these layers as well as limiting growth of dermal cells. It is 70–100 nm thick and contains type IV collagen, BM-40 (osteonectin or SPARC), laminin, nidogen and heparan sulphate proteoglycan (Table 2.6). It is presumed, based on in vitro studies of assembly, that basement membrane is composed of a lattice of type IV collagen that is associated with laminin, heparan sulphate proteoglycan and fibronectin. The amino acid sequences of Arginine-Glycine-Aspartic Acid, which are known to be specific for binding to certain cell types, are found on molecules such as laminin and nidogen. Anchoring fibrils composed of type VII collagen connect the basement membrane to the dermis. Type VII collagen molecules exist as antiparallel dimers of two triple helical subunits. Fibronectin, a dimer of two glycoprotein chains, is found near the basement

Table 2.6 Components associated with basement membrane*

Component	Function
Fibronectin	Cell and extracellular matrix attachment factor
BM-40 (osteonectin, SPARC)	Cell and extracellular matrix attachment factor
Heparan sulphate Proteoglycan	Connects cell surface to extracellular matrix
Laminin	Component of basement membrane
Nidogen	Cell attachment factor
Type IV collagen	Component of basement membrane
Type VII collagen	Connects basement membrane to dermis
Laminin	Component of basement membrane

* Geesin and Berg, 1991

54   Wound dressings and skin replacement

membrane. Cell matrix interactions are mediated by fibronectin since it has cellular and extracellular binding domains.

Dermis

Dermis is composed of collagen, elastic fibres and small amounts of proteoglycans (Figure 2.2). Type I, III, IV and V collagens are found in the form of fibres. The predominant forms of collagen in dermis are types I and III while types IV, V and VI are minor components (Table 2.7). All of these molecules are triple helical; however, the helical length and composition of each type varies. Types I and III collagens contain three chains with helical lengths of about 1015 amino acids. In addition, there are non-helical ends that are located at the carboxy and amino ends of the molecule. Type IV and V collagen molecules are somewhat different. The type V molecule has a

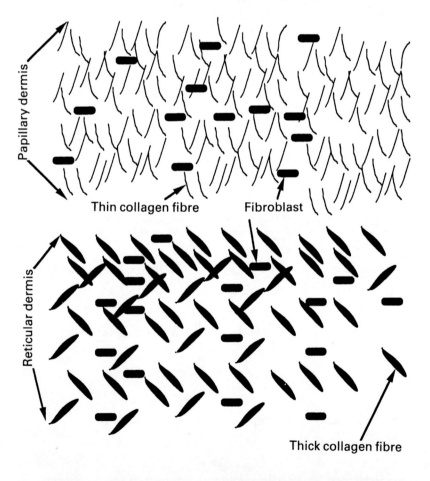

Figure 2.2 Diagram of extracellular matrix in the dermis.

Table 2.7 Collagen and other macromolecules found in dermis*

Macromolecule	Location
Collagen	
type I	Large diameter fibres
type III	Mixed with type I in small diameter fibres
type IV	Basement membranes
type V	Mixed with other types in fibres
Elastin	Combined with microfibrillar proteins in elastic fibres; forms amorphous core
Fibronectin	Cell attachment factor
Hyaluronic acid	Forms filament on which proteoglycans attach and aggregate
Microfibrillar proteins (fibrillin)	Form rim of elastic fibres
Proteoglycans	Attach to and surround collagen fibres
Vitronectin	Cell attachment factor

* adapted from Geesin and Berg, 1991

triple helix that is about the same length as that of types I and III; however, it has non-helical ends that are much larger. Type IV collagen differs from types I, III, and V in that it has sequences of Arginine-Glycine-Aspartic acid as well as other regions that do not form a tight triple helix. In addition, it has a higher molecular weight than types I and III.

Collagen in the dermis is known to interact with various other macromolecules including heparan sulphate proteoglycan, vitronectin, and fibronectin.

Elastic fibres are involved in the recovery of skin after mechanical loads are removed. Elastin is a highly insoluble protein that is composed of repeat amino acid sequences including the amino acids lysine, proline and glycine. Elastin is cross-linked through four lysyl residues to form an insoluble network which is believed to be the amorphous component of elastic fibres. Elastic fibres are also composed of microfibrillar proteins that form the outer core of elastic fibres. The ratio of elastin to microfibrillar components varies according to location within the skin. Recently fibrillin has been reported to be one of the molecules that is present in microfibrils (Geesin and Berg, 1991).

Proteoglycans are found attached to and surrounding collagen fibres in the dermis and are involved in the viscoelastic behaviour of skin. They may mediate interfibrillar slippage during the application of tensile loads.

Proteoglycans in skin exist in a number of physical and chemical forms including both dermatan sulfate and chondroitin sulphate proteoglycans (Table 2.8). Each form is characterized by a protein core to which glycosaminoglycan side chains are attached. Variations in size and amino acid sequence of the core protein as well as the length and type of sugars attached to the core protein lead to differences in the ability of PGs to bind to hyaluronic acid as well as differences in the ability of these molecules to self associate.

The small dermatan sulphate proteoglycans (molecular weight less than (100 000) called DS-PGI (biglycan) and DS-PGII (decorin) have been isolated from bovine fetal skin. Recent evidence suggests that DS-PGI and DS-PGII differ in primary structure (Choi *et al.*, 1989). Both DS-PGI and DS-PGII contain core proteins that have molecular weights of about 40 000. DS-PGI has two glycosaminoglycan chains while DS-PGII has only one chain (Choi *et al.*, 1989). A recent report suggests that only DS-PGII binds to type I collagen fibrils *in vitro* (Brown and Vogel, 1989) (Table 2.9). Substantial binding to type I collagen was noted for both intact small DS-PGII from tendon and core protein from which the glycosaminoglycan chain was removed.

Large proteoglycans have molecular weights in excess of 1 000 000 and contain chondrotin sulphate. In skin, unlike cartilage, large proteoglycans do not associate with link proteins and hyaluronan (HA) to form aggregates. Small proteoglycans also do not associate with link proteins or HA but are seen in the electron microscope bound to the d band of positively stained

Table 2.8 Types of proteoglycans (PGs) in dermis*

Type	Location
Chondroitin sulphate PG	Between collagen fibres
Dermatan sulphate PG	Attached to collagen fibres
Heparan sulphate PG	Embedded in cell membrane

* Scott, 1992 for a review

Table 2.9 Binding of small dermatan sulphate (DS) PG to type I collagen†

Molecule	Number core GAG* chains	Collagen binding
DS-PGI (biglycan)	2	–
DS-PGII (decorin)	1	+

* GAG = glycosaminoglycan
† Choi *et al.*, 1989; Brown and Vogel, 1989

collagen fibrils in tissues. Large proteoglycans are believed to fill the spaces between collagen fibrils and facilitate fibril sliding.

Hyaluronan (HA) (formerly referred to as hyaluronic acid or hyaluronate) is an unbranched polysaccharide that is found in low molecular weight form (less than 100 000) in the vitreous and high molecular weight form (greater than 1 000 000) in synovial fluid and other tissues. High molecular weight HA molecules behave like random coils in solution and occupy very large domains while low molecular weight HA behaves in a worm-like coil manner. A few reports suggest that high molecular weight HA forms fibrous networks that are visible in the electron microscope. Aggregation of HA into double helical and other forms has been postulated based on x-ray diffraction.

Adhesion glycoproteins in the extracellular matrix mediate interaction between cell cytoskeletal components and the fibrous components that provide a scaffold for tissues. Integrins are a family of transmembrane receptors (Hynes, 1987) present in the tissues that specifically bind to the amino acid sequence Arginine-Glycine-Aspartic acid which is sometimes abbreviated to RGD. RGD sequences are present in a number of extracellular matrix macromolecules including collagen, fibronectin and laminin. The integrin family consists of one of three different *beta* subunits which is associated with one of several *alpha* subunits. These receptors link extracellular matrix components to intracellular actin of the cytoskeleton (Figure 2.3) adapted, based on Ruoslahti (1991).

2.3 Mechanical properties of skin

The mechanical properties of skin are largely a result of the collagen and elastic fibre networks that form a scaffold upon which cells sit. The physiological functions of skin include providing a smooth barrier that protects internal organs from electrical and mechanical insult, loss of water and heat, and penetration of bacteria and other harmful stimuli. The surface layer of skin which appears creased under visual observation, is normally under a bi-axial pretension and pulls taut under normal physiological loads. If a square piece of the skin is cut within the plane, the skin edges will retract as a result of internal tension. In areas of the body where skin covers joints, it must be able to double its length on stretching to allow free joint movement. Therefore, the ability of skin to deform in a plane as well as to maintain its continuity when subject to forces both in the plane and perpendicular to the plane are of utmost importance.

The mechanical properties of skin to a first approximation are a consequence of the collagen and elastic fibre networks present as well as the proteoglycans that are found between neighbouring collagen fibrils (Silver and Doillon, 1989). The epidermis contributes very little to these properties except in areas of the body where the epidermis is thick, such as the palms of the hands and the soles of the feet.

58 Wound dressings and skin replacement

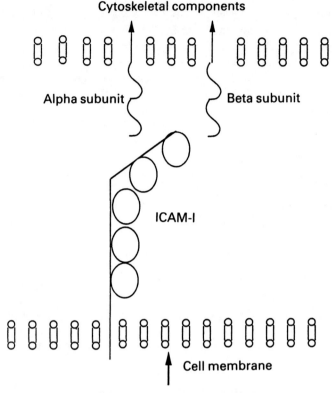

Figure 2.3 Schematic diagram of relationship between integrins and actin in cell membranes.

Collagen types I and III form mixed fibres in skin in cross-linked continuous networks that prevent premature mechanical failure. The collagen molecule by virtue of its inherent stiffness (Table 2.10) dictates the upper bounds of the modulus or stiffness of skin. The modulus of skin is determined by taking the ratio of change in stress required to cause a change of strain where stress is the ratio of force to the area over which it is applied and strain is the ratio of change in length to the original length (Figure 2.4).

A typical stress–strain curve for skin is shown in Figure 2.4 illustrating an increasing slope with increasing strain. The maximum slope of this plot for individual fibres from rat tail tendon is several thousand MPa (1 MPa is 10 N/m^2) (Figure 2.5). This value is very close to the value of 4000 MPa calculated from viscosity measurements of single collagen molecules (Nestler et al., 1983). This observation suggests that the stiffness of collagenous tissues is a consequence of the triple helical structure and approaches that of an individual collagen molecule in the dry state. In this

Table 2.10 Definitions of mechanical terms*

Term	Definition
Cross-sectional area	Specimen width times thickness
Stress	Force per unit cross-sectional area
Modulus (stiffness)	Slope of stress–strain curve (change in stress/change in strain)
Strain	Change in length/original length
Tangent modulus	Tangent to stress–strain curve
Toughness	Area under stress–strain curve

* Silver, 1987

state intermolecular and interfibrillar bonding is maximized. When intermolecular and interfibrillar slippage is possible, i.e. in wet tissues, energy is dissipated and as a result the stiffness falls to a level that is far below that of individual collagen molecules. Nature has designed a force dissipating

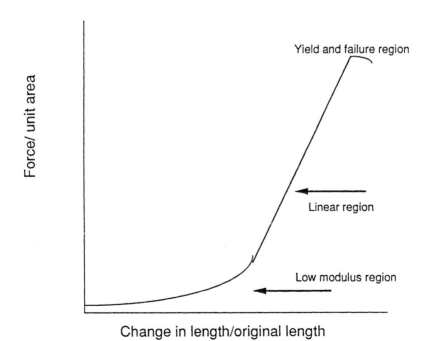

Figure 2.4 Diagram illustrating mechanical properties of generalized connective tissue.

60 Wound dressings and skin replacement

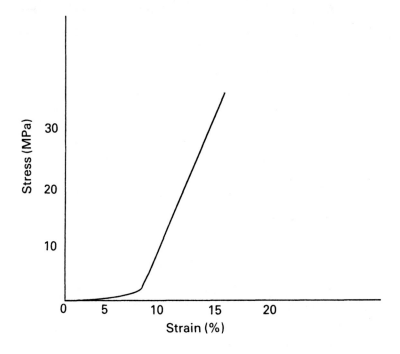

Figure 2.5 Stress-strain curve for an individual collagen fibre.

structure that can be somewhat pliant in soft tissues where hydration levels are high, or extremely rigid in bone and dentin where hydration is limited by mineralization.

Other factors that influence the mechanical properties of skin have been recently reviewed by Wasserman and Dunn (1991) and include the variation in thickness with location and age, anisotropy introduced by the direction of preferred orientation of collagen fibres in the skin, method used to measure the mechanical properties, rate at which skin specimens are stretched and the level of tissue hydration during mechanical testing (Table 2.11).

Stress–strain curves for wet skin have traditionally been analyzed in four parts (Figure 2.6). In phase I or the low modulus region, very small changes in stress result from fairly large strains. The region involves the removal of undulations and initial alignment of the three-dimensionally organized collagen fibres along the tensile load direction. This rearrangement is possible because the fibres in skin are in a non-woven fabric allowing neighbouring collagen fibrils to slide by each other.

Phase II of the stress–strain curve is characterized by recruitment of the collagen fibres into the load bearing network and is associated with an

Mechanical properties of skin 61

Table 2.11 Factors that influence the mechanical properties of skin*

Factor	Influence on tangent modulus
Location	Higher for skin from palm or sole
Orientation of specimen	Higher along Langer's lines
Rate of specimen deformation	Increased at higher rate of deformation
Sex	Different for male and female
Temperature	Varies
Thickness variation	Higher increased thickness
Tissue hydration	Higher with low water content

* adapted from Christiansen *et al.*, 1991

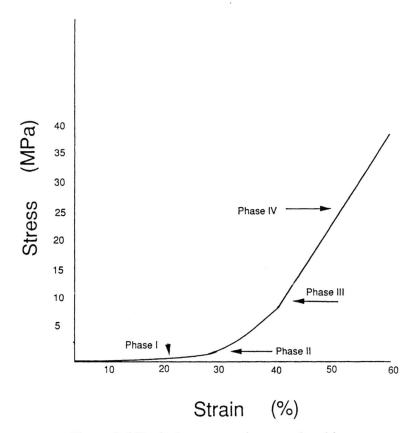

Figure 2.6 Typical stress-strain curve for skin.

increase in the modulus to about 16 MPa at a strain of about 60%. Linearity of the stress–strain relationship occurs at the point (phase III) where the collagen fibres bear the full load. Physiologically, skin is believed to operate in phases II and III since the normal pretension in skin probably accounts for enough strain to partially align the collagen fibres.

Failure of skin occurs in phase IV at stresses of between 7 and 12 MPa or 14 and 24 MPa if one corrects for the loss of cross-section that occurs as the specimen is stretched. At low strains, only about 50% of the total stress applied to skin is stored; however, at high strains the amount of elastically stored energy increases to 75% (Figure 2.7 adapted from Dunn and Silver, 1983). These values depend on the rate of deformation and reflect the viscoelastic behaviour of skin.

2.4 Repair of skin

Repair of skin involves a series of events that are initiated by mechanical, chemical, bacteriological, viral and other traumatic stimuli (Table 2.12).

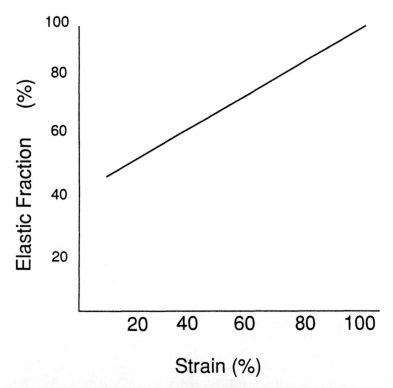

Figure 2.7 Diagram illustrating the fraction of elastically stored energy in skin stretched to different strains.

Table 2.12 Events that trigger skin repair*

Event	Effect
Bacteriological infection	Inflammatory response
Chemical burns	Degradation of extracellular matrix
Electrical burns	Tissue necrosis
Mechanical trauma	Vascular leakage and tissue swelling
Viral infection	Inflammatory response

* Silver and Parsons, 1991

These events lead to plugging of vascular leaks as well as filling in of tissue defects that arise as a result of tissue damage. Repair of dermis precedes repair of the epidermis. Dermal repair involves inflammation, immunity, blood clotting, platelet aggregation, fibrinolysis and activation of complement and kinin systems (Table 2.13). In the absence of a chronic inflammatory response, dermal wounds are repaired through deposition and remodelling of collagen to form scar tissue. Each of the phases of wound healing are discussed below.

Repair of the dermis occurs as a response to the disruption of blood vessels and injury to cells of the extracellular matrix (Silver and Parsons, 1991). Activation of blood clotting leads the formation of an insoluble fibrin network and activation of complement, kinin, and fibrinolytic systems required to clean tissue debris. These systems are cascades by which

Table 2.13 Biological systems involved in repair*

System	Function
Blood clotting	Prevents excess bleeding
Complement	Involved in lysis of foreign cells and vasodilation of vessels
Fibrinolysis	Removes blood clots
Immunity	Destroys foreign bacteria
Inflammation	Cleans up dead tissue
Kinin	Involved in vasodilation
Platelet aggregation	Plugs leaks in vessel walls

* adapted from Silver, 1987; Silver and Parsons, 1991

activated plasma proteins trigger vasoactivity, fibrin clot removal and destruction of foreign cellular material all of which are processes that are required before healing can be initiated (Figure 2.8).

Tissue repair involves inflammatory, proliferative, granulating and remodelling phases (Table 2.14). Initially, synthesis of hyaluronic acid and ensuing binding to fibrin that is deposited in a blood clot occur. This complex forms a matrix that is believed to play a role in the granulating and remodelling phases of wound healing. Fibronectin that is cross-linked to fibrin in the wound, promotes chemotaxis, migration and adhesion of inflammatory cells including polymorphonuclear leukocytes. Factors elaborated by inflammatory cells trigger proliferation and migration of cells that synthesize extracellular matrix as well as trigger continued influx of additional inflammatory cells. The first phase of wound healing therefore

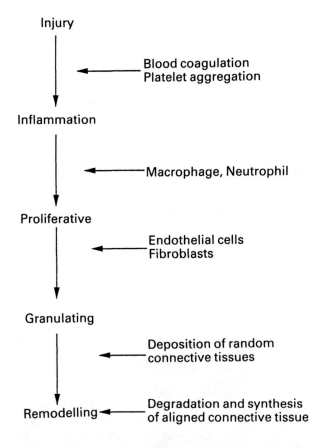

Figure 2.8 Schematic diagram illustrating events that precede healing.

Table 2.14 Phases of wound healing*

Phase	Events
Inflammatory	Influx of blood cells into wound area, removal of tissue debris and deposition of hyaluronic acid
Proliferative	Influx and division of connective tissue cells that synthesize new extracellular matrix
Granulating	Deposition of thin random collagen fibrils
Remodelling	Digestion of thin collagen fibrils and replacement by aligned large diameter fibrils

* adapted from Silver and Doillon, 1989

involves recruitment of inflammatory cells into the wound area and the initiation of removal of dead tissue by these cells.

Following the inflammatory phase of wound healing, is a period characterized by the proliferation of cells that form new blood vessels and extracellular matrix. Fragments of collagen as well as fibronectin in the blood clot are chemotactic to fibroblasts which synthesize types I, III and V collagens and proteoglycans. In the presence of an implant that biodegrades during the proliferative phase, or induces a chronic inflammatory response, inflammation and deposition of new extracellular matrix occur simultaneously. When the inflammatory response is prolonged, host tissue may be damaged resulting in enlargement of the wound and/or excessive deposition of scar tissue. The extracellular matrix laid down immediately after wounding is composed of thin randomly organized collagen fibrils and is referred to as granulation tissue.

During the the next phase of dermal wound healing, granulation tissue is remodelled by a process which involves phagocytosis of collagen fibrils. Another possible mechanism for removal of collagen fibrils involves release of interleukin 1 by macrophages which stimulates collagenase elaboration by fibroblasts. A number of enzymes that are active in degrading collagen types I and III have been identified including mammalian collagenase a metal dependent lysosomal enzyme. Random collagen fibrils are removed from granulation tissue and are replaced with orientated large diameter collagen fibrils that make up scar tissue.

Once the dermis is repaired with scar tissue, epidermal cells present at the wound periphery, in hair follicles or in other glandular structures found in skin, begin to migrate from the wound periphery within 24 hours in human epidermis. Epidermal migration is believed to be facilitated by factors such as fibronectin, epidermal growth factor, interleukin 1 as well as a smooth muscle cell factor. Activation of plasminogen activator and fibrinolysis enables epidermal cells to move through fibrin networks allowing migration below the desiccated portion of the blood clot and above the new extracellular matrix.

2.5 Incidence of skin wounds

Wound dressings and artificial skin are used to repair and replace areas of skin damaged by localized pressure (bed sores), burns, cancer excision sites, and complications of conditions including diabetes (diabetic skin ulcers) and insufficient cardiac output (venous stasis skin ulcers).

Skin wounds that require wound dressings or replacement of the entire thickness of skin have a number of etiologies. Between 11 and 12 million patients in the United States alone suffer from ulceration of the skin. One million people each year sustain burn injuries and 100 000 are serious enough to require hospitalization (MacMillan, 1984) (Table 2.15). In addition, there are about 600 000 cases of skin excision each year related to removal of skin cancers as well as cosmetic procedures. This translates into a wound care market of close to two billion dollars (not all of which involves only the skin) of which about 100 million is devoted to bandages, 300 million to sterile packings, 100 million to irrigating solutions and one billion to wound closures (sutures and staples) as tabulated in Table 2.16. The market for burn dressings is somewhat more limited and is about seventy million dollars a year in the US as is indicated in Table 2.17.

2.5.1 Pathophysiology and management of pressure sores

Decubitus ulcers, commonly known as pressure sores, are the consequence of reduced blood supply to the skin (Parish *et al.*, 1983). Several factors have been postulated to lead to occlusion of capillary blood flow in the skin that if

Table 2.15 Prevalance of skin wounds in the US

Type of wound	Number in US per year (million)
Burn	1.0
Severe burns	0.1
Skin excision	0.6
Skin ulcers	
Diabetic	3.7
Pressure sores	8.0

Table 2.16 Wound care marketing data

Product type	1989 Market (Million $)*
Bandages and dressings	97.0
Debridement	48.7
Hemostats	61.2
Irrigating solutions	126.3
Prep supplies	72.3
Sponges	95.3
Sterile packs	335.8
Suction and drainage devices	113.3
Wound closures	923.4
Total	**1,873.3**

* adapted from Biomedical Business International Vol. XII No. 9 September 18, 1989, Tustin, CA

Table 2.17 Burn dressing market

Type of dressing	Companies	Sales in million (year)

Biological
  Porcine skin
  Cadaver skin
  Amniotic membranes
	Genetic laboratories
	Human skin banks
	Hospitals
		10 (1985)*

Biosynthetic BioBrane	Woodroof laboratories	6 (1985)*
Synthetic	Winfield laboratories Smith & Nephew, 3M Squibb, Lohmann	56 (1985)*

Adapted from Biomedical Business International, Tustin, CA
* Vol. XI No. 5 May 10, 1988

uncorrected leads to skin cell death. These include

- pressures greater than 25 mm Hg,
- shearing forces,
- repeated injury,
- infection, and
- lack of cutaneous sensation (Parish *et al.* 1983).

Ulceration due to these factors occurs primarily in areas of the body where skin is compressed against bony areas when a person sits or lays down. Blood supply to the underlying muscle bed may also be an important factor in formation of skin ulcers and in some patients skin lesions may be secondary to muscle necrosis (cell death).

Ischemic skin is more likely to be damaged by normal and shearing forces acting on a bedridden patient. An external pressure of 100 mm Hg applied to the skin of animals for two hours can produce histological changes to muscle; however, the time required depends on the thickness of the fat layer beneath the dermis. Muscle subjected to previous mechanical insult shows degeneration at a lower pressure in shorter time periods. Therefore, ischemic injury to muscle and perhaps fat may be the stimulus that precedes necrosis of the dermis and epidermis (Parish *et al.* 1983). Inflammation that arises from muscle and fatty tissue cell death results in:

- blood clotting
- platelet aggregation
- immune complex formation
- accumulation of inflammatory cells
- activation of fibrinolysis, kinin and complement systems

Clinically, the first sign of formation of a pressure sore is redness (erythema) that is removed by pressure exerted by a finger which is placed over the area in question. The next stage in the progression of symptoms involves erythema that is not removed by pressure. This leads to:

- skin inflammation (dermatitis)
- superficial ulcer formation (wet areas of skin)
- uncontrolled deep ulcers, and
- erosion of dermis

The areas of the body where skin ulcers are commonly observed are:

- ankles
- buttocks (sacral areas)
- heels
- hips (iliac crest), and
- knees

The symptoms of each stage are associated with physical changes that occur in the skin (Parish *et al.* 1983).

- When the erythema is removed by pressure there is normally an *elevation in temperature* of the affected area as well as a colour change.
- When external pressure is removed from the area, the skin returns to normal colour and temperature within 24 hours. At the next stage, the *skin redness* is more intense, and *tenderness and pain* are common features of the lesion.
- Inflammation of the skin (dermatitis) is characterized by loss of integrity of the epidermis with resulting *scaling* and *fluid build up*. At this stage two to four weeks are required for healing if the underlying problem is *resolved*.

- Once the defect has eroded into the dermis and subcutaneous tissue, it takes on a pale red appearance and does not bleed very easily. Any black or dark coloured tissue present consists of *dead cells* (termed necrotic) and is normally removed by either enzyme treatment or surgical scraping with a scalpel.

Bacterial contamination of the ulcer along with compromised blood supply are two problems that must be corrected before healing can be accomplished. Both aerobic and anaerobic bacteria have been identified in pressure sores. Methods for estimating bacterial contamination in wounds have also been useful in predicting the duration required for wound closure.

Management and prevention of pressure sores is becoming a major challenge as the population ages. Non-specific measures include keeping the skin cool by using cold compresses or packs and application of a water repellent barrier (to prevent further contamination from urine and faeces) is recommended (Table 2.18). Steroid creams applied three times a day decrease inflammation. Once an ulcer forms, cleansing of wounds reduces the number of bacteria and allows host immunity to fight off an infection. Solutions such as saline, hydrogen peroxide, acetic acid and other chemicals have been used to wash away bacteria. Fluid exudate from the wounds can be controlled by use of polymeric beads composed of Dextran^{TM} or other hydroscopic material. However, these materials must be removed from the wound or else they can induce an inflammatory reaction. Removal (debridement) of necrotic tissue using enzymes such as collagenase, trypsin, fibrinolysin and papain or mechanical scraping are used to limit the infection since dead tissue is an excellent substrate for bacterial proliferation. Topically, 5-Fluorouracil applied as a cream facilitates removal of dead

Table 2.18 Techniques used to prevent and treat skin ulcers*

Technique	Purpose
Cold compress and barrier dressing	Reduce skin inflammation
Steroid cream application	Reduce skin inflammation
Saline, peroxide or chemical wash	Reduce bacteria count
Pack wound with hydroscopic material	Absorb wound fluid
Wound debridement	Remove necrotic tissue
Vapour permeable dressing application	Promote wound healing

* Eaglstein *et al.*, 1987; Braden and Bryant, 1990; Hutchinson and McGuckin, 1990

tissue over a period of about two weeks. Other methods for wound cleansing include the use of wet-to-dry dressings, hydrotherapy, and laser ablation.

Topical antibiotics are not particularly effective in disinfecting pressure sores because they do not normally penetrate the dead tissue. Contact dermatitis and systemic allergic reactions can occur with the use of topical antibiotics. Granulation tissue stimulation can be achieved by applying collagen, a collagen derivative or benzoyl peroxide to the wound three times a day until wound closure is achieved.

2.5.2 Management of burn wounds

Burn injuries that arise from exposure to thermal or chemical sources are characterized as 1° or superficial, 2° or superficial partial thickness burn, 2° or deep partial thickness burn, 3° full thickness, and 4°–5°–6° burns (Petro, 1983) (Table 2.19). 1° or superficial burns are characterized by loss of the epidermis resulting in redness, pain, swelling and blistering (Table 2.20). Within three to five days these wounds heal; however, itching can occur for several days. Superficial partial thickness or 2° burns result in loss of the epidermis and part of the dermis. They are characterized by skin redness and pain as well as blistering. The outcome of these burns is normal healing without scarring within two weeks. Pigmentation returns to normal and itching subsides within a few weeks. Deep partial thickness or 2° wounds result in loss of the epidermis and a large part of the dermis along with some skin appendages. Skin colour is red turning to white when pressure is applied and the hair hurts when plucked. These burns require greater than two weeks to heal and may form uncontrolled areas of scar tissue (hypertrophic scars). When these wounds heal pigment may be missing and itching prolonged. Skin grafting may be considered for these wounds. Full thickness or 3° burns result in loss of skin and its appendages. Skin is firm and stiff and hair does not hurt when plucked from these wounds. Skin grafting is recommended for patients with large wounds; pigmentation, sensation and itching are not normal for years after the wounds are healed.

Table 2.19 Types of burn injuries*

Type	Description
1° or superficial	Loss of epidermis
2° or superficial partial thickness	Loss of epidermis and some dermis
2° or deep partial thickness	Loss of epidermis and most of dermis
3° or full thickness	Loss of skin and its appendages
4°–5°–6°	Loss of skin, fat, muscle and bone

* Petro, 1983

Table 2.20 Healing of burn injuries*

Type	Healing pattern
1° or superficial	Redness, pain, swelling and blistering; healing in three to five days; treatment with aspirin
2° or superficial partial thickness	Redness, pain and blistering; healing in two weeks; wrap with dressing
2° or deep partial thickness	Red skin turning white when pressure applied; healing in greater than two weeks with some scarring; treat with anti-bacterial agent
3° or full thickness	Loss of sensation in skin; healing requires skin grafting; treatment with topical antibiotics and wound dressings
4°–5°–6°	Contracture of wound tissue around joints and some deformity; healing is prolonged

* Petro, 1983

In the case of 4°–5°–6° burns a loss of fat, muscle and bone is involved and requires immediate surgical debridement until all necrotic tissue is removed. Injury to muscle immediately causes contraction and deformity across the joint involved.

Treatment of burn wounds is based on the extent, depth, location and the complications that arise during the initial post-burn period. As a result of burning, a fixed number of cells are killed and additional cells are injured and may die. The zone of tissue necrosis that surrounds the burn area is in contact with a zone of injured cells that may become necrotic unless care is taken to correctly manage and limit further injury. The zone of injured cells without treatment shows a progressive decrease in capillary circulation within 24 hours of the burn (Table 2.21). Cooling the site of injury for 20 to 30 minutes with cold tap water limits inflammation and the associated tissue damage. Dermal circulation also reappears about 24 hours post-wounding and is promoted by keeping the wound wet and limiting infection.

Contamination of the necrotic tissue (eschar) by bacterial proliferation is common, and daily wound cleansing is required to prevent infection. Bacterial proliferation followed by invasion of skin lymphatics and vascular tissue can lead to a systemic infection and death in patients with large body surface area (BSA) burns. Treatment includes local antibiotic

Table 2.21 Events following burn injury*

Event	Timing
Cell injury and death	Immediately
Decrease in capillary circulation	Within 24 hours
Reappearance of capillary circulation	24 hours post-wounding

* Petro, 1983

therapy, systemic treatment with antibiotics, surgical removal of eschar and adjacent tissues.

First degree burns result from overexposure to sunlight or exposure to steam. They are usually treated with an anti-inflammatory agents such as a topical steroid and an analgesic such as aspirin (Table 2.20). Recovery normally takes place within several days.

In the case of superficial partial thickness second degree burns, where injury is limited to the epidermis and dermis, healing normally occurs within three weeks in healthy individuals. The blister that forms over these wounds adequately protects them from bacterial contamination. When the blister breaks, the wound should be washed and covered with petroleum jelly and then a gauze dressing that is held in place with a bandage. Areas of the body that are not easily dressed can be cleaned and treated with Bacitracin or an ointment containing Silvadene.

Deep partial thickness second degree burns are more difficult to manage since bacteria present in hair follicles can proliferate and contaminate necrotic tissue deep in the dermis. Gram positive organisms are important in burn wound contamination intially; however, gram negative organisms become important five days post-burning. Silvadene (silver sulfadiazene) and Betadine (povidene iodine) are used to treat these wounds alternately every two to three days to avoid development of resistance to any single agent. Wound care using topical agents is used for two to three weeks after which surgical debridement of the eschar followed by skin grafting is considered.

Full thickness third degree burns are debrided and prepared for skin grafting as early as possible to limit the possibility of infection. Care includes covering the wound to limit contamination from foreign debris and bacteria as well as excision and grafting of the wound. Bacterial counts below 10^5 per gram of tissue are acceptable and do not require immediate skin grafting. When bacterial counts exceed this threshold, excision followed by skin grafting becomes more prone to graft failure. Topical agents used (Rovee, 1991) to control bacterial proliferation include

- silver sulfadiazine
- povidone iodine

- mafenide acetate and
- silver nitrate

Materials used for control of water loss from burns include

- amnion
- skin homografts (cadaver skin)
- heterografts (pig skin) and
- film dressings (Hydron, Biobrane, Op-Site, Ivalone etc.).

2.5.3 Compromised wound healing

People who suffer from diabetes or have compromised heart function, are candidates for development of skin ulcers due to circulatory problems. Diabetes is a chronic disorder that affects carbohydrate, fat and protein metabolism. Defective or deficient insulin secretion results in poor glucose uptake by cells and hyperglycemia. As a result of impaired uptake, glucose is present in excessive amounts in the extracellular matrix and recent evidence indicates that collagen chemically reacts with glucose to form glycated product. One consequence of diabetes is premature arteriosclerosis chracterized by thickening of blood vessel walls; as a result, individuals with either diabetes or cardiac insufficiency develop skin ulcers that are difficult to heal. The compromised wound healing observed in these patients is thought to be a result of the vascular changes experienced by both groups of people.

2.6 Wound dressings

A wide variety of materials have been used as dressings for burns, skin donor sites, skin ulcers and other excisional sites. These include synthetic barrier dressings, animal and human tissues, reconstituted collagen and tissue culture produced 'artificial skin' (Table 2.22). The skin autograft is the gold standard for covering air exposed tissue; however, great progress has been made in developing materials such as synthetic polymeric film

Table 2.22 Types of wound dressings and skin replacements*

Type	Example
Biological	
Reconstituted collagen	Collagen sponges
Tissues	Skin grafts, dura mater, pericardium, amnion, placenta
Cell seeded collagen	Bell's skin equivalent, Yannas' collagen/GAG membrane
Synthetic	Hydrocolloid, foam, membrane

* adapted from Pachence *et al.*, 1987, Silver and Pins, 1992

dressings and biological tissues that are used to protect the wound for periods of days to weeks. Synthetic film dressings are used to limit moisture and heat loss as well as to prevent bacterial contamination for periods of up to weeks. Tissues, including amnion and skin from cadavers or pigs, can be used for a few days to protect the wound. Their use is limited because these materials stimulate the rejection process. Reconstituted collagenous materials do not stimulate rejection and can be seeded with cells to form a permanent skin replacement.

2.6.1 Temporary synthetic barrier dressings

It has been known for quite some time that epithelialization is accelerated by keeping wounds wet with a dressing that retains moisture. Comparatively, air-exposed wounds heal less rapidly (Winter, 1962). Based on this concept, a number of dressings have been designed to act as a barrier between the external and internal environments. The exact design of a barrier dressing depends on the application.

For burns, the design criteria (Rovee, 1991) include the ability of the dressing to

- adhere to the wound surface,
- control water transport,
- flexibly cover the wound surface, and
- be antiseptic and hemostatic (MacMillan, 1984)

Adherence to the wound surface is the most important criterion since this will reduce pain, limit infection and facilitate healing. Barrier dressings can be formulated to adhere tightly to the wound surface by presenting a velour, porous, or roughened surface or they can be smooth surfaces that attach loosely. The use of either of these types of dressings depends on the location of the wound and the preference of the surgeon or practitioner. A number of commercially available synthetic polymeric dressings are used to treat both burns and ulcers (Table 2.23). Many of these contain polymer films to which other components are attached; these dressings vary in their ability to transmit moisture. Moist wet wound healing that occurs when a polymer film dressing is used is preferred over healing when the wound is exposed to air. However, there is very little agreement over the vapour transmission rate of a film dressing that maximizes epithelialization without compromising dermal repair. Additionally, the use of occlusive films on deep skin ulcers can lead to systemic infection that if left untreated can lead to mortality.

Results of recent studies suggest that optimization of wound healing may be more complex than merely limiting water permeability of the dressing. During the first days of wound healing under occlusive film dressings, the exudate can build up or pool. Fluids within the wound bed act as an excellent source of nutrition for growth of bacteria and further inflammation. Jonkman *et al.* (1988) reported that re-epithelialization under a

Table 2.23 Types of synthetic dressings used to cover skin wound

Name	Composition	Supplier
Bioclusive	polyurethane + adhesive	Johnson and Johnson
Biobrane	nylon fibres embedded in silastic membrane coated with collagen derived peptides	Woodroof Labs
DuoDERM	polyurethane film + carboxymethyl cellulose + adhesive	ConvaTec.
Epigard	polyurethane foam laminated to outer sheet of polyethylene	Parke-Davis Co.
Hydron	poly(2-hydroxy-ethylmethacrylate)	Abbott Labs
IP-758	silastic membrane on nylon velour	Int. Paper Co.
Omniderm	acrylamide grafted onto polyurethane	Omikron Scientific
Opraflex	polyurethane + adhesive	Lohman GMBH & Co.
Op-Site	polyurethane membrane + adhesive	Acme United Corp.
Tegaderm	polyurethane + adhesive	3M
Vigilon	polyethylene oxide radiation cross-linked to polyethylene mesh support	C. R. Bard, Inc.

References: James and Watson (1975); MacMillan (1984); Behar et al. (1986); Jonkman et al. (1988)

poly(etherurethane) wound dressing with a high vapour permeability was significantly better than wounds treated with OpSite, an occlusive dressing, or those exposed to air. In contrast, Ksander et al. (1990) report that synthetic, adherent, moisture vapour-permeable dressings severely inhibited the deposition of granulation tissue and subsequent collagenous tissue when compared with air-exposed wounds in animals. Therefore, it appears that moisture vapour-permeable dressings lead to rapid granulation of shallow wounds.

2.6.2 Temporary biological dressings

According to Pruitt and Levine (1984), cutaneous allografts are the most frequently used effective biological dressing. These dressings have distinct advantages over synthetic dressings including (Miller *et al.*, 1967, Tavis *et al.*, 1978, Pruitt and Levine, 1984):

- adhesion to underlying wound bed
- reduction in bacterial population density of underlying wounds
- facilitated wound debridement
- reduction of pain
- increased capillary content of granulation tissue, and
- improved healing

Allograft skin is used for coverage of full thickness burn wounds after removal of necrotic tissues. The affected area is treated prior to autograft application for protection of second degree burns (Pruitt and Levine, 1984). If adherence of allograft skin to the wound bed is followed within 24–48 hours of application by revascularization, then the wound is ready for autografting.

Allografts are most commonly less than 0.38 mm thick and are harvested from patients who have died at the hospital from diseases not involving the skin. Fresh grafts have a seven to ten day life time when stored at 4°C. Lyophilized (freeze-dried) and frozen allografts have longer lifetimes. However, most allografts are removed prior to rejection and are replaced with an autograft from the host unless the patient is immunosuppressed or the allograft is modified.

The results of recent studies indicate that allograft rejection can be suppressed after treatment with cyclosporin and ribavirin at concentrations that do not cause kidney toxicity (Jolley *et al.*, 1988). A combination of these two drugs results in better skin allograft survival than is achieved with an optimal dose of cyclosporin. Rejection of a skin allograft is mediated by antigen-specific cytolytic T cells and requires the induction of target Ia alloantigens (which are coded for by the class II major histocompatibility complex) on epidermal cells (Rosenberg *et al.*, 1989). Burns treated with allogenic skin from which the epidermis was abraded after three to four weeks of implantation, and then seeded with autologous keratinocyte cultures, resulted in the reconstitution of skin with excellent textural and histologic qualities (Langdon *et al.*, 1988).

Amnion has been described in the literature as a burn dressing since the 1900s (Thomson and Parks, 1984 and Walker, 1984 for reviews) (Table 2.22).

The steps involved in use of amnion as a wound dressing include the following.

- Obtain amnion from placenta after delivery.

- Strip chorion and rinse in 0.25% sodium hypochloride and saline (Thomson and Parks, 1984; Walker, 1984).
- Monitor for two to three days for microbial contamination by incubating of an aliquot in a growth medium.
- Apply to wound and cover with mesh gauze and tubular netting or netting alone.
- Remove from wound after three days.
- Hold in place by a single layer of non-occluding gauze that is covered with ointment. A bulky outer dressing, gauze roll and a loosely applied elastic bandage (Walker, 1984) are then applied.

Porcine skin xenografts have been used as a burn wound covering as discussed by Pellet et al. (1984). They are believed to be less effective compared to skin allografts in reducing bacterial contamination of the underlying wound (Levine et al., 1976). Bacterial population density of less than 10^5 organisms per gram of tissue is recommended prior to the application of skin grafts (Pruitt and Levine, 1984)

To decrease the antigenicity and potential for infection, porcine skin is processed prior to clinical use (Pellet et al., 1984). Processing includes:

- removal of the epidermis and skin appendages such as hair (epidermal cells are antigenic),
- freeze-drying which minimizes the effects of enzyme degradation of the graft (freezing to $-15°C$)
- antigenicity of allogenic membrane components, and
- irradiation at 3.5 Mrad (decreases inflammatory response as well as kills bacteria).

Porcine skin that is used to cover dermal wounds, has an initial antibacterial effect which is promoted by lyophilization and irradiation. Genetic Laboratories of St. Paul, Minnesota supplies silver treated porcine skin under the tradenames of MEDISKIN + SILVER and EZ DERM™ which are used to treat full-thickness burns and partial thickness wounds, respectively for periods of two days or longer.

Treatment of porcine skin with enzymes (such as trypsin) to remove antigenic components leads to another classification of wound dressing. Oliver et al. (1972) reported the use of this approach to purify dermal collagen in xenografts. The results of their studies suggested that enzymatically treated xenografts were progressively lysed and replaced by granulation tissue even when covered by skin autografts and allografts. Results of later studies suggested that pre-treatment of trypsinized grafts with glutaraldehyde, demonstrated some permanence of the collagen fibril bundle architecture (Oliver et al., 1977). These studies are the foundation for later efforts to use biodegradable collagen as a dermal substitute as discussed below.

2.6.3 Biodegradable dermal substitutes

The biological dressings discussed in section 2.6.2 are temporary dressings that are replaced or removed prior to rejection by the recipient. They are chiefly composed of collagen, the primary structural protein found in mammalian tissues. Based on Oliver's work and work by Thiele (1964), a number of research groups isolated collagen from mammalian tissues and formulated it into cell-free xenografts. These materials, after cross-linking to mask the antigenic determinants, are not rejected but are biodegraded and replaced by host tissue. In a series of articles, Yannas and co-workers (Yannas and Burke, 1980; Yannas et al., 1980; Dagalakis et al., 1980) describe the physicochemical, biochemical and mechanical considerations that form the basis for the two-stage design of a bi-layer membrane which is useful as an experimental burn dressing. In stage I, the basic design parameters chosen were physicochemical and mechanical, including optimization of surface energy, modulus of elasticity, tear strength, and moisture flux rate (Yannas and Burke, 1980). In stage II, they suggested that biochemical constraints, including a very low level of antigenicity and optimum biodegradation rate without release of toxic products, are critical parameters. They chose collagen as a starting material because it is hydrophilic and is capable of biodegradation at controlled rates by varying the cross-link density. Previous clinical experience, based on the design of collagen-based sutures and other collagen devices, demonstrated that type I collagen was a weak antigen. Other advantages to its use include (Pachence et al., 1987):

- abundant sources of highly purified (medical grade) collagen,
- the ability to be reconstituted into high strength forms useful in surgery,
- the wealth of research literature on the characterization of collagen,
- improved processing techniques,
- introduction of several commercial collagen products,
- recent advances in use of collagen as a delivery system.

The use of glycosaminoglycans (GAGs), a polysaccharide tissue derivative from mammalian tissues, as the second macromolecular component of the membrane was based on additional considerations. These include modification of the mechanical and cross-link density of collagen for control of membrane biodegradation, and the open pore structure exhibited by collagen-GAGs composites. A later report (Yannas et al., 1980) detailed methodology for preparation of collagen-GAGs membranes with known composition. Reports indicated that these membranes protected dermal wounds from infection and fluid loss for over 25 days without rejection or manipulation. Control of chemical composition of these membranes was achieved by cross-linking with glutaraldehyde, or alternately, by dehydration at high temperature under vacuum. Appropriate use of the cross-linking treatment allowed separate study of changes in membrane composition due to elution of GAGs from changes in enzymatic degradation of the implanted membrane. Preservation of pore structure was best achieved when collagen-GAGs composites were freeze-dried (Dagalakis et al., 1980).

Variation in mean pore size was reported to be an important parameter. Subcutaneous implants which had virtually no pores larger than 5 μm were surrounded by dense fibrous tissue whereas implants with many pores larger than 50 μm showed little evidence for fibrous sac (capsule) formation (Yannas, 1981). Coating the collagen-GAG membrane with a layer of silicone rubber resulted in a bi-layer membrane that in an excised guinea pig model delayed the onset of contraction without affecting the final wound area reduction (Yannas, 1981).

Clinical studies by Burke et al. (1981) evaluated the use of the bi-laminate collagen dressing for excised burn wounds covering 15–60% of the total body surface area. Firm attachment to the wound bed was observed within minutes and early vascularization was also observed. When donor skin was available for autografting, the Silastic™ membrane was peeled off and a 0.1 mm graft was applied. Histologically, the implant was replaced with new dermis with some fibrous tissue present.

Chvapil (1982) has reviewed the work on synthetic wound dressings (including collagen), especially the affect of adding GAGs and chemical cross-linking agents. Cross-linking with glutaraldehyde results in internal cyclopolymerization and forms variable length polymers producing polymeric units that cross-link collagen. The bi-functional aldehydes react with amino, carboxyl, amide and other groups present on collagen. Speer et al. (1980) showed that glutaraldehyde is continuously hydrolyzed as monomer from cross-linked collagen and requires several weeks of exhaustive washing to remove. Ingrowth of cells into glutaraldehyde treated materials is reduced which argues against its use in cross-linking collagenous materials that are used as wound dressings. In addition to this problem, dissociation of GAGs from the collagen matrix at neutral pH and its release into the wound environment has also been cited as a factor that may need further consideration (Chvapil, 1982).

Ongoing studies on collagen-GAGs matrices include optimization of average pore diameter (Boyce et al., 1988), optimization of conditions for growth of human dermal keratinocytes (Boyce and Hansbrough, 1988) and maximization of cell proliferation (Matsuda et al., 1990).

Silver and co-workers (Silver et al., 1989a) have studied the use of type I collagen as a packing material for stage II and III skin ulcers. Their research demonstrated that a collagen sponge matrix enhances repair of animal wounds by organizing the spatial deposition of newly synthesized collagen and accelerating remodelling (Doillon et al., 1984; 1985). Results of clinical studies conducted by these investigators, indicated that the areas of skin ulcers in patients treated with collagen sponge matrix decreased by 40% during six weeks of treatment compared with no change in areas of control wounds (Doillon *et al.*, 1988). In a follow-up study, 12 out of 14 patients treated with collagen flakes manufactured by mechanically shearing collagen matrices, showed a 41% decrease in wound area after six weeks of treatment while only three out of seven patients treated with a collagen sponge matrix showed a similar wound area reduction (Silver *et al.*, 1989a).

2.6.4 Artificial skin

Recent success in development of biodegradable materials that actively participate in dermal wound healing as well as advances in expansion and differentiation of dermal and epidermal cells in tissue culture has led to the growth of 'artificial skin' (Silver and Pins, 1992). Growth of epidermal cells in culture and their use to cover wounds was reported by Billingham and Reynolds (1952). Freeman *et al.* (1974) reported that small pieces of rabbit skin could attach to support surfaces and proliferate to form layers of epithelial cells that propagate in tissue culture. Igel *et al.* (1974) extended these observations to report that autograft–allografts or autograft–xenografts were transplanted to large surface area wounds achieving essentially complete epithelial coverage within two to three weeks. Worst *et al.* (1974) reported on the growth of pure epidermal cells on collagen gels formed at the bottom of a silicon chamber and observed that at up to eight weeks after implantation the cells formed an intact, well-differentiated epidermis. Rheinwald and Green (1975) serially cultivated epidermal cells on feeder layers of 3T3 cells. Eisinger *et al.* (1980) presented evidence that human epidermal cells grown in vitro could be transplanted to the mouse and that growth and transplantation of such tissue continues in vivo. Bell *et al.* (1981) reported on the fabrication of a living skin equivalent consisting of dermal and epidermal components each made with cells taken from a potential graft recipient that were cultured on a contracted collagen matrix. The equivalent served as a substitute for skin in experimental animals after rapid vascularization. It inhibited wound contraction, and was immunologically tolerated. In a later study (Bell *et al.*, 1983), it was proposed that allograft cells cultured on a collagen matrix were tolerated because cells without class II antigens were selected during in vitro cultivation and these cells were used to form a replacement.

The above studies serve as the basis for the engineering of tissue cultured skins. Below we review the background to the genesis of this new field as well as its extension to other tissues.

Cell culture on collagen substrates

A variety of surfaces have been used as cell growth substrates. However, most of the non-biological surfaces act as passive physical supports and do not 'interact' with the cell surface. Data in the literature suggest that cells specifically recognize collagen substrates.

Table 2.24 Effects of extracellular matrix factors on cell growth on collagen

Matrix component	Initiator	Matrix or cell effect	Ref.
Heparin	human skin fibroblasts from foreskins	inhibition of contraction of Type I collagen gels	Guidry and Grinnell, 1987
Fibroblasts	release of fibroblast seeded type I collagen gels from tissue culture surface	retraction of pseudopodia, collapse of actin filaments, loss of cell surface fibronectin	Mochitate et al., 1991
Cell surface fibronectin	fibroblasts	cell surface fibronectin and not plasma fibronectin required for gel contraction	Asaga et al., 1991
B_1-integrin	fibroblast	B_1-integrin collagen receptors play critical role	Gullberg et al., 1990
Gel geometry	fibroblast cell body	tension exerted by cells leads to reorientation of collagen fibres	Klebe et al., 1989
Prostaglandin E_2	fibroblasts in collagen lattice	down regulation of collagen synthesis	Bell et al., 1984a
Collagen matrix	fibroblasts	fibroblasts observed to have large pseudopodia-like processes extending into collagen matrix	Elsdale and Bard, 1972
Collagen matrix	fibroblasts	spatial deposition of newly synthesized collagen follows alignment of collagen matrix	Doillon, et al., 1984

From Silver and Pins, 1992

Fibroblasts grown on collagen matrices appear to differentiate morphologically and biochemically. Cells grown on collagen adopt an elongated morphology and are observed to have large pseudopodia-like processes extending into a collagen matrix (Elsdale and Bard, 1972) (Table 2.24). In addition, the spatial deposition of newly synthesized collagen follows the orientation of collagen fibres in a reconstituted collagen matrix (Doillon *et al.*, 1984). Fibroblast cell bodies have been observed to exert tension that leads to reorientation of a collagen matrix (Klebe *et al.*, 1989) and to down regulation of collagen synthesis as a result of the release of the prostaglandin E2 (Bell *et al.*, 1984).

In 1979, Bell and co-workers (Bell *et al.*, 1979) showed that fibroblasts incorporated into a freshly prepared collagen gel differentiated and caused contraction of the lattice (Table 2.25). Previous studies by Karasek and Charlton (1971) and Freeman *et al.* (1974) indicated that skin cells could be grown on collagen substrates yielding a tissue-like product. This approach was extended by various groups to form what was termed a 'living skin equivalent' (Bell *et al.*, 1983).

Fibroblasts mixed with rat tail tendon collagen have been observed to contract collagen lattices (Bell *et al.*, 1979). Inhibition of contraction of collagen gels by fibroblasts occurs in the presence of heparin (Guidry and Grinnell, 1987) and the release of fibroblast seeded type I collagen gels is associated with retraction of pseudopodia, collapse of actin filament bundles and loss of cell surface fibronectin (Mochitate *et al.*, 1991). Other results indicate that cell surface fibronectin and not plasma fibronectin is required for gel contraction (Asaga *et al.*, 1991) and that β1-integrin collagen receptors play a critical role (Gullberg *et al.*, 1990).

These results suggest that fibroblast cell attachment, elongation and deposition of newly synthesized extracellular matrix on reconstituted collagen is associated with several cellular events and involves specific cell surface receptors. Since all tissues contain collagen, it is likely that cell-matrix interactions are important in regulating tissue turn over.

Tissue engineering
A number of tissues have been engineered by growth of one or more cell types on collagen matrices. These cells are derived from skin, liver, thyroid, cartilage, bone, pancreas, cornea, cardiovascular, adipose, mammary and nervous tissues. Below, we will briefly review progress in the area of skin replacement.

Skin For over twenty years, techniques for growing skin epithelial cells on collagen matrices in cell culture have been investigated. Karasek and Charlton (1971) reported growth of post-embryonic skin epithelial cells on a collagen gel while Worst *et al.* (1974) used rat tail tendon collagen as a substrate for perinatal mouse skin epidermal cells (Table 2.25). Freeman *et al.* (1974) demonstrated that expansion of the epithelial cell surface by a factor of 50 occurred within 7–21 days when rabbit skin epithelial cells were

Table 2.25 Growth of skin cells on collagen

Cell Type (s)	Matrix	Tissue Produced	Ref.
Post-embryonic skin epithelial cells	collagen gel	epidermis	Karasek and Charlton, 1971
Epidermal (perinatal mouse skin)	rat tail tendon collagen	epidermal cells cultured for 1–4 days in vitro	Worst et al., 1974
Epithelial (rabbit skin)	porcine skin	expansion of epithelial cell surface by a factor of 50 within 7–21 days	Freeman et al., 1974
Epidermal (human)	collagen film (Helitrex Inc.)	single cell suspensions plated on collagen film	Eisinger et al., 1980
Fibroblasts (human foreskin)	rat tail tendon collagen	fibroblasts condense a hydrated collagen lattice	Bell et al., 1979
Fibroblasts + epidermal cells	rat tail tendon collagen	epidermal cells cultivated on a fibroblast contracted collagen lattice	Bell et al., 1983; Bell et al., 1981; Bell et al., 1981a
Fibroblasts, epidermal cells and melanocytes	rat tail tendon collagen	exposure of skin equivalent to UV light irradiation for 14 days stimulated pigment transfer from melanocytes to keratinocytes	Topol et al., 1986

From Silver and Pins, 1992

grown on porcine skin. Studies by other workers (Eisinger et al., 1980) indicated that the exact geometry of the matrix was not critical for survival of epidermal cells.

Later, studies by Bell and co-workers (Bell et al., 1981, 1981a, 1986, 1989) demonstrated that co-cultures of fibroblasts, epidermal cells and melanocytes resulted in production of a skin equivalent that showed stimulated pigment transfer from melanocytes to keratinocytes when exposed to ultraviolet light.

Animal and clinical studies Extensive progress with growth of autologous and allogeneic cells on collagen matrices in vitro has led to the potential of growing tissues and organs for transplantation. Although the literature contains numerous references to in vitro studies, only in the area of skin replacement has this technology been extended to evaluation of the long-term effects of transplantation. Below, the literature on skin replacement using cell cultured materials is reviewed with special attention directed at evaluating the long-term effects.

Cells cultured without a substrate In 1980, Eisinger *et al.* (1980) developed a technique for producing large quantities of differentiated epithelial tissue in vitro from cell cultures of small punch biopsies. Observations made six weeks after application of skin substitutes to full thickness wounds created on mongrel dogs, indicated normal implant maturation. Histological analyses of punch biopsies, showed no evidence of lymphoid infiltration. Follow-up studies conducted four months after the initial surgery reported that the graft tissue appeared healthy.

Experiments conducted on split and full thickness wounds in a porcine model, evaluated the efficacy of autologous skin grafts (Alvarez and Biozes, 1984). After one month, grafts on split thickness wounds appeared to have regenerated rete ridges similar to normal skin. In contrast, grafts on full thickness wounds had contracted 85% and resembled scar tissue. Similar studies employing autologous grafts were conducted by Eisinger (1985), using a porcine model. A well vascularized, hyperplastic epidermis with fibroblasts aligning parallel to the surface between 8 and 12 weeks post implantation was reported based on histological analysis on full thickness wounds. After 13 weeks, the dermis appeared normal, as did the epidermis, although no sweat glands or hair follicles were present. The graft was observed to contract by as much as 25%.

Hefton *et al.* (1986) investigated the use of cultured epithelial autografts for the treatment of full thickness, chronic skin ulcers. Four of the six ulcers covered with the autologous graft produced full thickness epidermis which remained intact for ten months. Of the four ulcers successfully treated, three remained stable after 2 years although hair follicles were never observed. Similar success was reported in the case of a patient who had been burned over more than 99% of his body (Pittelkow and Scott, 1986). Cultured epithelial autografts were used to cover a large portion of the full thickness wounds; these grafts exhibited many characteristics of epidermal tissue one month after grafting. Ten months after grafting, the wounds had healed and the patient returned to work.

These results demonstrated the efficacy of cultured epithelial autografts. The primary drawback for use of autologous cells is the three to four week delay between hospital admission and grafting. During this time, the patient is susceptible to infection and the risk of thermal shock.

To decrease the delay time prior to grafting, research has been conducted on the efficacy of epithelial sheets produced from allogeneic cells. Some of the preliminary studies using cultured allografts were conducted on full thickness dog wounds by Eisinger *et al.* (1980). Results indicated that four months after implantation, the cultured allografts appeared healthy and morphologically similar to autografts. Hefton used a similar technique to graft split thickness wounds in humans (Hefton *et al.*, 1983). After nine months, the cultured allografts had been accepted with little contraction although no rete ridges or adnexal structures were observed. Hefton and co-workers futher hypothesized that cultured epithelial allografts were not rejected because HLA-DR markers were lost during culturing. Madden *et al.* (1986) extended the investigation of cultured allografts to treat second and third degree burns. Two years after the grafts had been applied, hypopigmented, flat, smooth skin replaced the split thickness wounds. In contrast, third degree burns excised to full thickness did not support the allografts but instead healed by contraction and re-epithelialization from the wound edge. Despite their apparent failure as full thickness wound covers, histological studies conducted nine months after grafting and morphological observations made after two years suggest that cultured allogeneic epithelia may be an effective treatment for split thickness skin injuries. Additionally, since they do not necessitate the extraction of painful punch biopsies from the donor, they may be prepared and stored in large quantities, readily available for patients whenever required.

Cells cultured on lethally irradiated fibroblasts (Table 2.26) Green and co-workers have pioneered a technique for culturing keratinocytes on a bed of lethally irradiated 3T3 fibroblasts. This technique has been investigated extensively to facilitate rapid skin cell expansion for skin replacement of full thickness burn injuries (O'Connor *et al.*, 1981; O'Connor *et al.*, 1984; Gallico *et al.*, 1984; Herzog *et al.*, 1988, Woodley *et al.*, 1988; Compton *et al.*, 1989, Petersen *et al.*, 1990) and epidermal nevi (Gallico *et al.*, 1989). These cultured autografts have been observed to form a differentiated and confluent epidermal layer within one month after implantation (O'Connor *et al.*, 1981, Gallico *et al.*, 1989). By the end of the third month, Langerhan's cells repopulated the tissue (Compton *et al.*, 1989; Petersen *et al.*, 1990), the keratinocyte layer matured and stratified (Gallico *et al.*, 1984; Herzog *et al.*, 1988; Compton *et al.*, 1989) and the formation of a dermal–epidermal junction initiated (Herzog *et al.*, 1988; Compton *et al.*, 1989; Gallico *et al.*, 1989). During this time frame, Merkel cells were identified returning to the tissue (Compton *et al.*, 1990). Rete ridges were observed as early as three months after surgery (Heck *et al.*, 1985), and repigmentation occurred between six weeks and twelve months (Compton *et al.*, 1989; Gallico *et al.*, 1989). Maturation of the anchoring fibrils and basement membrane

Table 2.26 Long-term effects of skin graft implantation

Graft type Cell type/matrix	Model	Duration of implant	Results	Reference
Auto-EC / None	Mongrel Dog-FTW	4 months	Graft Healthy	Eisinger et al., 1980
	Porcine-STW	1 month	Normal Skin Appearance	Alvarez and Biozes, 1984
	-FTW	1 month	Wound Contracted	Alvarez and Biozes, 1984
	-FTW	3 months	Normal Skin Appearance-*	Alvarez and Biozes, 1984
	Human-FTW	10 months	Graft Stable	Pittelkow and Scott, 1986
	-FTW	2 years	Graft Stable-*	Hefton et al., 1986
Allo-EC / None	Mongrel Dog-FTW	4 months	Graft Healthy	Eisinger et al., 1980
	Human-STW	9 months	Graft Stable-*	Hefton et al., 1983
	-STW	2 years	Graft Stable-*	Madden et al., 1986
	-FTW	2 years	Wound Contracted	Madden et al., 1986
Auto-EC / 3T3 Fibroblasts	Human-FTW	5 years	Graft Permanent-*	O'Connor et al., 1981
Auto-EC / 3T3 Fibroblasts Cryopreserved Allodermis	Human-FTW	1 year	Graft Healthy	Langdon et al., 1988
Allo-EC / 3T3 Fibroblasts	Human-STW	9 months	Graft Permanent-*	Faure et al., 1987
	-FTW	18 months	Graft Intact-*	Phillips et al., 1989
Auto-EC / Collagen Sponge	Guinea Pig-FTW	4 months	Similar to Autograft	Yannas et al., 1981; Yannas and Orgill, 1986
Auto-EC / Auto-Fibroblast Seeded Collagen Sponge	Human-FTW	7 months	Graft Intact	Carter et al., 1987
	Human-FTW	1 month	Graft Healthy	Hansbrough et al., 1989
Auto-EC / Auto-Fibroblast Seeded Collagen Gel	Rat-FTW	13 months	Graft Intact-*	Bell et al., 1981a; Bell et al., 1989
Auto-EC / Allo-Fibroblast Seeded Collagen Gel	Rat-FTW	2 years	Graft Healthy	Bell et al., 1984
	Human-FTW	18 months	Graft Stable	Sher et al., 1983
Allo-EC / Allo-Fibroblast Seeded Collagen Gel	Rat-FTW	7 months	Graft Intact	Bell et al., 1984
	Human-FTW	6 months	Graft Intact	Hull et al., 1990

Key: Auto-EC = Autologous Epithelial Cells Allo-EC = Allogeneic Epithelial Cells
* = No Adnexal Structures FTW = Full Thickness Wounds STW = Split Thickness Wounds
From Silver and Pins, 1992

occurred between eight months and two years after the initial procedure (Compton *et al.*, 1989; Gallico *et al.*, 1989), and by the end of five years, the cultured autografts appeared permanent (O'Connor *et al.*, 1984), contained elastin and extensive vasculature, lacked adnexal structures (Compton *et al.*, 1989) and contracted less than 20% (Gallico *et al.*, 1989). Although cultured epithelial autografts perform satisfactorily as long-term skin replacements, they require three to four weeks to be produced in vitro (Compton *et al.*, 1989). Furthermore, histological and morphological examinations (Herzog *et al.*, 1988; Woodley *et al.*, 1988; Petersen *et al.*, 1990) conducted five months after surgery suggested that the absence of a dermal interface between the graft and the wound contributes to graft fragility. These observations were confirmed by Compton *et al.* (1989) although further investigation by the same group indicated that the epidermal–dermal junction matured after one year stabilizing the graft. Petersen *et al.* (1990) did not report on observations beyond five months.

In order to provide a stable wound bed for the implants, cultured epithelial autografts produced on 3T3 fibroblasts have been grafted onto cryopreserved allografts debrided of their epidermal layers. The cryopreservation of the allograft is believed to mask its antigenicity, and the removal of its epidermis eliminates most of the HLA-DR antigens (Cuono *et al.*, 1986). This technique was applied to debrided burn injuries and within three months after grafting a normal basement membrane was observed and some melanocytes were present (Langdon *et al.*, 1988). Long-term follow-ups on the same patients indicated that between 11 and 12 months a mature dermis with epithelial interdigitations was observed suggesting the initiation of rete ridge formation. Additionally, the hypercellularity of the epidermis subsided and some hair follicles and sweat glands were present (Langdon *et al.*, 1988).

A similar technique was employed by Heck *et al.* (1985) although they replaced the allogeneic epidermis with autologous epidermal blisters instead of cultured sheets. Ten months after surgery, grafts were confluent and stable with no evidence of contraction or scarring. Although grafting autologous epithelial sheets onto allogeneic dermal tissue produces excellent textural and histological results (Langdon *et al.*, 1988), it still necessitates obtaining biopsies from the patient and conducting a second surgical procedure to close the wound.

In order to reduce the lag time prior to grafting, cultured epithelial grafts utilizing allogeneic keratinocytes have been investigated. The cells were cryopreserved for six months and cultured to confluence on 3T3 fibroblasts for at least two generations. Epithelial sheets were grafted onto split thickness wounds on humans. These skin substitutes have been shown to 'take' within one month while only inducing a mild inflammatory response (Faure *et al.*, 1986). Shortly thereafter, a multi-layered epidermis and Langerhan's cells have been identified at the graft site (Faure *et al.*, 1986;

Thivolet *et al.*, 1986). Within five months the split thickness cultured allograft formed an epidermal–dermal junction with anchoring fibrils and a lamina densa (Kanitakis *et al.*, 1987; Faure *et al.*, 1987); but even after nine months when the graft appeared to be a permanent cover (Faure *et al.*, 1987), rete ridges and adnexal structures were not observed (Thivolet *et al.*, 1986). Cultured epithelial allografts were also used by Phillips *et al.* (1989; 1990) to cover full thickness ulcer beds. Six months after grafting, 73% of these wounds healed with an apparently normal epidermis. Histologically, no signs of rejection were observed and the dermal–epidermal junction, although flat was shown to contain anchoring fibrils (Phillips *et al.*, 1990). Follow-up observations at 18 months showed that 88% of the grafts were still intact (Phillips *et al.*, 1989). These studies suggest that it is possible to cross major histocompatibility barriers to facilitate rapid and adequate long-term repair when extensive loss of skin occurs.

Cells cultured on collagen matrices Several groups have reported on the use of synthetic collagen sponges as scaffolds for generating cell seeded skin grafts. Yannas and co-workers (Yannas *et al.*, 1981; Yannas and Orgill, 1986) innoculated porous collagen sponges with autologous epidermal basal cells and placed the skin analogue on full thickness guinea pig wounds. Follow-up studies noted that wound closure was achieved in less than two weeks; a neodermis was generated in place of the collagen sponge within the first month. Four months after implantation, the cell seeded sponge could not be differentiated from a full thickness autograft.

The advantage of the cell innoculated collagen sponge is that it may be employed almost immediately after a punch biopsy has been removed and rapid wound coverage can be attained without a second surgical procedure. Yannas *et al.* (1981) as well as Alvarez and Biozes (1984) noted that the collagen sponge actively controlled wound contraction and reduced scar formation. One significant drawback to this technique is that wound closure was markedly prolonged when larger areas were grafted and therefore the density of the innoculated cells was decreased.

Hansbrough *et al.* (1989) adapted the protocol established by Yannas and co-workers (Yannas *et al.*, 1981; Yannas and Orgill, 1986) for treatment of burns by culturing the collagen sponge with autologous fibroblasts and basal cells prior to implantation. Although the time required to produce the tissue analogue was three weeks, it allowed for greater wound coverage while employing a similar quantity of harvested epithelial cells. Hansbrough *et al.* (1989) also noted from their study that the collagen sponge encouraged rapid fibrovascular tissue ingrowth, and within four weeks, anchoring fibrils, basement membrane and epidermal–dermal interdigitation was present within the implant.

Carter *et al.* (1987) cultured autologous keratinocytes on collagen sponges to treat full thickness wounds in patients suffering from epidermolysis bullosa. The authors noted that seven months after surgery, the grafts on two of the three patients in the study had remained intact and became partially repigmented. Additionally, it was noted that the collagen sponge facilitated handling of the otherwise brittle keratinocyte sheet.

These studies indicate that a cell innoculated/cell seeded collagen sponge can be used as an immediate skin replacement. The major advantage of this design is the reduction in time between hospital admission and grafting.

Bell et al. (1981, 1981a) employed rat tail tendon collagen seeded with autologous fibroblasts to produce a dermal equivalent. Subsequently, the dermal equivalent, composed primarily of an extracellular matrix and fibroblasts, was used to culture keratinocytes on a media which mimicked de novo skin (Bell et al., 1983). In addition to resembling a full thickness autograft, the bi-layered skin equivalent could be moulded to the contour of the wound and produced in large enough quantities to treat extensive skin injuries (Bell et al., 1981, 1981a). When implanted onto full thickness rat wounds, the graft produced a smooth pinkish epidermis (Bell et al., 1981, 1981a) with a woven vascularized dermal mat within the first three months (Bell et al., 1981, 1981a). The same implant analyzed for periods of up to 13 months was smooth and hairless, lacking sebaceous glands and was slightly thinner than normal skin. Although the autologous skin equivalent rapidly vascularized and induced long-term skin regeneration, a lag time of approximately three weeks was required before grafting of the animal.

In order to reduce the critical waiting period prior to grafting, Bell and co-workers (Sher et al., 1983) experimented with allogeneic fibroblasts for the dermal equivalent. Isografts showed no signs of rejection when implanted onto full thickness rat wounds (Bell et al., 1983; Sher et al., 1983). They blended with the host skin and histologically proved to consist of 50% host tissue after one year (Bell et al., 1984). At the end of the second year the dermis contained a regular collagen basket weave, contraction was less than 20%, and the graft was indistinguishable from host tissue. Allogeneic skin equivalents showed similar results when implanted for periods as long as seven months. To challenge the immunologic tolerance of the animals to allografts, a number of the implants were removed after one month and replaced with identical grafts. After seven months, these grafts indicated no sign of rejection (Bell et al., 1984).

Hull et al. (1990) investigated the use of a similar graft design for the treatment of full thickness burns. Employing a cryopreserved, allogeneic dermal equivalent bearing only class I major histocompatibility complex-antigens, a skin equivalent containing autologous keratinocytes was ready for grafting within seven days after the removal of the punch biopsy. This implant appeared smooth and resembled adjacent skin after eight months. Histologically, vascularized dermis and tightly packed collagen bundles were noted. After 18 months, the skin grafts composed of an allogeneic dermal equivalent and autologous epidermal layers remained stable. From these preliminary results, it appears that a cryopreserved allogeneic dermal equivalent may some day provide patients with a viable skin replacement that is stable for long periods of time and can be made available in less than seven days after the initial punch biopsy.

Nanchahal *et al.* (1989) investigated a living skin equivalent which required no lag time prior to grafting. This was accomplished by producing a graft consisting of allogeneic fibroblasts and keratinocytes which had been cryoproserved and subcultured to remove class II major histocompatibility complex-antigens. One month after the allograft had been implanted in full thickness burn wounds in humans, fully differentiated epidermal and mature dermal structures were noted. Further observations on the same grafts conducted six months post-implantation showed them to be intact with only one minor incidence of contraction.

Summary of artificial skin research Extensive research on the growth of autologous and allogeneic cells on collagen matrices has shown that it is feasible to grow a number of skin cells in culture (Table 2.26). Extension of this technology has occurred in the area of skin cell culture for the treatment of burns, ulcers and other defects. The advantages of autologous sheets of epithelial cells are their inherent simplicity and biocompatibility. A fibroblast feeder layer for these cultures facilitates culture handling and cell differentiation. Long-term clinical studies indicate that these grafts successfully facilitate the repair of full thickness skin defects. The primary problem with autografts is the lag time required for graft preparation prior to implantation. Cryopreserved allogeneic skin grafts alleviate this problem as well as the need for obtaining punch biopsies from the patient. Allograft sheets of epidermal cells effectively treat split thickness and full thickness skin defects. Graft fragility, a problem associated with autologous and allogeneic epithelial sheets has been linked to the lack of dermal interface between the graft and the wound bed.

Skin grafts produced on collagen sponges overcome the problem of implant fragility while at the same time inducing rapid dermal ingrowth. Cell innoculated collagen sponges initiate rapid wound closure with no lag time prior to grafting. The limiting factor for preparation of these grafts is the availability of autologous epithelial cells.

Recently, skin equivalents consisting of fibroblast seeded collagen gels overlaid with epithelial cells were investigated. When these implants are produced using allogeneic fibroblasts and epithelia, they prove effective in treating full thickness skin defects. Since these grafts require no autologous tissue, they may be produced in large quantities and cryopreserved until the time they are required for treating wound defects. Ultimately, the use of cryopreserved allogeneic cell cultured materials will have a significant impact on management of patients that experience organ and tissue failure. Current limitations not only include the intensive amount of work required to produce isolated cell cultures but also the lack of automated procedures for production of cell cultured tissues.

2.7 Summary

There are a number of materials that are commercially available and used as wound dressings, to cover burns and superficial skin ulcers. These materials in general accelerate healing by preventing heat and moisture loss from wounds. Deep skin ulcers that are normally contaminated with bacteria are best treated with dressings such as gauze that allow the drainage of fluid and penetration of oxygen into the wound. In a number of research orientated medical centres, facilities are available to culture autologous and allogeneic cells for grafting patients with burns and ulcers. However, this requires an intensive effort and is very costly. Researchers in the field believe that this approach can be applied at almost any medical centre via the use of frozen cell cultured allografts that are slowly thawed just prior to grafting. The slow rate of transfer of technology from the laboratory to the commercial sector in the past, somewhat dampens the hope that by the year 2000, large areas of skin can be grafted in most medical centres using technology that already exists today. To attain this goal a new breed of scientist/physician is required, who is comfortable with the rapid application of new technology in a highly complex medical decision making environment.

3.
Replacement of Skeletal Tissues

3.1 Introduction

Injury to the musculoskeletal system is caused by traumatic injury as well as the end-stage of diseases such as osteoarthritis and rheumatoid arthritis. These processes lead to impaired locomotion and high levels of pain and therefore must be surgically corrected. Tissue grafts and synthetic polymeric materials are used to repair damaged tendons and ligaments while joint replacement is achieved using primarily metals and polymeric materials. Fixation devices including bone plates and screws are used to reinforce bone fractures. These devices are made of metals, although some polymeric materials have been studied experimentally.

3.1.1 Tendon and ligament injury

Mechanical trauma to the knee is a problem faced by military personnel, labourers, factory workers, and athletes competing in contact sports. Development of protective devices has been intended to decrease the number of serious injuries; however, the efficacy of some of these devices is questionable. In cases where injury occurs to the tendons and ligaments of the knee, the use of autogenous tissue has led to the restoration of normal joint function (Zarins and Adams, 1988; Friedman *et al.*, 1985); however, the post-surgical recovery time is prolonged and other structures in the knee are weakened. In cases where a tendon or ligament is damaged but not completely torn, i.e. the Achilles tendon, immobilization leads to repair via the formation of scar tissue. However, the strength of scar tissue is lower than that of normal tendon and results in soft tissue structures that are biomechanically inferior to tendon and ligament (Frank *et al.*, 1983). Studies of biodegradable scaffolds that promote healing are needed to help workers in the field develop the next generation of tendon and ligament replacements that combine the qualities of biological tissues and synthetics.

In addition, replacement of the flexor tendons in the hand is another example where replacement with a synthetic substitute leads to improved repair. Clinically, tears in these tendons are repaired with sutures, and synthetic materials are used only as a gliding surface to prevent adhesions. Below, we will consider only tendon and ligaments of the knee since they have been studied in great detail in order to develop a replacement for the anterior cruciate ligament.

3.2 Anatomy and physiology of tendons and ligaments

The knee joint is a complex arrangement of extracellular matrix that allows vertebrates to walk. The knee contains three long bones, the femur, tibia and fibula, and a smaller bone, the patella (Table 3.1 and Figure 3.1) The bones are held together by ligaments to form a structure that flexes and translates. The energy required to flex and translate this structure is provided by muscular contraction and length changes in the appropriate muscles. Length changes are transferred to tendons as forces which results in translation and rotation of the bones of the knee.

3.2.1 Anatomy of the knee

Anatomically, the lower end of the femur is expanded and forms a curved surface which is covered with articular cartilage (Hall-Craggs, 1990). Cartilage-to-cartilage contacts between the femur and tibia occur at two separate locations that are separated by a groove that runs between the medial and lateral condyles of the femur (Figure 3.2). The tibia also has a groove in its surface where it comes in contact with the femur and within the groove (intercondylar notch) on the femur and tibia are found the anterior and posterior cruciate ligaments (Table 3.2). These ligaments hold the bones together. The fibula is attached to the femur with the tibial collateral ligament and to the capsule of the tibio-fibular joint. Capsules are composed of extracellular matrix and are sealed units that separate and surround the areas where two bones contact each other. Within the capsule is found synovial fluid that bathes the articular surface of each bone. This fluid facilitates relative motion of the component bones by maintaining a low co-efficient of friction between the two surfaces.

Fibrocartilage elements termed menisci are found attached to the intercondylar region of the tibia and increase the rigidity of the connection

Table 3.1 Bones of the knee joint*

Bone	Function
Femur	Bone in thigh that rests on tibia
Fibula	Bone in back of tibia
Patella	Bone in the tendon of the quadriceps muscle
Tibia	Bone in lower leg that supports femur

* Hall-Craggs, 1990

94 Replacement of skeletal tissues

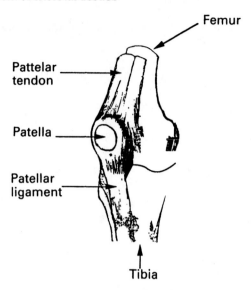

Figure 3.1 Diagram of knee structure.

between the bones in the joint and are involved in locking of the joint in the slightly hyperextended state.

The patella tendon/ligament is attached to the quadriceps femoris muscle and continues to form a connection with the patella bone and then as the patella ligament until it intersects with the tibia.

3.2.2 Physiology of the knee

The motion of the tibiofemoral joint has been recognized as a combination of translation and rotation for over 150 years. Muller (1983) gives a historical

Table 3.2 Ligaments and tendons of the knee*

Ligament (L) or tendon (T)	Function

cruciate (L)
  anterior
  posterior
	connects tibia to femur

patella (T)	connects quadriceps to patella continuing to tibia

collateral (L)
  tibial
  fibular
	connects tibia to femur
	connects fibula to femur

* Hall-Craggs, 1990

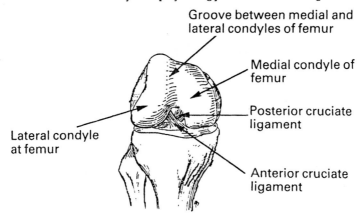

Figure 3.2 Diagram illustrating groove between medial and lateral condyles of the femur.

review of kinematics of the rolling–gliding principle on which the knee operates and credits the Weber brothers with the first description in 1836 of the rotational gliding and rolling (translation and rotation, respectively) in the tibiofemoral joint. Movement of the femur relative to the tibia during joint flexion causes changes in the contact points on both surfaces as motion proceeds. The basic kinematic principle of motion in the knee joint can be represented by the mechanism of the crossed four-bar linkage. A simple apparatus consisting of a sheet of paper on which two rods are hinged at one end can be used to represent the movement of the anterior cruciate ligament (ACL) and posterior cruciate ligament (PCL). The two hinge points lie on a line which intersects at a 40° angle the longitudinal axis through one of the points (Figure 3.3). One of the crossed rods is longer than the other. The length ratio is proportional to that of the length of the normal ACL divided by that of the PCL.

In an idealized model with only planar motion, during flexion, the cruciate ligaments should remain at a constant length and are radii that trace out small circular arcs during deformation (Muller, 1983). If the cruciate ligaments did not remain at a relatively constant length during normal deformation, then they would prematurely fail as a result of cyclic fatigue. With the tibia fixed, the end points on the femur lie on a circular line. The same is the case if the femur is fixed, the femoral end-point forms the centre of a circle. In this manner the rotation of the cruciate ligaments limit extension and hyperextension of the knee. Re-insertion of the ACL as a result of injury and surgical intervention may result in stretching of the ACL during flexion leading to premature failure. Anterior cruciate ligament deficiency results in excessive sliding of the femur posteriorly and contact with the posterior menisci, as they provide a decelerating force to the femur. This causes excessive wear of both the cartilage and the menisci.

96 Replacement of skeletal tissues

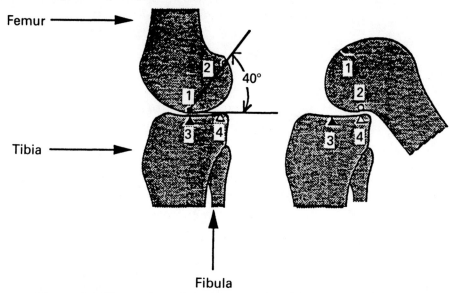

Figure 3.3 Illustration of the hinge points in the movement of the ACL. Adapted, based on Muller (1983) with permission of Springer-Verlag, Heidelberg.

The collateral ligaments, as is the case for the cruciate ligaments, can be ideally represented by a four-bar linkage. Again, as is the case for the cruciate ligaments, they follow a circular path during a hypothetical planar deformation. From this simple analysis the effect of failure of the collateral ligaments on the stablity of other structures in the knee can be evaluated.

3.3 Biochemistry and biophysics

The biochemical and biophysical structure of bone is discussed in chapter 7 and therefore the reader is referred to that chapter for a detailed discussion. Tendon and ligament are composed of water (60–65%), type I collagen (25–31%), type III collagen (2%), type V collagen (<1%), elastin (1–4%), cells (3–6%) and proteoglycans (1%) (Silver et al., 1992) (Table 3.3). Type I and III collagen in tendon are packed into quarter staggered arrays of molecules that exhibit a characteristic pattern with a 64–67 nm repeat distance when stained with heavy metals and viewed in the electron microscope (Silver and Doillon, 1989).

Much of our understanding of the self-assembly of collagen, in tissues and in vitro, has been a result of studying rat tail tendon collagen and its association. Tendon is a multicomponent cable-like element that cyclically transmits force in the absence of permanent dimensional changes. Since 1965, extensive study of tendons in the tails of rats has led to the development of a detailed model, down to the molecular level (Diamant

Table 3.3 Generalized composition of tendon and ligament*

Component	Composition
Cells	3-6%
Collagen	
type I	25-31%
type III	2%
type IV	<1%
Elastin	1-4%
Proteoglycans	1%
Water	60-65%

*adapted from Silver et al., 1992

et al., 1972; Elliot, 1965; Kastelic et al., 1978; Rowe, 1985). However, the structural models for different tendons and ligaments are not identical to those developed for tendons found in the tails of rats (Amiel et al., 1984; Brand, 1986; Danylchuk et al., 1978; Kennedy et al., 1974; Yahia and Drouin, 1989), which suggests that structure and, perhaps, function vary between sites.

Tendons in the tails of rats are composed of fascicles containing crimped, aligned collagen fibrils that are surrounded by a collagenous sheath, which was called the paratenon by Elliot (1965) and Rowe (1985), and endotendineum by McBride et al. (1985) (Table 3.4). In tendon fascicles, collagen fibrils laterally associate to form groups termed fibril bundles (Birk and Trelstad, 1986) which at the light microscopic level are seen as fibres (McBride et al., 1985) exhibiting diameters from several to hundreds of micrometres. Collagen fibril bundles are deposited within fascicles as discontinuous segmented structures (McBride et al., 1985; Birk and Trelstad, 1986) and are buckled into planes of wavy parallel fibrils that are misaligned with respect to neighbouring planes of fibrils (Niven et al., 1982). Collagen fibres are bundled together to form a fascicle. Recent evidence suggests that collagen fibrils branch and rotate and are not an ideal parallel aligned collagen network (Birk et al., 1989). Other connective-tissue sheaths that surround groups of fascicles are endotendon (also called peritendineum), which is continuous with the epitenon (also called epitendincum), and surrounds the entire tendon unit (Elliot, 1965; Rowe, 1985; Yahia and Drouin, 1989). Each of these connective-tissue sheaths, as well as the collagen fibrils of the fascicle, have different physical structures.

Epitenon is a coarse, translucent sheath that is composed of many layers of crimped collagen fibres in a criss-cross pattern (Rowe, 1985). Epitenon is continuous with the endotenon, which is also composed of layers of crimped

Table 3.4 Structural hierarchy of tendon and ligament*

Component	Size	Reference
Tendon/Ligament		
Tail tendon (rat)	300–500μm (diameter)	Kastelic et al., 1978
Extensor tendon (horse)	5.1 mm (diameter)	Abrahams, 1967
Anterior cruciate ligament		
(human-ages 48–86)	57.5 mm² (area)	Noyes and Grood, 1976
(human-ages 16–26)	44.4 mm² (area)	Noyes and Grood, 1976
Fascicle	>250μm (diameter)	Arnoczky, 1983
	20–40μm (diameter)	Rowe, 1985
	80–320μm (diameter)	Kastelic et al., 1978
Collagen fibre (fibril bundles)	up to 300μm (diameter)	Bear, 1952; Verzar, 1957
	1–20μm (diameter)	Danylchuk et al., 1978; Arnoczky, 1983
Collagen fibril	20–50 nm (diameter)	Rowe, 1985
	150–250 nm (diameter)	Danylchuk et al., 1978; Arnoczky, 1983
	0.05–0.5μm (diameter)	Kastelic et al., 1978
	318 nm (diameter)	Gotoh and Sugi, 1985
	189 nm (diameter)	Michna, 1984
	40 nm and 280 nm (diameters)	Parry and Craig, 1977
	185 nm (diameter)	Nokagawa et al., 1989
Crystalline domain	3.8 nm (diameter)	Hulmes et al., 1981

* Silver et al., 1992

collagen fibres in a criss-cross pattern. Paratenon is a loose multi-layered structure of finely crimped fibres composed of elastin and collagen (Rowe, 1985). In the paratenon, collagen fibres are aligned along the axis of the tendon. Collagen fibrils in the fascicle are larger in diameter than those of the paratenon (Rowe, 1985) and have been analyzed in detail by light microscopy, x-ray diffraction, and other techniques.

When viewed under polarized light, collagen fibres (fibril bundles in fascicle) in tendons in the tails of rats exhibit a characteristic series of light and dark bands, which Diamant *et al.* (1972) interpreted as arising from the periodic arrangement of collagen fibres along the axis of the tendon. Diamant *et al.* (1972) proposed that the collagen fibres change direction and exhibit a periodic fold or crimp. In tendons in the tails of mature rats, the distribution of the diameters of the collagen fibrils is bi-modal, with peaks at 70 and 280 nm (Parry *et al.*, 1978). Using x-ray diffraction, Brodsky *et al.* (1982) demonstrated differences in both the axial and the lateral structure of collagen fibrils in different tendons. These differences include the presence of interconnecting collagen filaments (Brodsky *et al.*, 1982), a helical twist within fascicular collagen (Amiel *et al.*, 1984) and a variable collagen fibril-bundle and fibre length (Birk *et al.*, 1989; Gotoh and Sugi, 1985; McBride *et al.*, 1988).

In addition to collagen, tendon contains hyaluronic acid as well as chondroitin sulphate and dermatan sulphate proteoglycans in various amounts, depending on the age of the animal (Scott *et al.*, 1981). Dermatan sulphate proteoglycan is found in orthogonal arrays around the collagen fibrils that compose the fascicle, and it binds specifically to the 'd' band of positively stained collagen fibrils (Scott and Orford, 1981). In contrast, hyaluronic acid and chondroitin sulphate are found in the extracellular matrix, loosely associated with collagen fibrils (Scott *et al.*, 1981). It is likely that proteoglycans facilitate sliding of collagen fibril bundles during tensile deformation and are involved in recovery of the original dimensions of the tendon after stress has been removed.

3.3.1 Microscopic anatomy of tendon and ligament
Ligaments are composed of dense aligned connective tissue in the form of multicomponent cable-like elements that dissipate energy in the absence of permanent dimensional changes. Much of the work on dense aligned connective tissue has been done on both tendons and ligaments because of their structural similarity. Extensive study over the last 25 years has led to a detailed structural model of these tissues down to the molecular level (Elliott, 1965; Kastelic *et al.*, 1978; Rowe, 1985). The structural models developed (Elliott, 1965; Kastelic *et al.*, 1978; Rowe, 1985; Amiel *et al.*, 1984; Brand, 1986; Danylchuk, *et al.*, 1978; Kennedy *et al.*, 1974; Yahia and Drouin, 1989; Cetta *et al.*, 1982) are not identical, suggesting species and site variations in structure and perhaps function. The structural and biochemical

components of dense aligned connective tissue are listed in Tables 3.3 and 3.4 (Elliott, 1965; Kastelic *et al.*, 1978; Rowe, 1985; Jimenez *et al.*, 1978; Bear, 1952; Frank *et al.*, 1988; Abrahams, 1967; Noyes and Grood, 1976; Arnoczky, 1983; Oakes and Bialkower, 1977; Gotoh and Sugi, 1985; Michna, 1984; Parry and Craig, 1977; Hulmes *et al.*, 1981; Nokagawa *et al.*, 1989; McBride *et al.*, 1985; Birk and Trelstad, 1986; Niven *et al.*, 1982; Birk, *et al.*, 1989; Parry *et al.*, 1978; Gotoh and Sugi, 1985; McBride *et al.*, 1988; Diamant *et al.*, 1972; Silver *et al.*, 1992; Mosler *et al.*, 1985).

Collagen in fascicles exhibits a characteristic series of light and dark bands which Diamant (Diamant *et al.*, 1972) interpreted as arising from the periodic arrangement of collagen fibres along the axis. They proposed that the collagen fibre changed directions and exhibited a periodic fold or crimp. The crimp period and amplitude for the ACL are 45–60µm and <5µm, respectively (Cabaud *et al.*, 1979).

In addition to collagen, fascicles contain elastin and proteoglycans in varying amounts depending on the age of the animal (Scott *et al.*, 1981). Dermatan sulphate proteoglycan is found in orthogonal arrays around the 'd' bands of collagen fibrils that compose the fascicle (Scott and Orford, 1981).

Some ligaments, such as the ACL, have additional levels of structural complexity. The aligned collagen network is twisted by about 180° from the femoral to tibial attachment sites and consists of anteromedial and posterolateral bands. The twist is superficial since it can be removed by allowing the femur to rotate relative to the tibia.

The design of an ACL replacement should take into consideration the normal structural hierarchy of ligament since the mechanical properties of this tissue are a consequence of the three-dimensional structure.

3.4 Mechanical properties of ligament

Ligaments are physiologically loaded along or close to the tissue axis and therefore uniaxial mechanical testing in vitro gives a reasonable approximation of the mechanical properties in vivo. It is, however, very difficult to predict the level of pre-stress existing in the tissue and therefore the exact operating range on the stress-strain curve is debatable. These tissues are in general viscoelastic and the stress at a fixed strain is therefore time dependent. For this reason the tabulation of a value for Young's modulus is not meaningful since the modulus and other material properties are dependent on the loading history and method of testing (Dunn and Silver, 1983; Fung, 1967; Fung, 1972).

The stress–strain curve for ligament is characterized by a non-linear toe region, a linear region and a non-linear yield and failure region (Figure 3.4 from Silver, 1987). The toe region is believed to reflect uncrimping of collagen fibres (Diamant *et al.*, 1972). In the linear region the collagen triple helix is stretched and interfibrillar slippage occurs (Mosler *et al.*, 1985).

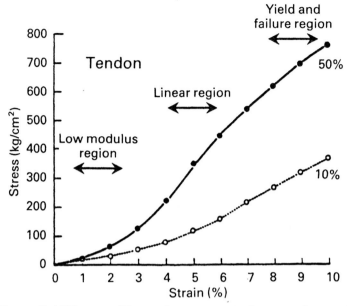

Figure 3.4 Diagram illustrating stress-strain curve for tendon.

Collagen fibres fail by fibril defibrillation during the yield and failure region (McBride et al., 1988).

The stress–strain properties in uniaxial tension are almost linear after an initial non-linear region, and are characterized by ultimate tensile strengths (UTS) and strains as high as 147 MPa and 70% for ligaments, respectively (Table 3.5) (Silver et al., 1992; Harkness, 1961; Woo et al., 1986; Yamada, 1970; Rogers et al., 1990; Barry and Ahmod, 1986; Vasseur et al., 1985; Kennedy et al., 1976; Viidik, 1987). The variation in values for these parameters in part reflects different testing protocols used in data acquisition. A variety of testing methods have been used to determine mechanical properties of ligaments.

The mechanical properties of femur-ACL-tibia complexes (FATC) have recently been reviewed by Woo and Adams (1990). When tested along the ACL axis they reported values for the ultimate load, linear stiffness and ultimate deformation of 1954 N, 292 N/mm, and 9.0 mm, respectively for FATC from younger donors and 642 N, 179 N/mm, and 5.8 mm, respectively for FATC from older donors (Table 3.6). Values for the ultimate load decrease exponentially between the ages of 20 and 100 (Woo and Adams, 1990). In comparison to these values, values for autograft tissues commonly used to replace the ACL range from 2900 N (patella tendon) to 249 N (quadriceps–patella retinaculum–patella) for ultimate load and 685 N/mm (patella tendon) to 118 N/mm (fascia lata) for stiffness (Woo and Adams, 1990) (Table 3.7).

Table 3.5 Stress–Strain Properties of Tendons and Ligaments*

Soft tissue	Maximum strength (MPa)	Maximum strain (%)	Elastic modulus (MPa)	Source
Tendon/Ligaments	55–83	6–8	–	human extensor
	60	10	700	cattle tendon
	11	5–8	430	human Achilles
	>100	10	500	–
	150–300	–	–	–
	49	9–10	625	rabbit MCL
	66	47	186	monkey ACL
	13.3–37.8	30–44	65–111	human ACL
	80–124			
	13–38	46–71	200–240	sheep ACL
	32–147	30–40	–	human ACL
	66	36–52	–	dog ACL
	13–66	47	–	–
		30–47	65–186	monkey ACL
	40–100	–	100–300	–
	30–100	–	1000–2500	–
	50–60	6–10	600–1400	–
	40–90	6–9	0.6–1.6 GPa	–

* From Silver et al., 1992

Table 3.6 Mechanical properties of femur-ACL-tibial complexes (FATC)*

Age group	Ultimate load (N)	Linear stiffness (N/mm)	Ultimate deformation mm
Young	1954	292	9.0
Old	642	179	5.8

* Adapted from Woo and Adams (1990)

A great deal of emphasis has been placed on the initial load bearing properties of ACL replacements and their fatigue properties. Biologic grafts initially have loads to failure that exceed (patella tendon) or come close to matching that of ACL. However, the failure load drops rapidly during the repair process. Synthetic polymeric replacements have excellent strength properties. Their use is limited only by fatigue failure. Ligament replacement with a material that has mechanical properties similar to ACL is desired; however, even autograft tissue initially loses strength and is able to bear ligament loads without failing. Therefore, strength is not the only criterion for successful ACL replacement. As discussed below, induction of deposition of repair tissue is as important.

3.5 Repair of Ligament

Ligament healing has been divided into three phases: inflammation, matrix repair and cellular proliferation, and remodelling or maturation. Inflammation occurs during the first 72 hours in which serous fluid begins to accumulate, surrounding tissues become edematous, and ligament stumps become increasingly friable (Viidik, 1990; Frank *et al.*, 1983). Leukocytes,

Table 3.7 Mechanical properties of biological grafts used to replace ACL*

Biological grafts	Ultimate load (N)	Stiffness
Bone – facia lata	628	118
Gracilis	838	171
Iliotibial tract	769	–
Patella bone	2734–2900	651–685
Patella-retinaculum-patella tendon	24–9–371	–

* Adapted from Woo and Adams (1990)

lymphocytes, monocytes and macrophages are actively engaged in this initial phase of healing. Unless chronic inflammation occurs, after 72 hours and until approximately six weeks after injury, matrix repair and cellular as well as vascular proliferation takes place (Viidik, 1990; Frank et al., 1983). In this second phase of ligament healing, vascular granulation tissue, stimulated by the presence of collagen breakdown products, is visible with fibroblasts predominating. Synthesis of extracellular matrix actively occurs resulting in a high ratio of type III to type I collagens with a cross-link pattern similar to embryonic tissues (Williams et al., 1984). The final phase of remodelling and maturation requires several months where the ligament matrix matures to a slightly disorganized and hypercellular tissue (Frank et al., 1983); however, this may be model and/or ligament specific. For example, the healing ligament maturation may not be achieved before 12 months in monkeys (Clancy et al., 1981), and only 50–70% of the original tensile strength is regained in rabbits (Frank et al., 1983; Woo et al., 1987). Healing of the ACL has been reported to be inhibited compared with the medial collateral ligament (Frank et al., 1983) and Achilles tendon, due to absence of revascularization (Kleiner et al., 1989).

Regardless of the cause of ligament injury, optimal healing of ligaments is achieved by maintaining continuity of the torn ligament fibres, and applying controlled functional stresses to stimulate the healing process via increasing collagen fibril diameters (Williams et al., 1984). However, the injured ligament must be protected from harmful stresses and overstress during the remodelling and maturation phases to avoid further permanent damage. Even under ideal conditions the crimp observed in the new ligament may differ from that observed in normal tissue (Goodship et al., 1985).

A transected ACL can be repaired if the ends are appositioned by sutures or wires and healing occurs by ten weeks post-surgery (O'Donoghue et al., 1966; O'Donoghue et al., 1971). When autografts are substituted for the ACL, transplanted grafts undergo a process of necrosis, revascularization, proliferation and remodelling (Arnoczky et al., 1982). Revascularization of autografts derives from the intrapatella fat pad and synovial tissues and occurs as soon as eight weeks post-implantation (Clancy et al., 1981) and is complete by about 20 weeks (Arnoczky et al., 1982). Revascularization progresses from the proximal and distal portions of the graft centrally (Arnoczky et al., 1982). After one year, autografts have 80% of the tensile strength and 52% of the maximum load prior to transfer (Clancy et al., 1981).

The success of bone–patella tendon–bone autografts as ACL replacements is a result of revascularization and subsequent remodelling leading to increases in the failure load of the neoligament. Although the maximum load decreases after autograft remodelling in animals, sufficient strength is achieved to prevent mechanical failure. Non-invasive evaluation of mechanical function is necessary to follow the progress of patients receiving ACL replacements.

3.6 Clinical evaluation of ligament function

Injury to the ACL of the knee has become a more common diagnosis in the past ten years because of an increase in athletic activities in the USA, an increase in diagnostic accuracy, and improvement in surgical techniques (Silver *et al.*, 1991). Lachman and other clinicians have contributed significant diagnostic tests that have helped to increase clinical diagnosis accuracy (Torg *et al.*, 1976). Marshall and others contributed newer ideas concerning the surgical techniques making it more reasonable to consider repair and/or reconstruction (Marshall *et al.*, 1982; Noyes *et al.*, 1983; Fox *et al.*, 1985).

With the dawn of magnetic resonance imaging and the newer arthroscopic techniques, the diagnostic accuracy and the surgical approach to the ACL has become more acceptable and successful.

Evaluation of the integrity of the ACL as well as a replacement has uniformly depended upon the clinical examination for the final decision. There are multiple physical examination tests described for each of the four ligaments of the knee. These tests vary in their sensitivity and application.

The clinical evaluation of the integrity of the ACL or a replacement begins with the Lachman test (Table 3.8). This test is performed with the knee flexed 30° and an anterior force exerted upon the tibia. If the examiner feels anterior translation without an endpoint, then the ACL or a replacement is considered to be disrupted. The value of the examination is that it can be performed with the knee flexed only 30°. This enables the examiner to make the evaluation without forcing the knee into the area of increased flexion and increased intra-articular pressure and associated pain. The test is most sensitive for disruption of the posterolateral bundle of the cruciate (Torg *et al.*, 1976).

Table 3.8 Typical diagnostic tests used to evaluate ACL function*

Test	State of knee	Condition	Results
Lachman	Flexed 30°	Anterior force Exerted	Anterior translation used as end point
Flexion rotation drawer test	Knee extended and flexed 10–30°	Tibia subluxed in extended position	Femoral rotation noted

* Silver *et al.*, 1991

The flexion rotation drawer test for the anterior cruciate is a modification of the Lachman. The leg is cradled in the examiner's hands and the knee is extended and flexed through a range from 15–30°. The tibia is subluxed in the more extended position and then reduced with the flexion. This movement can be observed, and the femoral rotation also noted (Noyes *et al.*, 1978).

The traditional anterior drawer test is performed in 90° of flexion and forms a part of the standard evaluation but is not as sensitive. This test is more sensitive for the anteromedial bundle (Larson, 1983).

The other rotational tests are most appropriate in the setting of the chronic anterior cruciate deficient knee. These tests require flexion and extension along with the internal rotation of the lower extremity with some form of valgus stress. The pivot shift, jerk, and Losee are the three variations (Galway *et al.*, 1972; Hughston *et al.*, 1976; Losee *et al.*, 1978).

Jacobsen and others attempted to standardize the knee ligament evaluations by combining the stress tests with roentgenographic documentation. Their findings certainly suggested that standardization was possible, but they were not entirely reproducible (Jacobsen, 1977).

This approach naturally led to the introduction of mechanical devices such as the KT-1000 arthrometer (Medmetric, San Diego, California) and the Genucom (Montreal, Canada). These machines represent an attempt to apply measurements to the previously established physical examinations. The KT-1000 applies a known anterior force to the tibia with the knee in the flexed position and, then, measures the displacement. The Genucom measures displacements of the tibia versus a neutral starting position with varus, valgus, anterior, and posterior forces applied. Thus, this device can theoretically be used to evaluate all of the ligaments and the associated capsular structures.

Initially, there was some enthusiasm for the devices; however, recent reports have indicated that there is a great deal of variation and lack of reproducibility from one exam to another (Bach *et al.*, 1990; Steiner *et al.*, 1990; Wroble *et al.*, 1990; Wroble *et al.*, 1990a).

Plain roentgenograms are not helpful unless there is an associated bone fragment with the cruciate disruption. Arthrograms were utilized for many years but did not have a very high sensitivity. Magnetic resonance imaging has added a great deal to the field, but the sensitivity has yet to be thoroughly evaluated.

At the present time, physical examination of the knee is still the most sensitive test for determination of the proper functioning of an ACL or an ACL replacement. The Lachman test is the most sensitive approach. The KT-1000 may have a place in the diagnostic evaluation but that still remains to be seen. Radiologic techniques are presently limited to magnetic resonance imaging, and this approach must still be further tested and compared.

3.6.1 Treatment of ligament rupture

In the clinical situation where ACL disruption is observed, it is then necessary to address the question of which patients are candidates for ACL replacement surgery. The patients are normally subdivided into those with open growth epiphyses and those who are already mature. Most authors agree that the skeletally immature should be treated more conservatively and that they should not undergo procedures that violate the growth plates for fear of a later growth irregularity and limb deformity (Lipscomb and Anderson, 1986).

In the adult knee one must establish the status of the medial and lateral meniscus. After disruption of the anterior cruciate, the menisci form the secondary restraints to anterior motion. If one or both of the menisci are injured, then the instability of the knee will be increased (Levy et al., 1989).

The acutely disrupted anterior cruciate is essentially a surgical problem because of the associated meniscal tears and the debris formed by the ligament itself. The primary problem is the approach to the ligament. If both of the menisci are normal, many groups debride the anterior cruciate and rehabilitate the knee. If one or both of the menisci are torn, then one must direct attention to the possibility of ligament repair or reconstruction (Feagin, 1988).

At the present time, primary repair of the anterior cruciate ligament is not popular. John Marshall's work was initially impressive but the long term follow-up of the primary repairs includes at least a 20% failure rate (Kaplan et al., 1990; Ferkel et al., 1988). The typical midsubstance tear divides the vascular supply and compromises the healing potential. Until surgical techniques can be significantly improved, the primary repair will remain questionable.

In patients where substitution is recommended, replacement can be accomplished using autografts or devices containing synthetic polymers. Since no medical device employing synthetic polymers is fully approved by the FDA, biological graft material is commonly used for substitution.

3.7 ACL Reconstruction using biological and synthetic materials

Successful reconstruction of the ACL using autogenous tissues including illiotibial band (Scott et al., 1985), semitendinosus and gracilis tendons (Cho, 1975), patella tendon (Jones, 1980; Johnson et al., 1984; Fried et al., 1985; Tillberg, 1977; Pattee and Friedman, 1988), and meniscus (Tillberg, 1977) have recently been reviewed (Pattee and Friedman, 1988; Newton et al., 1990) (Table 3.9). O'Donoghue et al. (1966; 1971) report that ACL reconstructions with illiotibial band tended to lose strength and stability with time. In contrast, repair of ACL with vascularized patella tendon showed

108 Replacement of skeletal tissues

Table 3.9 Tissues used to reconstruct ACL*

Tissue	Location
Illiotibial band	Tissue connecting muscle to tibia
Gracilis tendon	Tissue connecting superficial muscle in thigh to tibia
Patella tendon	Tissue connecting femur to patella
Semitendinosus	Tendon situated at posterior, inner aspect of thigh

* Pattee and Friedman, 1988; Newton et al., 1990

rapid revascularization (Clancy et al., 1981; Arnoczky et al., 1982) and revitalization in animals, and encouraging clinical results after a two year follow-up of 35 patients (Paulos et al., 1983). ACL reconstruction using meniscus does not result in neo-ligament formation and is not recommended (Walsh, 1972; Ferkel et al., 1988). Problems associated with the use of autografts include necrosis that occurs during the early post-operative period during revascularization (Clancy et al., 1981) and loss of normal structures that may compromise function.

When autograft material is unavailable either allografts, xenografts or synthetic implants have been used to restore joint function.

- Use of *fresh patella* allografts incited a marked inflammatory and rejection response (Arnoczky et al., 1986) while *deep-frozen grafts* appeared benign and underwent alterations similar to those observed in autografts (Arnoczky et al., 1986). At 18 months, Nikolaou et al. (1986) observed 90% of the control ligament strength obtained with a cryopreserved ACL allotransplant while Vasseur et al. (1987) observed loads of only 14% of the contralateral ACL.
- Jackson et al. (1987) reported the use of *freeze-dried* bone-ACL-bone allografts for ACL replacement and reported greater joint laxity and lower breaking loads compared to contralateral ACL controls. Freeze-dried allografts may fail due to a chronic intraarticular reaction, and their use as an ACL substitute is not recommended (Jackson et al., 1990).
- *Glutaraldehyde treated bovine tendon* (McMaster, 1985) as well as bovine pericardium (Chvapil et al., 1987) have been used as replacements for ACL. Preliminary clinical results with bovine ACL seemed positive (Abbink, 1988; Whipple, 1988); however, later studies reported cases of severe inflammation of the synovial lining that were associated with chemical treatment with glutaraldehyde, and their use in ACL reconstruction is not recommended (Dahlstedt et al., 1989; Good et al., 1989). On 7 May, 1987 the PreMarketing Approval (PMA) for ProCal

Bioprosthesis produced by Xenotec (Bovine ACL Xenograft) was noted 'not approvable' by the FDA Orthopaedic Panel (Whipple, 1988).

Although autografts and allografts have been reported to yield positive results in short-term follow-up studies, long-term results are not as promising. In addition, concerns such as

- sacrifice of normal joint structures
- viral contamination
- sterility

complicate the use of biological tissue grafts.

When biological grafts are not available, replacement of the ACL can be achieved using a number of medical devices that are conditionally approved for clinical use. A variety of synthetic materials have been evaluated as ligament implants including carbon fibre, (Integraft), poly(ethylene terephthalate) (Leeds-Keio ligament), poly(tetrafluoroethylene) (Gore-Tex ligament), and braided poly(propylene) (Kennedy Ligament Augmentation Device) (Table 3.10).

Jenkins and co-workers first demonstrated that pure carbon in a filamentous form had great strength and induced the formation of new tendon (Jenkins *et al.*, 1977). Later studies by Alexander and co-workers (Parsons *et al.*, 1984) showed that filamentous carbon fibres coated with absorbable polymer acted as a scaffold for deposition of new collagen and could be used to secure Achilles repair.

Based on the studies of Alexander and co-workers (Alexander *et al.*, 1981; Aragona *et al.*, 1981), a carbon-fibre stent coated with poly(lactic acid) was developed which was investigated in the repair of ACLs and other joint structures by Hexcel (Rusch *et al.*, 1988). On 19 June, 1986 the Orthopaedic and Rehabilitation Devices Panel recommended not to approve Hexcels PMA for this device because of concern over the fate of carbon particles (Table 3.11). They also noted that use of the device was not better than autogenous reconstruction (Ferl *et al.*, 1988).

Table 3.10 Devices used to replace ACL*

Name	Description
Integraft	Carbon fibre stent coated with poly(lactic acid)
Leeds-Keio	Polyethylene terephthalate braided material
Gore-Tex	Expanded poly(tetrafluroroethylene)
Kennedy Ligament Augmentation Device	Braided poly(ethylene)

* Ferl *et al.*, 1988

Table 3.11 Comments related to use of ligament replacement devices*

Device	
Integraft	Migration of carbon particles
Dacron™ Ligament Augmentation Device	Questions concerning effectiveness
Gore-Tex™	Early evidence of joint laxity
Kennedy Ligament Augmentation Device (LAD)	LAD successfully used in conjunction with middle third of patellar tendon, central two-thirds of prepatellar retinaculum and middle third of quadraceps tendon

* Rusch et al., 1988; Ferl et al., 1988

Replacement or augmentation of the ACL with Dacron™ has been studied by several investigators. Andrish and Woods (1984) studied Dacron™ augmentation of a patella tendon autograft and found that in only one of six cases did the augmented graft perform better than the unaugmented one. They concluded that the Dacron ligament stress shielded and weakened the autograft tissue. In contrast, Park et al. (1975) reported that use of high strength Dacron™ offered significant promise as an augmentation device.

Stryker developed a ligament replacement consisting of a porous tube of woven Dacron™ attached to woven tapes (Leeds-Keio ligament) that allowed tissue ingrowth and its clinical use was shown to follow a good post-operative course when used for ACL reconstruction (Fujikawa, 1988). This knee augmentation graft developed by Stryker was provisionally approved by the FDA for reconstruction of salvage patients who otherwise would require a total joint replacement. However, recently this ligament was removed from the market.

The Gore-Tex™ cruciate ligament prosthesis consists of a single long fibre of expanded poly(tetrafluoroethylene) that is wound into loops and the loops are joined to form a three-bundle braid (Bolton and Bruchman, 1985). Results of clinical trials using this ligament suggested that joint laxity occurs 12 months post-operatively (Stonebrook et al., 1988) and that ligament pre-conditioning may decrease the degree of laxity. A high strength ligament consisting of poly(tetrafluoroethylene) was evaluated in 130 patients by Bolton and Bruchman (1985). They reported that 129 out of 130 patients receiving this ligament showed improved knee stability at 15 months or less. The Gore-Tex™ cruciate ligament was approved by the FDA only for use in salvage patients on 19 June, 1986 (Ferl et al., 1988).

The Kennedy ligament augmentation device consists of a cylindrical prosthesis of diamond-braided poly(propylene) and is used in conjunction with the middle third of the patella tendon, central two thirds of the prepatellar retinaculum and middle third of the quadriceps tendon (McPherson et al., 1985). Results of clinical studies indicated that augmented transplants were stronger after two years than unaugmented ones (McPherson et al., 1985), and patients treated with augmented and non-augmented grafts show good clinical results. The Kennedy LAD PMA initiated by 3M was reviewed at the 31 October, 1986 FDA Panel meeting and was conditionally approved for human use as an augmentation device in the Marshall–MacIntosh procedure using the quadriceps tendon-prepatella tissue-patella tendon autograft (Ferl et al., 1988).

Goodship et al., (1985) evaluated the development of collagenous tissue around implants and concluded the presence of less extensible fibrous implants could adversely affect the morphology of the collagen induced within the implant. Collagen found within implants containing high stiffness materials was uncrimped whereas crimp was observed with implants containing lower stiffness fibres, including nylon and polyester. These findings, taken in conjunction with the findings that permanent synthetic polymers such as ultrahigh-molecular weight polyethylene (Chen and Black, 1990) do not possess adequate fatigue properties to replace the ACL, suggest that synthetic implants should be designed as temporary scaffolding structures and not permanent implants.

3.7.1 Biodegradable polymeric scaffolding materials

A number of biodegradable polymers including:

- collagen
- copoly(ether-ester)
- poly(carbonate)
- poly(ε-caprolactone)
- poly(dioxanone)
- poly(glycolic acid)
- poly(imino carbonate)
- poly(lactic acid)
- poly(orthoester)

have potential uses as temporary scaffolding devices in orthopaedic surgery (Daniels et al., 1990; Vert et al., 1984; Vainionpaa et al., 1987; Leenslag et al., 1987; Leenslag et al., 1987a; Cohn and Younes, 1988; Pulapura et al., 1990; Shieh et al., 1990; Durselen and Claes,1990). These materials have tensile strengths that range between 0.6 and 500 MPa and moduli between 10 and 6500 MPa. Biodegradation times of days to months are achieved using these polymers as well as co-polymers of these materials.

Cabaud and co-workers (Cabaud et al., 1982) reported the use of poly(glycolic acid), (PGA), for reinforcement of a transected dog ACL. The braided PGA reinforcement device provided excellent support for the healing ligament. At five weeks the repaired ACL had firmly attached the repaired ACL to the femoral condyle and the PGA ligament had resorbed (Table 3.12).

Parsons and co-workers (Shieh et al., 1990) report the characterization of a slowly degrading random co-polymer of dimethyltrimethylene carbonate and trimethylene carbonate (TMC). TMC fibre was reported to have a tensile strength of 500 MPa and tangent modulus of 5.4 GPa. In a rabbit Achilles tendon repair model, TMC fibres were still intact at 26 weeks and remained relatively inert in the host tissue, eliciting a minimal foreign body response.

It has been known since the 1950s that purified type I collagen molecules in acidic solution will self-assemble at neutral pH in the presence of ions, to form collagen fibres that have similar banding patterns when viewed in the electron microscope to those seen in collagenous tissues (Birk et al., 1991). Using this approach aligned type I collagen fibres have been reconstituted that have structures and mechanical properties similar to that observed for rat tail tendon fibres (Kato et al., 1991; Dunn et al., 1992). These fibres have been aligned and coated with uncross-linked type I collagen to form a biodegradable scaffold that mimics the acellular portion of tendon and ligament. This collagen scaffold has been studied after cross-linking the fibres with either glutaraldehyde or a combination of severe dehydration followed by cyanamide treatment (Kato et al., 1991). Results of preliminary studies, using an implant containing 225 collagen fibres, indicate that in both rabbit Achilles and ACL models cyanamide treated implants are biodegraded by ten weeks post-implantation and are replaced by neo-tendon and neo-ligament that is crimped (Kato et al., 1991; Dunn et al., 1992). Glutaraldehyde treated implants remain intact up to 52 weeks post-implantation and are encapsulated in a foreign body type of response as previously described (Durselen and Claes, 1990). Rapid increases in

Table 3.12 Use of biodegradable polymers for tendon/ligament replacement

Polymer	Application	Reference
Collagen	Achilles tendon and ACL	Kato et al., 1991; Dunn et al., 1992
Poly(glycolic acid)	Transected replacement ACL	Cabaud et al., 1982
Trimethyl carbonate	Achilles tendon	Shieh et al., 1990

neo-tendon and neo-ligament strength are observed in cyanamide treated implants between 4 and 20 weeks post-implantation (Kato *et al.*, 1991) suggesting that the repair tissue is capable of bearing increased loads as healing progresses. These results suggest that optimal healing of the ACL is achieved when a collagenous scaffold biodegrades between 10 and 20 weeks post-implantation. It is important to note that revitalization and remodelling of ACL autografts occurs by eight weeks and is complete by 20 weeks post-implantation, a time frame that is similar to that observed for reconstituted collagen implants.

3.8 Total joint replacement

The primary factor that leads to joint replacement is degeneration of the cartilage surfaces between long bones and the consequent pain that is experienced during locomotion. Clinically, this process is termed degenerative joint disease and can be diagnosed at its end stages by decreased intraarticular distances on an x-ray and extreme pain that occurs during translation and rotation of joint components.

Joint instability, due to excess laxity, is an aggravating factor but by itself does not lead to joint destruction unless cartilage erosion is extensive. Joint replacement, is also known as surface replacement arthroplasty, and involves substitution of artificial bearing materials that maintain their position relative to the bone and do not wear out during the life of the patient (Lewis and Lew, 1987). Replacement involves understanding the kinematics of joint motion, the loads normally borne by the joint, the materials available for construction of artificial joints and the interaction between natural and synthetic materials. Lewis and Lew (1987) have reviewed the mechanical requirements for total joint replacement and this information will only be summarized here.

Widespread use of joint replacement dates back to Charnley's pioneering work involving use of poly(methyl methacrylate) (PMMA) for fixation of the implant to the bone in the early 1960s (Charnley, 1965). In 1987 it was estimated that 287 000 hip and knee procedures were conducted each year (Biomedical Business International, vol 13, No. 3, 23 March, 1990). About 5% of all implants fail each year which has led to an effort to identify the critical factors that are reponsible for premature failure.

Major problems leading to implant failure include:

- loosening of components from bone with consequent pain and immobility;
- dislocation or other mechanical instability;
- infection; and
- restricted range of motion due to component impingement or ligamentous constraint (Lewis and Lew, 1987).

Of these, loss of interfacial contact between the implant and bone is the most frequently observed reason for clinical failure.

Most total joint replacements are composed of

- metal (either titanium–aluminium–vanadium or cobalt–chromium alloys),
- plastic (high molecular weight poly(ethylene) and cement (poly(methyl methacrylate).

The exact design characteristics of each replacement is dictated by the anatomy of each joint.

3.8.1 Total hip replacement (THR)

Hip replacement consists of a femoral component that is a ball mounted on a shaft and an acetabular component that has a socket into which the ball sits. Both cobalt–chrome and titanium–aluminium–vanadium alloys are used by different manufacturers for the femoral component as well as with high molecular weight polyethylene to cover the socket. Each manufacturer has several stem lengths and design types (e.g. long versus short stem, straight versus curved, etc.) that have evolved in parallel. Since the FDA does not have any performance standards for THRs, a side-by-side comparison of these designs is not available.

Although the first generation of hip replacements was associated with a high incidence of infection, improvements in operating room procedures and use of antibiotics after surgery substantially reduced the incidence of infection (Charnley, 1972). Early femoral component breakage was a result of

- suboptimal metal properties,
- prosthetic design problems and
- problems with cementing that led to stem breakage during the first five post operative years,
- femoral component loosening at seven to eight years and
- acetabular loosening at ten to fifteen years (Poss et al., 1988; Lewis and Lew, 1987).

The hip is the joint that is most frequently replaced. Problems encountered include loosening of the femoral stem. Potential failure of the acetabular component, the cup, is also possible. Design concerns for the bioengineer include:

- configuration of the femoral head and neck;
- fixation of the femoral stem;
- fixation of the acetabular component;
- wear of the articulating surfaces (Lewis and Lew, 1987).

The neck configuration has been modelled based on the normal anatomy with apparently adequate clinical results. Implant fixation for the femoral component is an ongoing problem. The stem is fixed to the bone typically with PMMA which creates a 'force fit' between the stem and collar of the implant, the cancellous bone at the top of the implant, the stem of the implant, and the cortical (compact) bone at the bottom of the implant. Analysis of system stresses include questions concerning:

- stem length;
- stem cross-sectional shape;
- stem material; and
- effect of a stem collar that transfers loads to the calcar bone (Lewis and Lew, 1987).

Experimental and theoretical studies suggest that the metal stem protects the bone near the collar from loading (or stress) (Oh and Harris, 1978; Hampton *et al.*, 1980) resulting in bone resorption and loosening of the cement that surrounds the implant. The degree of unloading depends on the stiffness of the material used for the stem. A high stiffness material will unload the calcar cortical bone in the presence or absence of a collar. As the stiffness of the stem is decreased, the loading on the calcar bone increases; in the presence of a collar the loading is increased further.

The acetabular component has been studied to some degree to determine if a metal backing is desirable to reinforce the high density poly(ethylene) cup. Lewis and Lew (1987) conclude that the literature suggests that a metal-backed cup should have lower bone and cement stresses than a plastic cup alone; however, these authors did not state whether the differences in stresses would be enough to favour one design over another.

3.8.2 Total knee replacement (TKR)

The design of a total knee replacement is somewhat more complicated than a hip because of the complex loading pattern of the knee. The tibial component of the total knee replacement is fixed in the cancellous (spongy) bone of the tibia.

Black (1989) recently reviewed the requirements for sucessful total knee replacement. The femoral component consists of a fairly thin, rigid shell with an attached fixation system to bone. In some cases, a central mechanical stabilizing element is present. The geometry of the femoral shell requires a stiff, high strength, low-wear-rate material, which is typically metal. The fixation system may be either a PMMA cemented type or a biologic ingrowth type. The tibial portion consists of a broad plateau covering the tibia, after the bone of the subchondral plate is removed. In most designs, a composite, consisting of a stiff metal tray supporting a polymeric or fibre reinforced polymer, is used.

The femoral component is fixed to the cortical bone of the femoral shaft. Fixation is achieved using PMMA cement and therefore loss of fixation leads to mechanical failure. Because the tibial component of the total knee is rigid and sits on a compliant foundation, i.e. the bone, loading near the edges results in beam tilting and the development of tensile forces at the bone-implant interface (Lewis and Lew, 1987). Since repeated tensile loading of a brittle material (PMMA) is more likely to cause failure than repeated compressive loading, failure is enhanced at the PMMA–bone interface.

Lewis and Lew (1987) summarize the design parameters for total knee replacement as follows:

- Metal components generally give lower bone–cement interface tensile stresses.
- Lower PMMA tensile stresses due to the bending load being concentrated on the metal.
- Separated medial and lateral implant components result in higher bone compressive stresses and bone–cement interface tensile stresses.
- Fixation post and its geometry can alter the stresses within the system (Lewis and Lew, 1987).

3.9 Materials used in total knee replacement

Replacement or restoration of knee components damaged by osteoarthritis or mechanical trauma has proceeded along different paths (Walker, 1989). Resurfacing components in the form of tibial plates, were introduced by a variety of different workers. This approach demonstrated that metallic resurfacing components were stable on bone for long periods. For more serious problems, metallic hinges with intramedullary stems for fixation were developed, however, this approach resulted in limited motion, patellar pain, bone resorption, loosening, bone fracture around the implant stem tip and infection. Later devices consisted of cemented metal-plastic replacements that initially showed a high loosening rate and inadequate fixation. These problems were later overcome and the tibial plastic was enclosed in a metal tray for improved fixation.

TKR utilizes a limited number of metallic alloys including cobalt-base and titanium-base (e.g. Ti6Al4V) alloys (Black, 1989). Cobalt-base alloy combined with ultra high molecular weight poly(ethylene) (UHMWPE) remains the contact surfaces of choice despite some adverse effects on biocompatibility described below. Bone cements utilize *in situ* curing PMMA or PMMA/poly(styrene) filled with barium sulphate for identification by x-ray.

Mechanical problems associated with THR include:

- creep of the UHMWPE component due to high stresses;

- wear of the polymeric contact surface due to adhesion of the polymer surface to the metal, and particulate deposition (bone, PMMA, ingrowth coatings) between the gliding surfaces;
- fatigue of UHMWPE due to repeated loading;
- fretting of UHMWPE and titanium-base alloys as a result of contact with bone.

Other problems encountered include corrosion of cobalt-base and titanium-base alloys and fatigue separation of tibial coating elements from their base.

3.9.1 Biological response to THR and TKR

In the absence of infection, wear debris stimulates a foreign body response characterized by infiltration of inflammatory cells at the interface between the implant and host tissue. At the bone–PMMA interface a fibrous capsule containing inflammatory cells is observed. In porous implants soft tissue may penetrate pores as small as several micrometres while hard tissue forms within pores that are ten to one hundred times greater in size (Hunderford and Kenna, 1983; Cook et al., 1985). Loosening of the tibial element is the primary limit to the lifetime of a TKR (Knutson et al., 1986; Hansen and Rand, 1988). Tibial loosening has been associated with a phagocytic response to wear particles including PMMA and UHMWPE as is the case for THR (Willert and Semlitsch, 1977; Pizzoferato, 1979; Maguire et al., 1987). Recruitment and activation of inflammatory cells leads to release of prostaglandin E_2 and other interleukins and lysis of bone (Chambers, 1980; Goldring et al., 1983).

Adverse reactions to unpolymerized PMMA have been well documented including hypotension (Dandy, 1973; Ritter et al., 1984). Immune responses to cobalt-alloy THR components (Waterman and Schrik, 1985), metal sensitivity as a result of metal release (Cracchiolo and Revell, 1982) and tumour formation after THR (Gillespie et al., 1983) have been reported.

Use of PMMA bone cement

The problems associated with use of bone cement, including implant loosening and bone lysis secondary to cement fragmentation, have led to considerable research to improve the strength of the bone–implant interface. Radiographically, the incidence of loosening of the femoral component was reported as approximately 20% by five years post-implantation and 30% by ten years. Acetabular loosening was reported as minimal even after ten years; but approximately 24% of these components showed evidence of radiographic loosening by 12–15 years post-implantation. One study reported that only $\frac{1}{3}$ of the loose acetabular components are actually identified radiographically (O'Neill and Harris, 1984).

Changes in prosthesis design and the manner in which the cement is prepared have improved the strength of the bone–cement–implant interface. Advances in femoral stem design have occurred as a result of recognition that high stresses in the bone cement were responsible for failure. To decrease the stresses in the bone cement, the femoral stem should be made of a superalloy and have a broad medial border without sharp corners. In addition, increases in stiffness of the acetabular reconstruction would have a beneficial effect in reducing peak stresses in the acetabular bone cement, in the trabecular bone in the supra-acetabular region, and in the medial wall of the acetabulum. This has been achieved using a metal backing for the acetabular component.

Use of a cement gun for introducing cement (Harris, 1975) coupled with use of cement in a low viscosity state (Krause *et al.*, 1982) provide excellent penetration. Pre-coating the metal with methylmethacrylate strengthens the interface and may reduce the effect of saline immersion. A minor degree of surface roughness also enhances interfacial shear strength.

Improved cementing techniques for the femoral component has increased the fatigue life of bone cement. This is achieved by reducing the porosity of cement using either centrifugation (Burke *et al.*, 1984) or vacuum mixing (Wixon *et al.*, 1985).

3.10 Summary

Successful clinical repair of the ACL is routinely accomplished using autografts of bone–patella–bone complexes. Although this procedure requires a second surgical site and sacrifices other soft tissue structures in the knee, it results in revascularization and subsequent neo-ligament formation. Although the strength of the autograft initially decreases, the higher initial value of the load to failure for the patella tendon compared to the ACL prevents failure until a neo-ligament can provide mechanical stability. Revitalization of these implants occurs by eight weeks and is complete under normal conditions by 20 weeks post-implantation.

The mechanical properties of the autograft can be enhanced in the presence of a ligament augmentation device (LAD); however, the device must be designed to support but not stress shield the neo-ligament. If the full load is borne by the LAD then it will ultimately fail due to fatigue and will require an additional surgical procedure. Successful use of bone–patella–bone allografts have been reported, although additional handling problems are associated with removal of viral and cellular contaminants associated with these materials.

Neo-ligament formation, that is associated with use of auto and allografts, is a result of the chemotactic properties of collagen, derived peptides released from the graft material as it biodegrades. These peptides stimulate angiogenesis and wound healing, ultimately resulting in neo-ligament formation. The graft acts as a biodegradable scaffold stimulating wound healing.

Combining the advantages of autografts and LADs a new generation of ACL replacements can be achieved. Autografts possess scaffolding materials that stimulate revitalization and repair while synthetic polymers have high strengths. The next generation of ACL replacements is likely to contain scaffolding materials in addition to high strength biodegradable fibres analogous to LADs. The function of the LAD is to mechanically reinforce the device transferring at least 50% of the mechanical load to the scaffolding material by the time revascularization is complete (approximately ten weeks). The scaffolding should promote deposition of normal tendon and ligament (dense aligned connective tissue) and may contain peptides that are chemotactic for microvascular, inflammatory and other connective tissue cells including fibroblasts. By combining the advantages of autografts and high strength synthetic fibres, a new generation of materials is possible that has the advantages currently found by using autograft tissue in combination with LADs.

In the area of total joint replacement a number of classical materials including HMWPE, cobalt-chronium and titanium-aluminium-vanadiun alloys are used extensively. Although some ceramic materials are under development they are not used extensively in the US. Problems associated with total joint replacement include component loosening at the bone, infection, mechanical instability and restricted range of motion. Problems with loosening of cemented components has led to the development of devices that are fixed to bone by porous ingrowth.

4.

Biomaterials Used In Ophthalmology

4.1 Introduction

Ophthalmology is a field that has rapidly advanced as a result of the development of new techniques and materials (Table 4.1). For instance correction of vision using contact lenses has been accomplished since the 1960s and will eventually be replaced using a procedure in which a biomaterial and laser surgery are used to change the curvature of the cornea. Viscous solutions containing large molecules are used during surgical procedures to protect the cellular linings of the eye chambers and to allow insertion of intraocular lenses. These lenses are used to replace natural lenses containing cataracts. Polymer solutions are used to replace the fluid contained in the posterior eye chamber to force the retina backward and maintain its position after surgery. Scleral buckling materials are used to indent the retina inward toward a site of retinal detachment.

Biomaterials are an important component of the procedures that are used to improve and maintain vision. The gradual ageing of the population has made it important to continue to develop new materials to maintain the highest level of correction as well as to solve problems that to this date remain the subject of extensive research investigation. In this chapter we will

Table 4.1 Devices incorporating biomaterials used in ophthalmology

Device or procedure	Medical application
Contact lens	Correct vision
Intraocular lens	Replace lens containing cataracts
Epikeratoplasty	Change corneal curvature and correct vision
Scleral buckling materials	Indent detached retina
Viscous polymer solutions	Insertion of intraocular lenses, cataract removal and maintain retinal position

review the materials that make up normal structures of the eye as well as those that are used as replacements.

4.2 Anatomy of the eye

The eye is contained within the bony orbit in the skull and is held in the socket in the rear by extrinsic eye muscles. The eyeball is approximately spherical and has a diameter of about 2.5 cm. It contains three layers including the fibrous outer coat, vascular middle coat and light sensitive innercoat (Figure 4.1, Table 4.2).

The outer fibrous coat consists of the sclera (white portion) which is continuous with the cornea (transparent portion). Sclera (Table 4.3) is composed of stroma containing collagen fibres that run parallel to the surface of the eyeball and elastic fibres that form a network (diFiore, 1981). In comparison, the cornea is composed of outer layers of squamous epithelium that are on top of a layer of columnar cells. The columnar cells rest on a basement membrane that is in contact with Bowman's membrane that separates the cellular epithelial layers from the underlying connective tissue or stroma. The stroma makes up the bulk of the cornea and contains lamellae composed of aligned collagen fibrils and rows of flattened corneal fibroblasts. Neighbouring lamellae are approximately orthogonally aligned. The inner surface is lined with low cuboidal

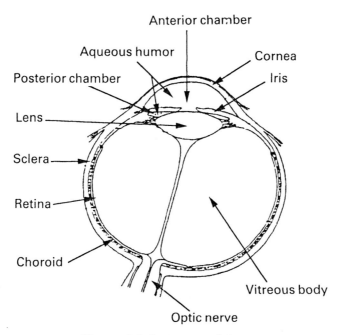

Figure 4.1 Anatomy of the eye.

Table 4.2 Structural composition of the eye*

Component	Function
Anterior chamber	Separates cornea from lens and iris
Aqueous humor	Aqueous fluid filling anterior chamber
Choroid	Vascularized membrane attached to retina
Cornea	Clear layer that protects lens
Iris	Controls amount of light entering the eye
Lens	Focuses light on retina
Optic nerve	Transmits electrical impulses to brain
Posterior chamber	Separates iris and lens
Vitreous body	Chamber at rear of eye near retina

* di Fiore, 1981

epithelium which sit on another basement membrane termed Descemet's membrane. Recently it was suggested that fibres 27.5 nm in diameter were seen crossing into stromal lamellae from Bowman's layer while in comparison fibres 22.3 nm in diameter appeared attached to the anterior surface of Decemet's membrane.

In the back of the eye, is a vascularized thin pigmented membrane, the choroid, that supports the retina. The retina is a light sensitive membrane lining the internal surface that transduces light intensity and colour into electrical signals. The choroid consists of the suprachoroid, vascular layer, choriocapillary layer and the glassy membrane (Bruch's membrane) (Table 4.4).

The suprachoroid consists of layers of fine collagen fibres mixed with elastic fibres, fibroblasts and cells termed chromatophores. The vascular layer contains large blood vessels with large chromatophores residing between the vessels in the loose connective tissue. In the choriocapillary layer, large capillaries are embedded within fine collagen and elastic fibres.

Table 4.3 Structure of cornea and sclera*

Element	Composition
Sclera	Stroma containing collagen and elastic fibres
Cornea	Stroma containing lamellae of aligned collagen fibrils
Bowman's membrane	Membrane which separates outer epithelial layer of cells and inner stroma
Descemet's membrane	Membrane that lines inner surface of cornea

* di Fiore, 1981

Table 4.4 Layers found in choroid*

Layer	Components
Suprachoroid	Collagen and elastic fibres, fibroblasts and chromotophores
Vascular	Large blood vessels and chromotophores
Choriocapillary	Large capillaries embedded in collagen fibres
Glassy membrane	Layer in contact with retinal pigmented epithelial cells

* di Fiore, 1981

The glassy membrane lies adjacent to the outermost layer of the retina containing pigmented epithelium.

In addition to the pigmented epithelium, the retina contains rods and cones in the outermost nuclear layer, axons of the rods and cones in the outer plexiform layer, nuclei of bipolar cells in the inner nuclear layer, synapses between axons of bipolar cells and dendrites of ganglion cells in the inner plexiform layer, multipolar neuron cell bodies and neuroglia cells in the ganglion cell layer, vertically and horizontally directed axons of ganglion cells in the nerve fibre layer and axons of the ganglion cells that converge to form the optic nerve. Light that passes through the cornea impinges on the pigmented cells and thereby stimulates photoreceptor cells, the rods and cones. Rods are sensitive to dull light and give vision of movement and shape. Cones are sensitive to bright light and are receptors of colour and sharp outline. Photostimulation of these cells results in the production of nerve impulses that are conducted to the brain via the optic nerve.

Light passes through the cornea and the anterior and posterior chambers, aqueous humor, the lens, the vitreous body and then impinges on the retina. The aqueous humor fills the anterior and posterior chambers of the eye and carries nutrients to the avascular cornea and lens. An intraocular pressure of about 24 mm Hg is maintained by continuous production and drainage of fluid. The lens lies between the posterior chamber and vitreous body. It is a transparent structure composed of protein that is stretched into an oval shape by suspensory ligaments.

4.3 Biochemistry of eye structures

Eye structures including the cornea, sclera, lens and vitreous body are composed of collagenous tissue that contains other macromolecules such as the crytstalline proteins of the lens. Although many eye tissues contain type I collagen, post-translational modification of type I collagen varies between different tissues of the eye. For this reason much research has been conducted to understand the biochemistry of components that make up the structures in the eye.

4.3.1 Cornea

Collagen accounts for over 70% of the total solid content of the cornea. The major collagen type found is a type I collagen that has a similar primary amino acid sequence found in other tissues but differs in the extent of post-translational glycosylation. Although the type I collagen molecule accounts for most of the material found in the orthogonal plywood type arrangement (Freeman, 1982), other collagen types including II, III (Praus et al. 1979), V (Davidson et al., 1979) and VI (Linsenmayer et al., 1986) have been reported in cornea. Antibodies to type VIII collagen have been reported to recognize enzyme resistant fragments from Descemet's membrane and the lattice collagen in that tissue may be a member of a novel class of long-spacing fibrils (Sawada et al., 1990).

Recent studies indicate that collagen types I and V are assembled together within single fibrils (heterotypic fibrils) in the corneal stroma (Birk et al., 1988). One consequence of the formation of these fibrils may be the regulation of the thin corneal fibril diameter and regular spacing, a condition that is essential for maintaining corneal transparency.

Structural studies on type I collagen show that the molecule is similar to type I collagens from other sources (Freeman, 1982); however, the level of hydroxylysine glycosylation (collagen contains hydroxylysine derived complexes with mono and disaccharides) is higher than in other tissues (Freeman, 1982). Although this high level of glycosylation may cause a larger intermolecular spacing, no evidence is available to support a direct relationship between sugar content and narrow (25–35 µm) fibril diameters.

In addition to collagens, corneal stroma contains proteoglycans. It has been estimated that 5% of of the corneal stroma is composed of glycosaminoglycans, the sugar component of proteoglycans (Maurice, 1969). Proteoglycans are known to be present in the gap region in the quarter-stagger packing arrangement of collagen molecules in this region (Meek et al., 1986).

4.3.2 Sclera

Sclera is a supporting element that protects intraocular structures from mechanical injury as well as providing enough rigidity to maintain a fixed intraocular pressure. About 80% of the dry weight of this tissue is composed of collagen fibrils and fibres with fibril diameters ranging from 30–300 µm (Freeman, 1982). In addition, elastic fibres are seen between the bundles of collagen fibrils.

Scleral collagen is composed of about 94% type I and 6% type III (Freeman, 1982). In some species, such as avian, other associated structures contain collagens such as type II (Trelstad and Kang, 1974).

4.3.3 Vitreous body

About 80% of the eye is occupied by the vitreous body, a gel like material. The vitreous is mostly water containing thin diameter type II collagen fibrils surrounded by a matrix of hyaluronic acid and other material. Electron microscopic studies have revealed the characteristic D-period in collagen fibrils isolated from vitreous (Snowden and Swann, 1980). Although the physical structure of vitreous type II collagen fibrils is similar to that observed in type II fibrils from cartilage, chemical differences have been reported (Snowden and Swann, 1980).

Hyaluronic acid (HA) is a linear polymer of D-glucuronic acid and N-acetylglucosamine that has a molecular weight that has been determined as low as 77 thousand for vitreous to 14 million for synovial fluid (Silver and Swann, 1982). Cleland and Wang (1970) determined that HA molecules from vitreous with molecular weights in excess of 10^5 had properties similar to that of molecules that form random coils in solution. In comparison, molecules with molecular weights less that 10^5 behaved as worm like coils. Other studies suggest that low molecular weight HA molecules may more effectively interact in solution as compared to high molecular weight HA (Silver and Swann, 1982).

4.3.4 Lens

The lens is surrounded by a layer of basement membrane and therefore contains

- the collagens,
- cell attachment factors and
- proteoglycans characteristic of this tissue.

In addition, it contains a class of unusual proteins termed the **crystallins** that are uniquely arranged to result in transparency (Tardieu and Delaye, 1988). A decrease in lens transparency leads to cataract formation and a resultant loss in vision.

The crystallins consist of globular particles of alpha-crystallins containing 40–55 copies of A and B sub-units. Each of the sub-units has a molecular weight of about 20 000. Beta-crystallins form dimers to octomers while gamma-crystallins are monomers with a molecular weight of about 20 000.

4.4 Mechanical properties of ocular tissues

Tensile stress–strain curves have been measured for cornea and sclera for humans and animals by Yamada (1970). For persons 29–79 years of age, the stress–strain curve is characterized by an increasing slope (strain 0–8%) until it becomes constant in the linear region (strain about 11%). The tensile strength and strain at failure for cornea are about 4.8 MPa and 14.8%, respectively (Table 4.5). In animals, the tensile strength is as high as 5.5 MPa and the strain at failure as high as 32%. In comparison, the ultimate

Table 4.5 Mechanical properties of ocular tissues*

Tissue	Ultimate tensile strength (MPa)	Ultimate strain (%)
Cornea (human)	4.8	14.8
(animals)	5.5	32
Sclera (human)	6.9	20

* Yamada, 1970

tensile strength and strain at failure of human sclera are about 6.9 MPa and 20% respectively, which is similar to that reported for animals. The similarity of mechanical properties of these tissues reflects the high content of collagen and lack of fibre orientation along the tensile axis during mechanical testing.

4.5 Corneal wound healing

Processes such as physical trauma or infection can lead to the loss of transparency of the cornea and result in visual impairment. For this reason insertion of any material into the eye can have profound effects on vision. Inflammation can be induced by either of these stimuli and result in the accumulation of neutrophils at the site of injury. Activation of plasminogen and generation of complement factor 3a lead to chemotaxis of additional neutrophils. Release of collagenase and subsequent degradation of the stroma appear to be related to plasminogen activation.

Healing occurs through the deposition of scar tissue that unlike normal corneal stroma contains large diameter collagen fibrils. Freeman (1982) observed that corneal scar tissue contained a high content of type I collagen similar to normal cornea; however, type I trimer was synthesized at the expense of type V collagen.

4.6 Viscoelastic solutions

Solutions of macromolecules in a solvent, termed viscoelastics by workers in the field, have unique properties (Table 4.6) including high zero shear viscosity, the ability to shear thin and to protect delicate tissue structures. They protect cells from mechanical damage, maintain and create tissue spaces, separate and lubricate tissues, allow manipulation of tissues while limiting mechanical damage and prevent and control cell movement and activity (Balazs, 1983).

In the 1950s viscoelastic solutions were introduced as vitreous substitutes and in the 1970s they were used for the first time in anterior or segment surgery (Benedetto, 1992). Use of viscoelastics has made it possible to

Table 4.6 Function of viscoelastic solutions*

Property	Function
High viscosity	Allows delicate manipulations of instruments; protects eye structures
Shear thinning	Easily introduced through a syringe
Surface active	Coats intraocular lenses and corneal endothelium

* Benedetto, 1992

perform a 5.0 mm continuous circular capsulotomy or phacoemulsification or insertion of a foldable intraocular lens into the capsular bag.

The optimum properties (Balazs, 1983; Liesegang, 1990) of a transparent viscoelastic solution include:

- ability to coat cellular linings
- biologically inert and non-toxic
- high zero shear rate viscosity
- low resistance to aspiration
- low surface tension
- no elevation of intraocular pressure
- rapid clearance from eye
- sterilizable and pyrogen-free
- thixotropic (shear thins)

Viscoelastics are used for

- insertion of intraocular lenses,
- during corneal transplantation, in cataract, corneal, glaucoma, trauma, and vitreo-retinal surgery, and
- as a tear substitute (Liesegang, 1990 for a recent review)

Polymeric materials used in formulating viscoelastics include:

- hyaluronic acid (HA)
- chondroitin sulphate (CS)
- polyacrylamide
- hydroxypropylmethyl cellulose (HPMC)
- collagen and mixtures of these materials

The purpose of this section is to review the physical properties of viscoelastics and to evaluate what is known concerning the long-term effects associated with their use.

4.6.1 Vitreous humor hyaluronic acid

Since the vitreous humor of the eye is composed primarily of hyaluronic acid (HA), it was proposed by Balazs (1960) that a viscous solution of HA was a logical replacement for this material. This molecule was recently renamed hyaluronan to better reflect its chemical structure. Although this concept was simple, it took an additional 15 years for the purification of non-pyrogenic, non-antigenic, and non-inflammatory material that was suitable for use in the eye (Balazs, 1983). Since that time, HA has been the 'gold standard' for viscoelastics and therefore many viscoelastics have been designed based on the properties of solutions of high molecular weight (in excess of 10^6) ultrapure HA. Below the properties of HA solutions that have been the basis for development of several other viscoelastics are reviewed.

HA is a polymer of N-acetyl-D-glucosamine and D-glucuronic acid linked together with $\beta(1-4)$ glycosidic bonds containing disaccharides linked together with $\beta(1-3)$ bonds. Thirty years ago it was known that HA from vitreous humor was polydisperse since it contained a distribution of low (77 000) and high molecular weight (1.7×10^6) molecules (Laurent et al., 1960). High molecular weight HA chains (two to five million) were used to prepare viscoelastic solutions (Balazs, 1983) with high zero shear viscosities that showed dramatic viscosity reduction at high shear rates. Shear thinning (thixotropy also termed pseudoplasty) of HA molecules is dependent on their large molecular domains and molecular flexibility and is related to network forming capabilities.

Commercial viscoelastics containing high molecular weight HA are prepared at concentrations of 1%–3% (Table 4.7) in phosphate buffered saline containing ions such as 0.146 N NaCl, 0.34 mm NaH_2PO_4, 1.5 mm Na_2HPO_4 at pH 7.2. HA molecular weights of $2-4 \times 10^6$ were reported to give kinematic viscosities (viscosity divided by density) between 100×10^3 and 30×10^3 cSt (Balazs, 1983) at zero shear and about 100 at a shear rate of greater than 1000 sec^{-1} (Liesesgang, 1990) demonstrating the shear thinning behaviour of this molecule.

When HA solutions were used in the anterior chamber of the eye, the intraocular pressure was found to peak in three hours and return to normal in 24 hours (Balazs et al. 1972). In the owl monkey model, with an intact anterior cortical gel, HA is eliminated by 120 days. If the cortical gel is damaged this time decreases to three to six days. From these early studies it was apparent that complete viscoelastic clearance from the eye and from the body may take up to several months even under normal conditions. Complications associated with viscoelastic clearance from the eye have increased the morbidity associated with their use.

4.6.2 Types of viscoelastics

A number of macromolecules besides HA have been used as viscoelastics including chondroitin sulphate (CS), collagen, hydroxypropylmethylcellulose (HPMC) and other cellulose derivatives and polyacrylamide (Silver et al., 1992a for a review). All of these molecules except collagen and

Table 4.7 Physical properties of ophthalmic viscoelastic solutions

	Composition	Molecular weight (Daltons)	Osmolality (mosmol/kg H_2O)	Dynamic viscosity (cps)	Viscosity at shear rate 1000 (Vs1000)	Vs0/Vs1000	Contact angle (degrees)
Amvisc	1% Na Hyaluronate	1.0E+06	318	35 000	110	909	60
Amvisc Plus	1.6% Na Hyaluronate	2.0E+06	340	–	–	–	70
Chondroitin SO_4 50%	50% Chondroitin SO_4	2.5E+04	1050	10 000	12 000	1.4	–
Healon	1% Na Hyaluronate	4.3E+06	302	40 000	110	3600	60
Healon GV	1.4% Na Hyaluronate	5.6E+06	–	2 000 000	–	–	60–70
HPMC	2% hydroxypropyl-methylcellulose	1.0E+06	–	5000	240	23	50
Occucoat	2% hydroxypropyl-methylcellulose	8.6E+04	285	–	–	–	60
Ocugel	2.75% hydroxypropyl-methylcellulose	1.0E+05	–	–	–	–	–
Orcolon	4% polyacrylamide	1.0E+06	340	10 000	350	100	20
Viscoat	3% Na Hyaluronate + 4% Na Chondroitin SO_4	5.0E+04	325	40 000	310	130	52
Vitrax	3% Na Hyaluronate	5.0E+05	–	40 000	–	–	–

Silver et al., 1992a

polyacrylamide are polysaccharide derivatives and exhibit the conformational freedom that allows them to form random coils in solution. Collagen is a triple helical protein that exhibits a high chain stiffness at neutral pH. The physicochemical characteristics of each of these macromolecules are reviewed below.

Hyaluronic acid
HA as stated above, is a polymer of the monosaccharides β-D-glucuronic acid and β-D-N-acetyl-galactosamine (Table 4.8). The basic conformation of β-D-glucuronic acid is the $^4C_1$ or C1 chair conformation based on x-ray diffraction studies of β-D-glucuronic acid and N-acetyl-D-glucosamine (Silver, 1987 for background material). Theoretical free energy calculations indicate that the C1 chair conformation of glucose and glucose derivatives is more stable than the boat conformation. Other free energy calculations indicate that β-D-glucose residues linked into chains via repeat of β (1–2), (1–3) or (1–4) linkages, restrict rotation of each sugar residue to about 4% of the theoretical area of a conformational plot (Sathyanarayana and Rao, 1971). This observation indicates that polysaccharide chains containing only β(1–2), (1–3) or (1–4) linkages are rigid. In comparison, plots for combinations of (1–3) and (1–4) linkages in HA appear to centre around the extended conformation of (0°,0°) with a rotational flexibility of about 50° (Silver, 1987). These data suggest that the HA molecule has inherent flexibility because of the mix of β(1–3) and β(1–4) linkages.

Although HA molecules are inherently flexible, based on the conformational freedom of the backbone, the inherent molecular flexibility is complicated by the formation of hydrogen bonds between the uronate carboxylate and acetamide NH groups (Heatley and Scott, 1988). Hydrogen bond formation theoretically stiffens the chain backbone under low shear conditions while, under high shear states, breakage of these bonds would lead to shear thinning. However, shear thinning may also involve breakage

Table 4.8 Structural hierarchy of hyaluronic acid*

N-acetyl-D -glucosamine and D-glucuronic acid linked via β (1–4) and β (1–3) glycosidic bonds

C1 chair conformation

Rotational flexibility of about 50^0

Hydrogen bond formation between uronate carboxylate and acetamide amide groups

Molecular dispersion in solution for molecular weights less than 350 000

Saturated network structure for molecular weights in excess of 1 600 000

---

* Silver *et al.*, 1992

of bonds between different molecules that form a network structure. Such a structure has been visualized by electron microscopy (Scott *et al.* 1991). Recent studies suggest that HA molecules exhibit network forming behaviours that are related to the chain molecular weight, and therefore also the solution viscosity. Yanachi and Yamaguchi (1990) reported that HA solutions with viscosity-average molecular weight of less than 35×10^4 are molecularly dispersed in solution while in comparison, solutions containing molecules with viscosity-average molecular weight, 160×10^4 or above, exhibited a saturated network structure. Electron microscopic (EM) evidence for formation of extensive branched structures discussed above is generally consistent with this data (Scott *et al.*, 1991); however, the exact relationship between the structures seen by EM and those implied based on solution studies remains to be proven. For this reason, shear thinning of HA may involve both hydrogen bond formation within a molecule as well as between molecules. This would result in a decrease in molecular flexibility and explain the viscosity changes that are observed for HA in solution.

Biological properties of HA that have been cited as helpful in its use as an implant or biomaterial include the following.

- HA is associated with cell proliferation and migration (Toole and Trelstad, 1971; Pratt *et al.*, 1975)
- Specific HA binding sites are present on limb cells that are modulated during differentiation (Knudson and Toole, 1987)
- Low concentrations of HA can mediate cell aggregation (Pessac and Defendi, 1972; Forrester and Lackie, 1981)
- HA and its receptors are involved in cell-to-substratum adhesion (Alho and Underhill, 1989)
- HA and fragments as small as N-acetyl-D-glucosamine have been shown to stimulate chemotactic and phagocytic functions of neutrophils (Hakansson and Venge, 1987)
- HA inhibits neutrophil adhesion (Forrester and Lackie, 1981)
- HA suppresses humoral response to different antigens (Delmage *et al.*, 1986)

Operationally, sodium HA solutions have been shown to coat and protect the corneal endothelium during animal surgery as well as to protect the endothelium against cell loss incurred by contact with intraocular lenses (Bahn *et al.*, 1986). Exogenous HA has been shown to bind to corneal endothelial cells, with the binding affinity related to the molecular weight (Madsen *et al.*, 1989).

Hydroxypropylmethylcellulose (HPMC)

HPMC is a derivative of cellulose, a polysaccharide found in wood and other natural structures. Cellulose is a polymer of β-D-glucose and forms an extended structure based on x-diffraction data (Blackwell, 1982). The chains are extended in ribbon like conformations, with two sugar rings

132 Biomaterials used in ophthalmology

repeating every 1.03 nm. Treatment of cellulose with alcohols or ketones results in derivatives that have reduced hydrogen bonding potential. Replacement of hydroxyl by methyoxy groups is achieved up to 29% of the time and by hydroxypropyl groups up to 8.5% of the time in a typical raw material (Liesegang, 1990).

HPMC solutions contain a range of concentrations from 0.5–5% of polymer in a physiological salt solution (i.e., 0.49% NaCl, 0.075% KCl, 0.048% $CaCl_2$, 0.03% $MgCl_2$, 0.39% sodium acetate and 0.17% sodium citrate pH 7.2). A 2% solution has a low shear viscosity of about 4 000 cps for polymer chains with an average molecular weight of 86 000 (Liesegang *et al.*, 1986).

Results of clinical studies indicate that either solutions containing 2% HPMC or those containing 1% of high molecular weight HA helped maintain the normal shape of the anterior chamber and facilitated anterior capsulotomy and nuclear expression in extracapsular cataract extraction with posterior chamber lens implantation (Liesegang, 1990). Patients treated with HA solutions had a larger increase in intraocular pressure during the early post-operative period than did patients treated with solutions of HPMC (Table 4.9). Endothelial cell loss nine weeks after surgery was similar with either of these viscoelastics. Endothelial cell counts for eyes treated with solutions containing HPMC were reported to be similar to values obtained with non-operated eyes (Fechner and Fechner, 1983) suggesting that endothelial cells are protected by use of this viscoelastic during lens implantation. Results of other studies indicate that the loss of endothelial cells may be somewhat higher with solutions containing 1% as opposed to 2% HPMC (Aron-Rosa *et al.*, 1983) and that corneal endothelium is only minimally protected using solutions containing only 0.4% HPMC (MacRae *et al.*, 1983) (Tables 4.10 and 4.11). Clearly all viscoelastics studied protect against damage to corneal endothelium better than saline solution.

Chondroitin sulphate (CS)
CS is a polysaccharide derivative (glycosaminoglycan) with a repeat unit containing β-D-glucuronic acid and β-D-N-acetyl galactosamine. It is very similar to hyaluronic acid except for modification of the position of a hydroxyl group and the addition of sulphate groups to the galactosamine residue. CS is normally attached to a protein core to form a proteoglycan (PG) monomer in tissues and forms high molecular weight aggregates. Protease treatment of PGs and chromatographic separation of the product leads to isolation of individual CS chains. Commercial preparations have molecular weights of about 25 000, far below values reported for HA solutions (Liesegang, 1990). Low values of the molecular weight require high concentrations to yield viscous CS solutions; however, CS solutions do not show shear thinning in a similar manner to solutions containing HA. Solutions of 20% or 50% CS have been used to create products with

Table 4.9 Intraocular pressure observed using viscoelastics

	PreOp press. (mm Hg)	Low (high) press. (mm Hg)	Study duration	Time at max. press. (mm Hg)	Comments
BSS		18 (28)	1–48 hrs	6 hrs	monkey
BSS		15 (21)	1–48 hrs	3 hrs	rabbit
20% CS		17 (50)	1–48 hrs	2–3 hrs	rabbit
20% CS		25 (58)	1–48 hrs	3–4 hrs	monkey
1% HA	22–28	25 (43)	1–48 hrs	1–4 hrs	two different vol.
1% HA		17 (48)	48 hrs	4 hrs	rabbits
1% HA		25 (70)	48 hrs	2 hrs	monkey
1% HA	16.0	19.3 (28.8)	3 hrs – 1 wk	6 hrs	
1% HA	15.94	14.11 (18.00)	1 day – 9 wks	1 day	
HA	18	22.04 (46.82)	2–48 hrs	16 hrs	Conc. unreported
3% HA & 4% CS	14	18.5 (28.4)	3 hrs – 1 wk	6 hrs	
HA & CS	18	22.14 (35.54)	2–48 hrs	16 hrs	Conc. unreported
2% HPMC	15.79	13.75 (16.91)	1 day – 9 wks	1 day	
1% and 2% HPMC		25 (34)	1–5 days	1 day	

Taken from Silver *et al.*, 1992a
* BSS = Balanced Salt Solution

Table 4.10 Endothelial cell damage observed using sodium hyaluronate and mixtures with chondroitin sulfate

	Amount (ml)	Animal	Testing technique	Measurement technique	% Damage	Comments
1% HA (MW = unreported)	0.12–0.15	Rabbit	Lens abrasion	Light microscope	10.1	
1% HA (MW = 3.8×10^6)	0.25	Rabbit	Phacoemulsification*	Computer photo scan	6.1	46.7 sec to emulsify
1% HA (MW = 3.8×10^6)	0.20	Rabbit	Lens abrasion	Light microscope	14.8	
1% HA (MW = 2.0×10^6)	0.20	Rabbit	Lens abrasion	Light microscope	14.5	
1% HA (MW = 1.7×10^6)	0.25	Rabbit	Phacoemulsification*	Computer photo scan	5.9	34.2 sec to emulsify
3% HA & 4% CS	0.25	Rabbit	Phacoemulsification*	Computer photo scan	2.3	48.6 sec to emulsify
3% HA & 4% CS	0.20	Rabbit	Lens abrasion	Light microscope	15.0	

Taken from Silver et al., 1992a
*Lens emulsified at 80% Power and Ultrasound for 2 min.

Table 4.11 Endothelial cell damage observed using hydroxypropylcellulose, methylcellulose, chondroitin sulfate and balanced salt solutions

	Amount (ml)	Animal	Testing technique	Measurement technique	% Damage	Comments
Air Bubble		Human	Laser capsulotomy	Unknown	8.0	
BSS	0.12–0.15	Rabbit	Lens abrasion	Light microscope	48.1	
BSS	0.20	Rabbit	Lens abrasion	Light microscope	48.5	
10% CS	0.12–0.15	Rabbit	Lens abrasion	Light microscope	23.2	
20% CS	0.12–0.15	Rabbit	Lens abrasion	Light microscope	9.5	
0.4% HPMC	0.12–0.15	Rabbit	Lens abrasion	Light microscope	34.0	
2% HPMC	0.25	Rabbit	Phacoemulsification*	Computer photo scan	2.2	44.8 sec to emulsify
2% HPMC	0.20	Rabbit	Lens abrasion	Light microscope	11.5	
1% Methylcellulose		Human	Laser capsulotomy	Unknown	25.3	

Taken from Silver *et al.*, 1992a
*Lens emulsified at 80% Power and Ultrasound for 2 min.

moderate viscosity; however, even solutions with these viscosities fail to reproduce the high zero shear viscosity of high molecular weight HA solutions (Arshinoff, 1989) (Table 4.12). Although a 20% solution of CS was reported to be nontoxic to corneal endothelium, this solution caused a marked decrease in corneal thickness because of its high osmolarity (MacRae *et al.* 1983) (Table 4.11). CS and high molecular HA solutions were observed to elevate intraocular pressure when injected into the anterior chamber (MacRae *et al.* 1983) in one study; however, in another report, postoperative monitoring of intraocular pressure revealed only normal pressures (Harrison *et al.*, 1982) (Table 4.9). Elimination of CS solutions from the anterior chamber was reported to occur in less than 40 hours (Harrison *et al.*, 1982).

Polyacrylamide
Polyacrylamide is a derivative of acrylic acid and therefore is generically an acrylic polymer. It is free radical polymerized in solution to form high molecular weight material (Rodriguez, 1982). Acrylics have similar backbone chemical structures to derivatives of ethylene and therefore the chains have an inherent degree of flexibility due to the carbon-to-carbon bonds. The large side chains prevent crystallization of this polymer as well as increase the hydrophilic nature of the molecules.

Commercial solutions of polyacrylamide used as viscoelastics contain molecules with an average molecular weight of 1×10^6 (Liesegang, 1990) (Table 4.7). The high molecular weight as well as the flexibility of the molecules provides some shear thinning behaviour similar to HA solutions of the same molecular weight (Liesegang, 1990). Animal studies using this polymer as a viscoelastic have been reported (Roberts and Peiffer, 1989).

Collagen
Collagen is a protein that is characterized by the presence of a triple-helix of varying lengths. There are at least 14 different genetic types of collagen that have been isolated from tissues (Van der Rest and Garrone, 1991). Type I, II and III collagens form highly organized fibrils that provide mechanical support to both soft and hard tissues (Christiansen *et al.*, 1991). Type IV collagen is characterized by interrupted sequences of amino acids that form a triple-helix. From solution studies this molecule has been characterized as significantly more flexible than collagen types I, II and III (Birk and Silver, 1986).

A recent review cites the use of several different approaches to using collagen solutions as viscoelastics (Liesegang, 1990). The problem with use of a protein solution, in the eye particularly collagen, involves the potential for chemotaxis of connective tissue and other cells that results from the release of collagen derived peptides (Postlethwaite *et al.*, 1978).

4.6.3 Rheological properties of viscoelastics

The ability of a solution to shear thin when stress is placed on it is a desirable property as it pertains to the injection of viscoelastic material through small gauge cannulas and tissue manipulation. Solutions of high molecular weight HA exhibit this behaviour. Solutions of low molecular weight HA (less than 50 000) are similar to pure solutions of CS in that they have no pseudoplastic character. Solutions of short chain molecules such as Vitrax, Occucoat and Ocugel, similarly exhibit less pseudoplastic behaviour (Table 4.12). Solutions that do not shear thin require significant force on the syringe plunger to express the solution from the tip of the cannula. This can decrease control of precision movements during microscopic surgery. A combination solution such as Viscoat, while exhibiting some of the properties of a pure hyaluronic acid solution, is less pseudoplastic than a pure solution of HA because of the presence of CS.

The ability of a viscoelastic solution to manipulate tissue, i.e. maintain space, is directly related to its viscosity when at rest. The higher its viscosity at rest (Healon GV has the highest) the greater the tissue manipulation capability. Thus, as a viscoelastic passes through a small gauge cannula, it is liquid-like because it is being subjected to high shear. As it exits the cannula, shear immediately drops to zero and the solution becomes very viscous, more solid and gel-like, resists flow, occupies space, and exerts a force on or displaces tissue.

The rheological properties of viscoelastic solutions that are relevant to their use in ocular surgery have been recently reviewed (Arshinoff, 1989; Liesegang, 1990) and will only be briefly presented here (Table 4.12). These parameters include viscosity, shear thinning, percent elasticity and surface coating ability. The viscosity of a solution is its resistance to flow which for non-Newtonian fluids is shear rate dependent. The shear rate for insertion of a lens coated with a viscoelastic solution has been estimated to be 2–5 sec^{-1} while that for removal of the viscoelastic via aspiration from the eye has been estimated at 1000 sec^{-1} (Arshinoff, 1989).

Table 4.12 Rheological parameters relevant to viscoelastic design*

Parameter	Clinical relevance
Cohesiveness	Tendency of viscoelastic molecules to stick together
Percent elasticity	Ability to maintain shape
Surface tension	Ability to coat ocular structures
Thixotropy	Shear thinning during flow, pseudo plasticity
Viscosity	Resistance to flow

* Arshinoff, 1989; Liesegang, 1990

The viscosity and shear thinning of macromolecular solutions depend on several molecular parameters including the molecular shape and shape factor, the nature of the interactions between polymer molecules and the interactions between polymer and solvent molecules (Silver,1987). The ratio of the solution viscosity in the presence of macromolecule (SV) to that in its absence (SVo) is dependent on the volume fraction of polymer (Vp) and the shape factor (SF) as given by Newton's law of viscosity, equation (1). The shape factor for spheres is 2.5 while it is proportional to the axial ratio raised to the power of 1.8 and 1.00, for cigar shaped molecules and discs, respectively (Silver, 1987).

$$SVo/SV = (1 + SF \times Vp) \qquad (1)$$

Therefore, the axial ratio goes up much more rapidly for rod-shaped molecules than for molecules that form spheres (random coils) for a fixed molecular weight. For this reason the viscosity of rod-shaped molecules is higher than that found for molecules that form random coils. In addition, macromolecules such as HA and type IV collagen that collapse under flow conditions (Silver, 1987) shear thin by a decrease in the axial ratio leading to a decrease in viscosity. Dynamic flow conditions are likely to break secondary bonds that exist under static flow conditions. Both collagen and HA have been shown to form interactions under zero shear solution conditions (Silver and Birk, 1984; Silver and Swann, 1982) which is another factor complicating their flow behaviour.

When the viscosity of commercial viscoelastics is compared (Table 4.7) it is clear that at low shear rates (2 sec^{-1}) only solutions containing HA molecules have viscosities as high as 40 000 cps. At high shear rates (1000 sec^{-1}) the viscosities of all commercial viscoelastics range from 110–350 cps. Therefore, after examining this data it appears that the molecular weight of the HA component should be at least 500 000 to have a significant thixotropic effect.

Viscoelastic solutions have properties of fluids (viscosity) which act to dissipate energy while the properties of solids including elasticity, lead to energy storage. Typically, the elastically stored energy results in conformational changes that are reversible such as a decrease in the randomness or increased compaction. Based on a recent report (Arshinoff, 1989), the highest percent elastic storage of a viscoelastic solution is found for solutions with HA molecules with molecular weights over 1 000 000.

At times, it is necessary to completely aspirate viscoelastic material from either the anterior or the posterior chamber. Such conditions might arise when a patient is known to have glaucoma or a traumatic injury to the anterior segment that might produce trabecular clogging from intraocular debris. In such instances, solutions of polymers of extremely long chain length should be considered because the entanglement of individual molecules makes them more cohesive and easier to aspirate. Aspiration forces are transmitted throughout the solution as if the individual polymer molecules were attached to one another, allowing for complete removal of the viscoelastic.

Solutions consisting of smaller molecules, heterogeneous solutions containing two components or solutions consisting of molecules of different structure and length (i.e. Viscoat, AmVisc Plus, Occucoat, Ocugel, and Vitrax) are less likely to be aspirated completely during surgery because they are less cohesive. When suction is applied, fracturing of these solutions takes place because of the decreased interaction of individual molecules, leaving part of the gel behind.

When such a viscoelastic solution coats the endothelium, problems may occur with visualization. An irregular interface forms at the viscoelastic-aqueous juncture, which may cause unwanted glare from light scattering. This phenomenon is occasionally seen with Viscoat and Occucoat.

Cohesiveness is a property by which a material resists fracture into small droplets that can be removed by aspiration during ocular surgery. Solutions containing high molecular weight HA, aspirate easily because they have high cohesion. A high degree of cohesiveness may not be optimal for the surgeon especially if he or she wishes to remove only a small fraction of the viscoelastic at one time. In addition, it has been suggested that too much cohesion can lead to blockage of the trabecular meshwork and associated elevation of intraocular pressure (Liesegang, 1990). It is the latter problem, that leads to blockage of the trabecular meshwork, that is associated with adverse effects.

Another aspect of the physical evaluation of viscoelastic solutions includes the determination of the surface coating ability. Due to the incomplete bonding that occurs at material surfaces, good adhesion (coating) normally occurs when macromolecules in solution are attracted to the surface in question. Solutions with low surface tension tend to coat better because there are less repulsive forces to be overcome.

Surface coating in anterior segment surgery should prevent damage from irrigation or endothelial touch. Ideally, a viscoelastic agent would form a thin coating on the intraocular lens (IOL), the instruments, and the endothelium. A solution's ability to coat a surface is often confused with its viscosity. Viscous solutions often appear to adhere to surfaces. While it is generally true that viscous solutions are unlikely to flow from a surface when applied, this does not necessarily mean that there is an interaction between the viscous material and the surface. Whether or not a given solution coats a surface depends on the solution's surface tension and its interaction with the solid surface it is intended to coat. Viscosity is not a property that applies to surface spreading or coating. When an aqueous solution of viscoelastic polymer interacts with a hydrophobic surface such as a poly(methylmethacrylate) (PMMA) IOL, the lower the solution's surface tension the greater the spreading of the solution on the IOL surface. Thus, solutions with low surface tension (e.g., Viscoat and Occucoat) are able to coat IOLs and instruments to a greater degree than solutions with high surface tension (e.g., Healon or AmVisc Plus) (Benedetto, 1992). The surface tension of a solution is directly related to the contact angle. Contact angles for viscoelastics are given in Table 4.7.

It is not understood how the surface tension of a solution affects endothelial coating because the surface properties of the corneal endothelium have yet to be well characterized. Clinically, solutions such as Viscoat, Occucoat, and Vitrax form an endothelial coating visible under the operating microscope. Whether this coating is present as a result of surface spreading of viscoelastic molecules on the endothelium or weak molecular interactions, such as hydrogen bonding, is not known. It is known that the corneal endothelium possesses a 1200 Å glycocalyx that extends from its surface. It is possible that viscoelastic molecules bind to this structure, and in fact this may be the binding site on the endothelium reported for Healon. Yet, clinically Healon does not appear to coat the corneal endothelium. In addition, a solution's cohesive properties also play a role in the ability of a solution to form a grossly visible endothelial coating. Protection of the endothelium from irrigation damage by viscoelastic coating has recently been reviewed in the literature (Benedetto, 1992).

4.6.4 Surgical requirements for viscoelastic solutions

The ability of a viscoelastic solution to maintain the deepness of the anterior chamber during surgery has been suggested to reflect its elasticity (Liesegang, 1990). This is consistent with a report that sodium hyaluronate was better able to maintain the deepness of the anterior chamber compared to HPMC, which has a lower molecular weight and therefore elasticity (Miyauchi and Iwata, 1986).

Another function of a viscoelastic solution is to act as a physical boundary in which manipulations can occur without risking injury to surrounding tissues. In the presence of a high viscosity viscoelastic that is gel like, manipulations can be done with precision without fear that a slight movement will result in mechanical trauma to neighbouring tissues such as the corneal endothelium. In addition, a material that has low cohesiveness allows for slow controlled aspiration of material. Unfortunately, this combination of properties is not currently available in a commercial product.

4.6.5 Long-term effects of viscoelastics

When viscoelastic solutions are placed in the eye, they are cleared in an unmetabolized state by filtration through the trabecular meshwork. Although it is not completely understood, the elevated intraocular pressure that occurs in the presence of viscoelastic solutions is thought to be due to the solution's molecular configuration as well as its viscosity. Large globular molecules that do not deform easily and are larger than the pore size of the trabecular meshwork could theoretically block the exit of aqueous material and cause elevated intraocular pressure. In contrast, a molecule that deforms easily might be able to exit the eye even though its size is larger than that of the trabecular pores. Solutions made of rigid, rod-like molecules that are smaller than the trabecular pore size could also cause significant outflow obstruction similar to a log jam in a flowing river.

To avoid intraocular pressure elevations, it is advisable to aspirate viscoelastic solutions from the anterior chamber as completely as possible. This can be accomplished by using a solution that is highly cohesive (i.e. has a high molecular weight HA). Furthermore, injecting a balanced salt solution into the anterior chamber dilutes other viscoelastic solutions and disperses the individual molecules, lessening the likelihood of trabecular obstruction. Because of a viscoelastic's tendency to increase intraocular pressure, many surgeons prescribe short-term antiglaucoma medication following their use.

Elevation of intraocular pressure has been attributed to three factors:

- impeding fluid outflow through trabecular meshwork
- extracataract extraction, and
- tight suturing during wound closure

Several investigators have determined that high molecular weight HA solutions injected into the anterior chamber caused a postoperative increase in intraocular pressure (Aron-Rosa et al., 1983; MacRae et al., 1983; Embriano, 1989). A summary of the data reported on post-operative intraocular pressure is given in Table 4.9. It has been theorized that the effect of ocular hypertension associated with high molecular weight HA is due to mechanical resistance in the trabecular network. Hyaluronidase, an enzyme normally present in the anterior segment, is incapable of rapidly clearing the trabecular meshwork because of the large amounts of HA forced into it (Passo et al., 1985). Thus, fluid outflow through the trabecular meshwork is diminished. It has also been reported that the intraocular pressure increases after extracapsular cataract extraction when saline is used to reform the anterior chamber. This result has been explained as a swelling of the trabecular meshwork and breakdown of the blood-aqueous barrier (Passo et al., 1985). Other investigators have discovered lysed zonular material causing a blockage in the trabecular meshwork, thereby, increasing intraocular pressure (Sears and Sears, 1974). It has also been shown that surgical technique, more specifically, tight suturing during wound closure, may cause structural distortion of tissue and edema, thus, inducing elevated intraocular pressure (Berson et al., 1983; Haimann and Phelps, 1981).

It is unclear whether the effects of ocular hypertension are due to one or both of these theories. In either case, however, elevated intraocular pressure is a serious though usually temporary, side effect of intraocular surgery. It is imperative that intraocular pressure be controlled for several reasons. It has been demonstrated that an increase in intraocular pressure is associated with patient post-operative discomfort (Haimann and Phelps, 1981). Various analgesics have been used to counteract pain. A second, more important reason for controlling intraocular pressure is to prevent permanent nerve damage. Most eyes can withstand intraocular pressures of 30–40 mm Hg for several hours with no permanent damage (Haimann and Phelps, 1981). Patients, however, with a compromised blood supply to the anterior optic nerve, can suffer nerve damage with even moderate increases in intraocular pressure (Haimann and Phelps, 1981). Elevated intraocular pressure can be treated post-operatively with drugs such as acetazolamide. Normal intraocular pressure is typically achieved 72 hours after surgery and drug therapy can be terminated.

Several studies have compared the different effects of ophthalmic viscoelastics on intraocular pressure. In general, it has been concluded that higher molecular weight viscoelastics have a greater tendency to cause post-operative ocular hypertension than do lower molecular weight viscoelastics. Several studies have shown Healon™, to cause an increased post-surgical intraocular pressure (Polack *et al.*, 1981; Berson *et al.*, 1983; Packer *et al.*, 1989). It is unclear whether removal of Healon, after ocular surgery has been performed, will alleviate elevated postsurgical intraocular pressure. Other high molecular weight viscoelastics, such as Viscoat and AmVisc also lead to elevated postsurgical intraocular pressure (Liesegang, 1990, Liesegang *et al.*, 1986). Investigators have determined that lower molecular weight viscoelastics, such as Occucoat (comprised of low molecular weight HPMC), do not exhibit postsurgical intraocular hypertension (Fechner and Fechner, 1983; Aron-Rosa *et al.*, 1983).

In at least one case, blindness was reported in two patients after use of polyacrylamide viscoelastic that may have been associated with microparticles of the polymer. These microparticles may have caused an increase in intraocular pressure. This same problem may be encountered with other viscoelastics if they are stored for long periods of time during which polymer precipitation can occur.

Although some data exists in the literature on the short-term increases in intraocular pressure observed with high molecular weight HA solutions, the long-term effects of this transient increase have not been quantitatively assessed. In addition, it is clear that use of viscoelastics helps prevent loss of corneal epithelium during ocular surgery; however, no data is available in the literature to indicate what are the long-term effects of endothelial cell loss.

Furthermore, it remains to be demonstrated that loss of even a small percentage of corneal endothelial cells is not associated with an increased probability of long-term morbidity.

4.7 Intraocular lenses

Loss of transparency of the lens or its capsule due to cataract formation results in loss of vision and sometimes blindness. Replacement of such a lens with a synthetic intraocular lens (IOL) dates back to 1949 (DeVore, 1991 for a review). Since then about ten million IOLs were implanted, nearly all of which were composed of poly(methyl methacrylate) (PMMA). In 1990 about 1.4 million of these devices were implanted in the US.

IOLs consist of an optic portion through which light passes along with loop or attachment regions. The optical portion of the IOL is composed of PMMA; however, other materials such as poly(hydroxyethylacrylate) (PHEMA) and silicone have also been used (Table 4.13). The attachment component has been fabricated using metals, nylon, glass, poly(imide) and polyethylene. Included in the polymer portion are antioxidants, ultra violet light absorbers and other agents to retard the decomposition of the lens.

Placement of IOLs in either the posterior or anterior chambers have been described. Although most (98%) IOls are placed in the posterior chamber, anterior chamber placement is also reported (DeVore, 1991). Posterior placement of the IOL in the capsular bag from which the opaque lens has been removed can be achieved if the bag is protected during emulsification of the lens. When anterior chamber placement is used, the lens is attached to the iris to prevent movement. Anterior chamber IOls are most frequently used after vitreous loss or rupture of the posterior capsule (Apple *et al.*, 1987).

Apple *et al.* (1984) reviewed the complications associated with use of intraocular lenses. The major advantages of anterior chamber fixation include: implantation after either intracapsulary or extracapsulary cataract extraction; the ability to perform secondary implantation; and dislocation of the lens would be minimized. Frequently, failure of IOls were a result of problems associated with fixation. Anterior chamber placement of the lens requires rigid fixation to the iris, or any movement may result in contact with the corneal epithelium, which will result in cell loss.

Table 4.13 Components of intraocular lenses*

Component	Composition
Optical portion	PMMA, poly(hydroxyethylacrylate), silicone
Loop	Metals, nylon, glass, poly(imide), poly(ethylene)
Retarders	Antioxidants, UV absorbers

* DeVore, 1991

Complications of IOL use may be due to surgical techniques, IOL design or the inability of some eyes with pre-existing disease to tolerate an implant. The major problems associated with anterior chamber lenses is the poor quality of manufactured lenses with respect to sharp optic and attachment components.

4.7.1 Tissue response to IOLs

Biological responses to PMMA lenses have been reported as long as 30 years after implantation. Results of these studies indicate that even PMMA lenses induce a foreign body-type encapsulation with fibrovascular tissue (Rummelt et al., 1990) (Table 4.14). Other reports suggest that the membrane that surrounds the implant is coated with cells and cell aggregates including foreign-body giant cells (Sievers and Von Domarus, 1984). PMMA lenses have been shown to remove iris epithelium which could lead to a foreign-body giant cell reaction (Burnstein et al., 1988). Another study (Galin et al., 1982) examined the activation of complement components and IOL coating with antibodies. Their results indicated that PMMA did not activate C3 and C5 complement components but did become coated with IgG aggregates, an event that may trigger complement activation.

Another aspect of PMMA biocompatibility is the release of free monomer from implanted lenses. Galin et al. (1977) examined the effects of monomer on toxicity to rabbit kidney cells and on tissue when implanted into the rabbit eye. They reported that rabbit kidney cells showed no response up to a monomer concentration of 2% and that at concentrations as high as 3.7% no response was observed in the rabbit eye. This level exceeds the 0.5% level used as a manufacturing specification for IOLs in the industry (DeVore, 1991).

Soft IOLs have been fabricated using poly (hydroxyethylmethacrylate) (PHEMA) and some short-term data is available in the literature on biocompatibility. In one study a six month follow-up on 50 hydrogel implant PHEMA lenses was reported to show improved compatibility over PMMA lenses (Percival, 1987) while a second study followed 106 patients for up to

Table 4.14 Biocompatibility of PMMA IOLs*

Reaction	Histological Description
Foreign body	Encapsulation with fibrovascular tissue, giant cells
Cell detachment	Loss of iris epithelium
Immune response	IOLs coated with IgG aggregates

* Rummelt et al., 1990; Sievers and Von Domarus, 1984; Burnstein et al., 1988; Galin et al., 1982

two years. In another study no adverse reactions related to use of the lenses were reported (DeVore, 1991).

Silicone flexible lenses can be folded for insertion through incisions and induce less damage to corneal endothelium than is reported for PMMA (Herzog and Peiffer, 1987; Burnstein *et al.*, 1988). Insertion of silicone lenses without folding was reported to decrease endothelial cell loss compared to that observed when the lenses were folded (Levy and Piscano, 1988).

Loop materials tested besides PMMA include nylon and poly(propylene). Nylon was used in loop materials in the 1950s and 1960s (DeVore, 1991) until it was demonstrated that polymer degradation and breakage occurred (Kronenthal, 1981; Apple *et al.*, 1984). In addition, it was subsequently replaced by other polymers including poly(propylene).

Although concerns have been expressed about using poly(propylene) in the eye, the clinical evidence concerning its possible degradation is mixed (Table 4.15). Drews (1983) reported microcracks on poly(propylene) loops within three years of implantation. Similar surface changes were reported by Apple and co-workers (1984). Results of other studies failed to confirm the presence of surface microcracks on poly(propylene) loops (Royer and Montard 1981; Mobray *et al.*, 1983).

Biocompatibility of poly(propylene) was reported by several groups of investigators. This polymer was found to activate complement by two groups (Galin *et al.*, 1982; Tuberville *et al.*, 1982). Tuberville *et al.* (1982) showed that poly(propylene) was capable of generating activity for human polymorphonuclear leukocytes. Apple *et al.* (1984) suggested that implantation of this polymer may lead to propagation of a complement-induced mechanism leading to tissue reactions.

4.8 Contact lens materials

Materials placed in direct contact with the cornea to correct vision have been used for over twenty years. These polymers include:

Table 4.15 Biocompatibility of poly(propylene)

Observation	Reference
Microcracks	Drews (1983), Apple *et al.* (1984)
No surface microcracks	Royer and Montard (1981), Mobray *et al.* (1983)
Activation of neutrophils	Tuberville *et al.* (1982)
Activation of complement	Apple *et al.* (1984)

- cellulose acetate butyrate
- PMMA
- poly(2-hydroxyethyl methacrylate)
- siloxan methacrylates
- silicones

(Refojo, 1982; McDermott and Chandler, 1989). Polymethylmethacrylate (PMMA) was the first material used for contact lenses because if its superior optical properties. However, because of its chemistry and rigid chain structure the oxygen permeability of this material is low. Oxygen transport to the cornea is achieved via tear fluid circulation. Since the provision of delivery of sufficient oxygen to the cornea is of primary concern in the development of contact lenses, this has led to the development of soft contact lenses which allow oxygen diffusion through the lens (Lippman, 1990 for a review).

Although oxygen diffusion through gels is greater than through rigid polymers, it is decreased as the lens thickness increases and with increasing time of wearing. In addition, negatively charged surfaces as well as those with pores are vulnerable to deposition of lipomucoprotein from the tear film, and growth of fungi and bacteria. It has been the later problems that have led to the development of rigid gas permeable materials (Table 4.16).

4.8.1 Rigid gas-permeable (RGP) materials

A number of RGP materials including silicones, fluorosilicone acrylates and fluorocarbons have been developed as contact lens materials (Table 4.17). Silicone was identified as material that provided a high oxygen diffusion coefficient. However, the hydrophobicity of this polymer led to interaction with insoluble tear components, preservatives in lens solutions and lipids (McDemott and Chandler, 1989).

Table 4.16 Advantages and disadvantages of soft and hard contact lenses*

Type	Advantage	Disadvantage
Soft-permeable	High oxygen permeability	Deposition of lipomucoprotein and bacterial growth
Rigid non-permeable	Optical properties	Low oxygen permeability
Rigid gas-permeable	High oxygen permeability	Accumulation of surface deposits

* Lippman, 1990

Table 4.17 Types of rigid gas-permeable contact lenses*

Polymer	Observation
Acrylate with microscopic holes	Increased permeability
Fluorinated methacrylate or pyrolidone	Reduced corneal swelling for as long as 60 days
Silicones	Interaction with insoluble tear components and preservatives in lens solutions
Silicone-methacrylate derivatives	Oxygen transmission not high enough for extended wear

* Lippman, 1990

Modification of silicone polymers to increase the hydrophilicity without interfering with the oxygen permeability was achieved by co-polymerizing methylmethacrylate and alkylsiloxanylmethacrylate into a silicone acrylate polymer (Lippman, 1990). Although silicone acrylates show less tendency to accumulate deposits, they still do not have sufficient oxygen transmission for extended wear (Rosenthal, 1985).

Addition of fluorinated monomers to silicone acrylates resulted in another generation of lenses that were free of the undesirable surface characteristics of the silicone acrylates. However, the oxygen permeability of this material and the corneal swelling observed after sleeping was unchanged by this modification.

Other polymers were produced containing fluorine co-polymerized with methylmethacrylate and n-vinyl pyrrolidone. Fluorine atoms replace hydrogen atoms in this poly(perfluoroether) polymer backbone thereby decreasing the resistance to oxygen diffusion. Extended wear studies as long as 60 days showed reduced corneal swelling with these lenses (Moore, 1989).

Another approach to increased oxygen permeability of polymeric materials has been to increase the diffusion of oxygen by creating small channels in a lens material. The permeability of hard acrylic lenses has been increased by creating microscopic holes in the lens using an excimer laser (Lippman, 1990). The long-term utility of this approach still needs to be evaluated.

4.8.2 Problems associated with extended wear lenses

As our society searches for ways to increase the amount of leisure time, an effort has been made to limit day-to-day manipulations associated with lens usage. Several publications have pointed out the increased frequency and severity of the extended use of contact lenses (Schein *et al.*, 1989; Poggio *et al.*, 1989). Problems associated with extended use of lenses include (Franks *et al.*, 1988):

- corneal abrasions
- hypersensitive reactions
- hypoxia
- infections
- toxicity

The risk of all complications was 2.2 times higher for soft lenses than for hard lenses with use of PMMA lenses giving the lowest risk. The risk associated with daily use of soft lenses was two times that of use of PMMA lenses while that of use of extended wear soft lenses was 6.8 times greater.

The risk of development of ulcerative keratitis using soft lenses was 10–15 times greater for those who wear their lenses on an extended basis (Schein *et al.*, 1989). This risk was estimated in another report to be 4.1 per 10 000 for daily use of soft lenses compared to 20.9 per 10 000 for extended wear (Poggio *et al.*, 1989).

4.9 Eye shields

Several commercial products are available in the form of thin films that are used after corneal surgery to protect the eye. These materials are composed of collagen in the form of a clear, pliable, thin film 0.0127–0.071 mm thick in a spherical shell shape with a diameter of 14.5 mm and a base curve of 9 mm. Post-treatment, collagen eye shields are used for relief of discomfort. Shields are used in treatment of:

- basement membrane associated disease
- cataract extraction
- corneal abrasion resulting from trauma
- corneal abrasion resulting from contact lense use
- epithelial defects
- neutrophilic ulceration
- penetrating keraplasty
- recurrent erosion

and other diseases that cause inflammation. Once applied to the eye, the shield absorbs fluid from the ocular surface and begins to dissolve. The dissolution time is dictated by the extent of cross-linking. Shields with dissolution times of 24, 48 and 72 hour are available. Oxygen transmission studies indicate that collagen shields behave like hydrogel contact lenses that contain 63% water (Weissman and Lee, 1988).

Since the introduction of the eye shield, ophthalmologists have begun to evaluate its use to prolong the delivery of drugs to bacterial and fungal infections. Slatter *et al.* (1982) reported the use of ocular inserts soaked in gentamicin to prolong the release of this drug. They found that gentamicin

Table 4.18 Prolonged delivery of drugs using collagen eye shields*

Drug	Application
Amphotericin	Bacterial infection
Gentamicin	Bacterial infection
Tobramicin	Bacterial infection
Antiviral agent	Viral infection
Antifungal	Fungal infection
Dexamethasone	Anti-inflammatory

* Unterman et al., 1988; Hobden et al., 1988; Willey et al., 1991; Schwartz et al., 1990

concentrations achieved 24 hours after insertion approximated the minimum inhibitory concentration (Table 4.18). Unterman et al. (1988) and Hobden et al. (1988) studied the retension of tobramicin sulphate by collagen shields. They found that shields made of porcine collagen placed in solutions containing either 40 or 200 mg/ml of tobramycin for five minutes resulted in antibiotic concentrations in the corneas and aqueous humor samples that exceeded the mean inhibitory concentration for most strains of Pseudomonas at one, four and eight hours post-application (Unterman et al., 1988). In addition, the collagen shields were as effective in reducing the number of viable bacteria per cornea as 4% tobramycin drops applied every 30 minutes over a four hour period (Hobden et al., 1988). Over a nine hour period, the addition of four drops of 4% tobramycin to shields in situ was as effective as exchange with a new shield rehydrated in 4% tobramycin (Hobden et al., 1988). Delivery of antiviral (Willey et al., 1991) and antifungal agents (Schwartz et al., 1990) have been described in the literature.

4.10 Other ocular materials

Materials are used in a number of other applications in ophthalmology including:

- artificial tears
- correction of corneal curvature
- scleral buckling materials
- vitreous replacements

Keratoconjunctivitis sicca is a dry-eye syndrome characterized by either decreased tear formation and/or flow (Holly and Lemp, 1977). Symptoms range from mild ocular discomfort to severe ocular pain that result in decreased vision and extreme uncomfort in the presence of light.
  Tear substitutes commonly employed contain

- methylcellulose

- polyvinyl alcohol
- hyaluronic acid (HA) and
- chondroitin sulfate (CS)

(Lemp, 1973; Lemp et al., 1975; Norn and Opauski, 1977; Limberg et al., 1987; Nelson and Farris, 1988). In a controlled, double-masked, randomized study in patients with moderately severe dry-eye syndrome, an unpreserved solution containing 0.1% sodium HA was compared against a preparation containing 1.4% polyvinyl alcohol and 0.5% chorobutanol (Nelson and Farris, 1988). Although the mean tear film osmolarity improved in both study groups, the degree of cellular metaplasia did not change significantly. In another study, solutions containing CS, HA and mixtures of CS and HA were compared to polyvinyl alcohol and polyethylene glycol. The results of the latter study indicated that no formulation was preferred by a majority of patients with dry-eye syndrome (Limberg et al., 1987).

Retinal detachment from the underlying pigment epithelium results in loss of its light sensitivity. The retina along with the pigment epithelium may also detach from the choroidal layer. Since the choroidal blood vessels bring nurtients to these tissues, the retina must be in close apposition to the choroid to maintain its photosensitivity. Scleral buckling is a surgical procedure whereby the sclera is indented inward at the site of retinal detachment.

The buckling is achieved by implanting a material in a pocket dissected in the sclera or by suturing the implant on the sclera. A number of materials including

- acrylic hydrogels
- cadaver sclera
- fascia lata
- gelatin
- poly(ethylene)
- poly(vinyl alcohol), and
- silicone rubber

have been used (Refojo, 1986).

Injections of silicone oil and HA into the vitreous cavity have been used in cases of retinal detachment to force the retina gently back toward the choroid and maintain its position post-operatively. The use of silicone injections for management of retinal detachments has been reported by Scott (1981) and Lean et al. (1982). Complications associated with use of silicone oil include emulsification of the fluid into droplets which can penetrate the subretinal space. Silicone retinopathy is caused by displacement of phospholipids in the cell membranes which damages affected retinal cells (Mukai et al., 1972). Complications associated with use of silicone injections require removal of this fluid several months after surgery.

HA has been used as a vitreous replacement. In healthy, young monkeys, much of the hyaluronic acid disappears within about three weeks (Balazs et al., 1972). Clinical observations have been reported using HA as a vitreous replacement (Pruett et al., 1977; Pruett et al., 1979).

Epikeratoplasty is a procedure developed to modify the curvature of the cornea to correct vision in the absence of corrective lenses or contacts. Epikeratophakia is a procedure that uses corneal tissue that has been lathed to individual patient specifications (Werblin and Klyce,1981), lyophilized, and vacuum-sealed for storage. The surgeon adds saline to rehydrate the tissue, removes the central epithelium from the patient's cornea, excises a portion of the cornea and then sutures the lyophilized tissue onto the patient's cornea. This procedure has been used to treat patients that lack a natural lens, are near sighted or farsighted, or have a protruded cornea.

Clinical studies reporting use of epikeratophakia for keratoconus indicate that all but two patients (in a study of 177 eyes) showed improved vision after this procedure (McDonald et al., 1986). Epikeratophakia for correction of near sightedness resulted in 98% of the desired correction in 12 eyes in one study (McDonald et al., 1985) and 120 patients equalled or improved pre-operative best corrected visual acuity (McDonald et al., 1987).

Problems associated with use of human lathed tissue include:

- less than optimum attachment to cornea (Binder and Zavala, 1987),
- difficulties in lathing (Barrett and Moore, 1988),
- prolonged recovery time to achieve optical clarity,
- optical changes associated with remodelling, and limited amounts of human tissues (Thompson et al., 1991).

Many of the problems associated with use of human tissues may be ameliorated by use of synthetic materials (McDonald, 1988; Thompson et al., 1991).

Thompson et al. (1991) review the requirements for a synthetic material to use in epikeratoplasty including

- optical clarity
- supports epithelial spreading
- permeable to nutrients and metabolites
- biocompatible and
- stable.

Potential materials identified by these authors include collagen, collagen co-polymers with synthetics, coated synthetics and bioactive synthetics.

4.11 Summary

Ophthalmology employs the use of a large number of materials for correction of vision, intraocular lense replacement, correction of the curvature of the cornea, indentation of a detached retina, insertion of intraocular lenses and for cataract removal. Each of these applications requires knowledge of the properties of ocular tissues as well as selection of materials that are biocompatible and produce the desired changes in the eye. This chapter has reviewed the materials of choice and the complications that are asssociated with use of each medical device.

5.
Cardiovascular Implants

5.1 Introduction

Although major advances in the treatment and prevention of heart disease have been achieved in the last two decades, diseases of the cardiovascular system contribute to about 20% of the fatalities in people between the ages of 36 and 74. Atherosclerosis, a process affecting the large and medium-sized diameter muscular arteries, especially the aorta, coronary arteries and cerebral arteries, is a major cause of death. In addition, valvular leakage results in insufficient cardiac output thereby making even moderate exercise difficult. Atherosclerotic vessels as well as leaky heart valves are routinely replaced by materials that are synthetic or of natural origin.

According to Biomedical Business International (Vol XII, No 3., March 20, 1989) the estimated vascular market in the US amount to about $100 million per year. The majority of these grafts are for reconstruction of peripheral vascular ($61 million), aortic ($14 million), arterio-venous ($14 million) and other vessels ($14 million) (Table 5.1). They also report that about 145 000 valvular implant units are used each year in the US (Biomedical Business International Vol XII, No. 13, August 10, 1987). Of these implants about 50% are mechanical while the other 50% are bioprosthetic (composite biological and prosthetic).

5.2 Physiology and anatomy of vessel wall and heart valve

The aorta is the major elastic vessel in the body. Its structure is similar to that of other vessel walls and can be used as a model of the trilaminate

Table 5.1 Estimated US market for vascular grafts*

Graft	Market
Aortic	14 M
Arterio-venous	14 M
Other	14 M
Peripheral vessels	61 M

* Biomedical Business International Vol. XII, No. 3, March 20, 1989

structure that is characteristic of soft tissue found vessels. Aortic valve is composed of connective tissue in a similar manner to vessel wall. Below we discuss the physiology and anatomy of each of these structures. The structure and function of the aorta and heart valves have been recently reviewed (Silver *et al.*, 1989; Thubrikar, 1990) and the reader is referred to these references for the details.

5.2.1 Aortic valve

The aortic valve is a composite structure consisting of flexible leaflets that are connected to the aortic wall via structures termed sinuses (Figure 5.1). The valve is located between the left ventricle and the aorta and it functions by allowing blood flow out of the ventricle and into the aorta without backflow (regurgitation). The aortic valve is one of four valves that separates the four chambers of the heart. The chambers include the right atrium and ventricle and the left atrium and ventricle. The valves in these chambers are the tricuspid, pulmonary, mitral and aortic as listed in Table 5.2.

During ejection of blood from the ventricles, the aortic and pulmonary valves remain open and the mitral and the tricuspid valves remain closed, and during ventricular filling, the aortic and pulmonary valves remain closed and the mitral and tricuspid valves are open. The heart valves open and close

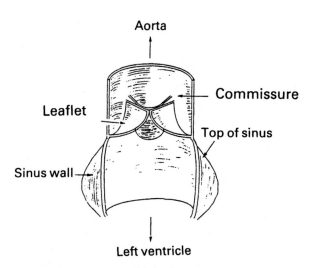

Figure 5.1 Diagram showing aortic valve in the closed position illustrating the sinus wall, top of sinus and commissure. The leaflets are positioned in the centre of the valve and prevent backflow of blood from the aorta into the left ventricle when the valve is closed. This Figure was adapted based on Thubrikar (1990).

Table 5.2 Valves and their characteristics†

Chambers	Valve	Characteristics
Right atrium-right ventricle	Tricuspid	Atrioventricular*
Right ventricle-pulmonary artery	Pulmonary	Semi-lunar**
Left ventricle-aorta	Aortic	Semi-lunar**
Left atrium-left ventricle	Mitral	Atrioventricular*

*atrioventricular valves are attached to the heart muscle by means of papillary muscle and fibrous cords.
**semi-lunar valves have their leaflets in the shape of a half moon and do not attach to the myocardium
†adapted from Thubrikar, 1990

over several billion times in a period of about 70 years, providing a mechanism by which blood can be appropriately pressurized and distributed for oxygenization and distribution to tissues and organs. Valvular leakage reduces the efficiency of the heart's pumping ability and ultimately leads to decreased tolerance for exercise of any kind. Because the left side of the heart experiences higher pressure than the right side, diseases of the mitral and aortic valves are more likely to lead to exercise related symptoms.

The aortic valve has been studied in the most detail and therefore will be presented as a model. It consists of three leaflets that open and close during heart contraction and expansion, and three sinuses that are cavities behind the leaflets. At the lower boundary, the sinuses become continuous with the left ventricle, and at the upper boundary they become part of the ascending aorta. The sinuses merge together at what is termed the commissures and continue into the aorta while the leaflets come together when the valve is closed and are described by the line (line of coaption) that describes the leaflet interface. The three sinuses and leaflets are present in an area that has a diameter that is greater than that of the aorta. From the external view, they each balloon out and form intersecting arcs. The surface of the leaflet, in contrast, is curved in only one direction facilitating changes in curvature that are associated with opening and closing of the valve.

The maximum mechanical stresses experienced by the valve occur at points of maximum flexion which include the point of leaflet attachment and the line at which leaflets come together (line of coaption). Additional stresses occur in a valve that has two or four leaflets because of the change in dimensions that occurs while these valves open and close. As pointed out by Thubrikar (1990), for a valve to create a circular opening the circumference ($2\pi R$) is about six times the radius (Figure 5.2) which is about the total length of the free-edges of the three leaflets when the valve is closed. In other words, the leaflets do not have to stretch or increase their free edge distance as they go from the open to closed positions.

156 Cardiovascular implants

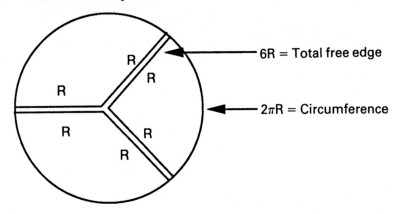

Figure 5.2 Diagram illustrating that a trileaflet valve has a total free edge of 6R which is approximately equal to $2\pi R$ the circumference. This enables the valve to open and close with a minimum of strain introduced on the valve leaflets. This Figure was adapted based on Thubrikar (1990).

Various measurements have been used to characterize the geometry of normal aortic valve. Assuming that the three valves are identical and can be superimposed on each other by rotation, a simple set of nomenclature has been developed to describe valve geometry (Figure 5.3). These include radius of the bases (Rb), radius of commissures (Rc), valve height (H), angle of the free edge to the plane through the three commissures ϕ, angle of the bottom surface of the leaflet to the plane through the three commissures α, coaption height at centre (Cc), commissural height, commissural height (Hs), and radius of the outermost wall of sinus (ds). Dimensions of the adult human aortic valve are Rb=11.3 to 14 mm, H= 15.7 to 19.8 mm, ϕ = 25 to 37° and α = 15 to 27° (Swanson and Clark, 1974).

5.2.2 Microscopic anatomy of aortic valve

The leaflets are composed of two layers of tissue, the fibrosa and spongiosa, that consist of dense and loose connective tissue, respectively (Gross and Kugel, 1931) (Table 5.3). At the aortic surface of the leaflet the fibrosa is most apparent. The alignment of collagen fibrils are similar to that observed in tendons and ligaments. Collagen fibrils in the fibrosa run mainly parallel to the edge of the leaflet which attaches to dense connective in the aortic wall (annulus fibrosis). The alignment is somewhat decreased in the centre of the leaflet. Some cross-weaving of layers of collagen fibrils are observed providing resistance to bi-axial stresses. The fibrils are 30–50 nm in diameter and account for the flexibility of this tissue. Proteoglycan filaments similar to those seen in tendon appear to link neighbouring collagen fibrils. Leaflets are anchored to the aorta by dense connective tissue.

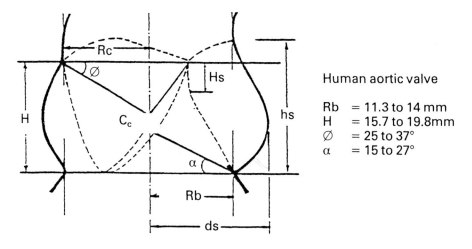

Figure 5.3 Schematic diagram of aortic valve showing leaflet and the parameters that are used to characterize its performance. The parameters are Rb (radius of base), Rc (radius of commissures), H (valve height), α (bottom surface angle of leaflet), φ (free edge angle of the leaflet), Hs (height of commissure), hs (su=inus height), ds (radius of outermost wall of sinus) and Cc (coaption height). Some of these parameters are given for human aortic valve based in Thubrikar (1990).

Beneath the fibrosa is the the spongiosa. The collagen fibres in this layer are highly separated and are orientated in the radial direction. The spaces between the collagen fibres are filled with water and proteoglycans providing a soft spongy feel. Fine elastic fibres appear to run among the collagen fibres. Fibroblasts in the spongiosa contain slender processes and large numbers of

Table 5.3 Structural components of aortic valve*

Component	Structural component
Fibrosa	Upper layer collagen fibrils run parallel to the edge of leaflet cross-weaving of layers of collagen fibrils 30–50nm in diameter
Spongiosa	Lower layer contains collagen fibres oriented in radial direction with fine elastic fibres

* Gross and Kugel, 1931

158   Cardiovascular implants

6–8 nm filaments, reported to be actin. Collagen fibres stressed by leaflet deformation transfer this stress to fibroblasts within the tissue via actin filaments (Deck, 1990).

The sinusese are similar in structure to the aortic wall in that they are composed of three layers; the intima, media and adventitia.

5.2.3 Physiology and anatomy of vessel wall

The aorta is the major conduit that distributes oxygenated blood to the various tissues and organs of the body (Silver *et al.*, 1989 for a review). It acts as an auxiliary pump by maintaining blood pressure by virtue of its elastic retraction during filling of the right ventricle. The ability of the aorta to withstand the shear and normal stresses imparted by the blood over many heart cycles is a consequence of the connective tissue networks

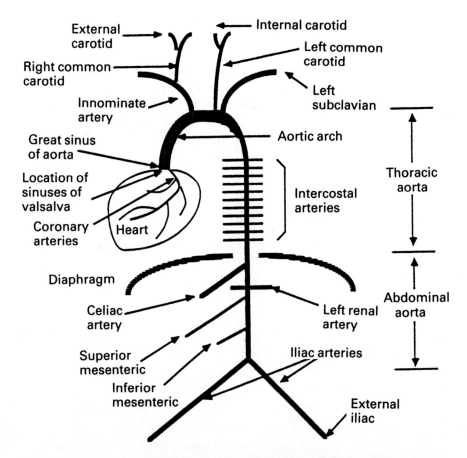

Figure 5.4 Schematic diagram of the aorta and it branches. The aorta consists of the arch, the thoracic, and the abdominal portions.

and cells which provide structural support. In addition, the changes in connective tissue structure that occur during normal ageing as well as those associated with genetic and acquired disorders modify the mechanical properties of aortic tissue.

The aorta is an inverted U-shaped tube that has one leg longer than the other (Figure 5.4). It contains numerous branches that are sites of blood flow disturbance and therefore influence the mechanical properties of aortic tissue (Table 5.4). The aorta commences at the upper part of the left ventricle where it is about 2.5 cm in diameter and ascends (ascending portion of the aorta) a short distance, arches backward in the chest cavity (arch of the aorta), then descends on the left side of the vertebral column. The aorta then passes through an opening in the diaphragm and enters the

Table 5.4 Aortic structures and their function*

Structure	Function
Aortic Arch	
Carotid arteries	Supply blood to head and neck
Coronary arteries	Provide blood flow to ventricular areas of heart
Sinuses of Valsalva	Prevent regurgitation of blood into cavity of ventricle
Subclavian arteries	Supply blood to upper extremities
Thoracic Aorta	
Intercostal arteries	Supply blood to chest area
Abdominal Aorta	
Celiac artery	Divides into gastric, hepatic and splenic arteries that supply the stomach, liver and spleen
Common illiac arteries	Supplies blood to lower extremities
Inferior mesenteric artery	Supplies blood to part of colon and rectum
Lumbar arteries	Supplies blood to back
Renal artery	Supplies blood to kidney
Superior mesenteric artery	Supplies blood to most of length of small intestine

* adapted based on Silver *et al.*, 1989

abdominal cavity (abdominal aorta) and terminates opposite the lower border of the fourth lumbar vertebra, where it divides into the right and left common iliac arteries.

The aorta just above it commences, is enlarged, and contains three valves (sinuses of Valsalva) that prevent regurgitation of blood into the cavity of the ventricle. At the union of the ascending aorta and the arch, the diameter increases (great sinus of the aorta) and the wall bulges outward. This portion of the aorta is contained within the pericardium that surrounds the heart and together with the pulmonary artery is contained in a membrane that extends from the surface of the heart.

There are several branches of the aorta; however, only the right and left coronary arteries that connect to the right and left ventricular areas of the heart branch off of the ascending aorta at the sinuses of Valsalva. Branches in the arch include right innominate artery, right common carotid, left common carotid and left subclavian. The carotid arteries supply blood to the head and neck via internal and external branches of these vessels, while the subclavian arteries supply blood to the upper extremities.

Branches of the thoracic aorta include the intercostal arteries that supply blood to the chest area. Abdominal aortic branches include the celiac artery that divides into the gastric, the hepatic, and the splenic arteries that supply blood to the stomach, liver, and the spleen, respectively. The superior mesenteric artery supplies blood to most of the length of the small intestine. The inferior mesenteric artery supplies part of the colon and the greater part of the rectum with blood. Renal arteries supply blood to the kidney, while the lumbar arteries, which are similar to the intercostal arteries, arise from the back of the abdominal aorta. The abdominal aorta divides into the two common iliac arteries (right and left common iliac arteries) that supply blood to the lower extremities.

Analysis of the mechanical properties of the aorta is complicated by this pattern of branches. In addition, it is known that the wall microstructure differs at least with respect to the collagen and elastic tissue content in the ascending and descending portions of the aorta.

Macro and micro structure of the aortic wall

The aortic wall of animals is similar to other vessels, since it contains three layers: the intima, the media, and the adventitia. The intima extends from the blood vessel wall interface to a layer of elastic tissue, termed the internal elastic lamella, which is about 100 μm in diameter (Bloom and Fawcett, 1975).

Intima

Endothelial cells are seen in contact with the blood and form a continuous lining of flat elongated, polygonal cells that align with the flow direction (Flaherty *et al.*, 1972). Endothelial cells rest on a basement membrane (basal lamina) composed of collagen type IV, proteoglycans, and laminin, which forms a continuous bond between these cells and the connective tissue matrix. The basement membrane provides a cushion that allows bending and changes in diameter associated with changes in blood pressure. Beneath the basement membrane are bundles of interlacing collagen fibres.

The intima in healthy young individuals is very thin and plays an insignificant role in the mechanical properties of the aorta. The intima thickens with age and the circumference increases (Clark and Glagov, 1979), affecting mechanical properties. A variety of different collagen types are found in the intima, including types I, III, IV, V, VI, and VIII (see Tables 5.5 and 5.6) (Merrilees et al., 1987; Murata et al., 1986; Ross, 1986; Keene et al., 1987; Chung et al., 1976; Benya and Padilla, 1986; Labat-Robert et al., 1985); Morton and Barnes, 1982). In addition, fibronectin (Labat-Robert et al., 1985), proteoglycans (Merrilees et al., 1987; Bartholomew and Anderson, 1983), and hyaluronic acid (Bartholomew and Anderson, 1983) are macromolecules that contribute to intimal structure.

Media
The mechanical properties of the aorta primarily reflect the thickness and structure of the media. Low-strain mechanical response of the aorta is a result of the extension of the elastic lamellar units found in the media. The media in humans is about 2.5 μm thick (Bloom and Fawcett, 1975) and contains 50–65 concentric layers of elastic lamellar units that consist of smooth muscle cells, elastic fibres, and collagen fibres. The smooth muscle contains a layer of cells that are surrounded by a common basement membrane and a closely associated group of collagen fibrils that tighten about the cell as the media is brought under tension (Orlandi et al., 1986). A series of attachments occur between smooth muscle cells and elastic fibres; wavy collagen fibres are woven between the layers of elastic fibres and smooth muscle cells. The auxiliary pumping ability of the aorta is believed to be associated with the elastic fibre network found in the media, while the collagen fibre meshwork prevents overdilatation and failure of this tissue (below). The collagen content is higher and the elastic fibre content is lower in the thoracic compared with the abdominal aorta (Fischer and Llaurado, 1966), For this reason the thoracic aorta is more compliant than the abdominal aorta.

Elastic fibres in the media are composed of an amorphous elastic core (Zarins and Glagov, 1987) containing a rim of microfibrillar protein (Fanning et al., 1981; Goldfischer et al., 1983) (Table 5.5). The media contains collagen types I, III, IV, and V, (Zarins and Glagov, 1987; Keene et al., 1987; Labat-Robert et al., 1985; Chung and Miller, 1974; Gay et al., 1976; Leushner and Haust, 1985) however, types I and III are the primary mechanical elements, since they are co-distributed throughout the large fibrils. Proteoglycans are found attached to collagen fibrils (i.e. dermatan sulphate), (Bartholomew and Anderson, 1983; Volker et al., 1986) in soluble complexes with hyaluronic acid (chondroitin sulphate) (Alavi and

Table 5.5 Macromolecular components of normal aortic wall

Component	Location
Intima	
Orientated endothelial cells	Blood interface
Collagen	
Type I	Subendothelial matrix
Type IV	Basement membrane
Type VI	Connects intima and subintima
Type VIII	Associated with endothelial cells
Fibronectin	Subendothelial matrix
Proteoglycans	
Dermatan sulphate and chondroitin sulphate	Subendothelial matrix
Heparan sulphfate	Associated with endothelial cell surface
Hyaluronic acid	Subendothelial matrix
Media	
Smooth-muscle cells	Circumferential lamellar unit
Collagen types	
I and III	Co-distributed in large- and small-diameter fibrils
Type IV	Smooth-muscle cell basement membrane
Type V	Pericellular coat attached to smooth-muscle cell membrane
Elastin	Amorphous core of elastic fibres
Microfibrillar protein	13.7 nm (diameter) microfibrillar component on periphery of elastic fibres
Fibronectin	Spread throughout media associated with elastic fibres
Proteoglycans	
Dermatan sulphate	Attached to collagen fibrils
Chondroitin sulphate	Soluble complex with hyaluronic acid
Heparan sulphate	Associated with smooth-muscle cells
Adventitia	
Collagen	Large-diameter fibrils
Proteoglycans	Decreased levels associated with collagen fibrils compared to media and intima

From Silver *et al.*, 1989

Moore, 1987), and attached to smooth muscle cells (heparin sulphate) (Contri *et al.*, 1985). Biochemical components found in the media are summarized in Table 5.5, including microfibrillar protein and fibronectin.

Table 5.6 Macromolecular components of atherosclerotic aortic wall

Component	Change observed
Intima/media	
Endothelial cell	Continuous loss of endothelial cell lining
Collagen	
Type I	Increased quantity throughout intima
Type III	Co-distribution with fibronectin
Type VI	Increased levels in plaque
Type IV	Increased levels associated with smooth muscle
Type V	Increased levels in intima plaques
Smooth muscle cells	Associated with plaques
Proteoglycans (PG)	Increased levels of chondroitin sulphate (PG) with lipid deposition, decreased levels of chondroitin sulphate-PG that bind to hyaluronic acid
Macrophages	Associated with lipid and plaque

From Silver *et al.*, 1989

Aortic structure has been studied extensively in animals such as rodents and the pig. In contrast to the well-defined elastic lamellar unit (Clark and Glagov, 1979) seen in these models, the ultrastructure in man is more complex. In addition to elastic lamellar units that contain solid elastic elements, spaces between these units contain thin streaks of elastin in close contact with smooth muscle cells (Dingemans *et al.*, 1981). Smooth muscle cells have no observable connections with collagen fibres (Dingemans *et al.*, 1981) in man. This may reflect differences due to ageing, since biopsies from human aortas tend to be from older patients that exhibit varying degrees of atherosclerosis.

Roach (1983) has observed that the ultrastructure of elastin is varied depending on the location within the media. Scanning electron microscopy showed that elastin on the intimal side of the media was in the form of fenestrated sheets, while on the adventitial side it was in a fibrous network form. These observations confirm the structural complexity of the media.

Table 5.6 lists the changes that occur in the macromolecular components of the intima and media associated with atherosclerosis. The atherosclerotic process begins by the accumulation of lipid thickening of the intima (Zarins and Glagov, 1987). During this process the intima begins to resemble the media, since smooth muscle cells are seen along with increased amounts of collagen (Table 5.6), especially type I (Labat-Robert *et al.*, 1985; Morton and Barnes, 1982). Cells such as the macrophage are also seen in plaques, as well as lipid droplets. At long-term, when viewed under polarized light, the human intima exhibits a layer of birefringent collagen similar to the network seen in scar tissue, which may explain the increased stiffness of the aortic wall associated with age (Kalath *et al.*, 1986). Proteoglycans are found in the plaque regions in higher than normal concentrations; however, there is a decrease in proteoglycans that associate with hyaluronic acid (Alavi and Moore, 1987; Wagner, 1985).

Adventitia
The boundary between the media and the adventitia is easily identified as the external elastic lamellar unit, while the outer limit of the adventitia is continuous with the surrounding connective tissue. The adventitia consists of fibroblasts, large-diameter collagen fibrils, and associated proteoglycans. It normally does not contribute extensively to the mechanical behaviour except in tethering the aorta to the surrounding tissues.

5.3 Anatomy and physiology of blood components

Normal blood contains cellular elements, proteins and other macromolecules as well as water, ions and a variety of low molecular weight materials. Normal blood flow requires a careful balance between activation of blood components to prevent excessive bleeding and continual activation of blood components that results in blood clotting, platelet aggregation, blockage of a vessel and embolism formation. Below we present the components that are involved in these processes and their role in the design of surfaces that are intended for use in the cardiovascular system.

5.3.1 Blood cells

Cells make up about half of the volume of blood while in comparison the other half is composed of water (35%), albumin (1–2%), fibrinogen (about 0.2%), ions (less than 1%) as shown from inspection of Table 5.7 (Williams, 1987). Albumin is present in blood to maintain the osmotic pressure and passively control blood volume. Fibrinogen is a protein involved in the blood clotting and prevents excessive bleeding when a vessel wall is injured.

Red blood cells (RBCs) make up about 45% of the volume of blood. Their function is to carry oxygen to the tissues and return carbon dioxide to the lungs. Changes in osmotic pressure or mechanical trauma can cause a shape change and release of haemoglobin, the oxygen carrying protein in RBCs. Contact with artificial or natural surfaces can result in red cell haemolysis reducing the blood's ability to effectively transport oxygen.

White blood cells are found in low concentrations in the blood; however, they are present in tissues and in a system of vessels termed lymphatics. The lymphatics irrigate tissues involved in production of immune cells, termed lymphoid tissue. The lymph nodes are an example of lymphoid tissue that serves as a reservoir of immature white blood cells involved in immune responses termed lyphocytes. B cells are precursors

Table 5.7 Composition of human blood*

Substance	Vol., %	Physical characteristics
Water	35	MW = 18
Proteins		
Albumin	1–2	MW = 69 000
Fibrinogen	0.2	MW = 34 000
Ions	less than 0.5	<100
Cells		
Red blood cells	45%	Biconcave disc, 8 × 1–3 μm
White blood cells	<1%	Spherical, 7–22 μm (Dia.)
Platelets	<1%	Disc, 2–4 μm (Dia.)

* Modified based on Williams (1987)
Dia. = Diameter
MW = Molecular weight

to antibody producing cells while T cells enhance or inhibit the development of antibody levels in the blood. T cells are also involved in cell mediated rejection of foreign cells or transformed cells. Leukocytes containing membrane bound granules filled with hydrolytic enzymes include macrophages (monocytes), neutrophils (polymorphonuclear leukocytes), basophils, and eosinophils. These cells are involved in reactions to materials that lead to biodegradation of implants.

Platelets are cells lacking nuclei that contain granules. They are involved in limiting bleeding when a vessel is cut or when placed in contact with a foreign surface. Upon activation, platelet structure changes from disc like to spherical and release of the contents of the granules occurs stimulating the aggregation of platelets.

5.3.2 Plasma proteins

Blood contains a number of soluble proteins that are involved in cellular nutrition, transport of hormones, minerals and other molecules as well as in regulation of a number of biological control systems. Of these components albumin at about 40 g/l represents the most abundant protein. It is synthesised in the liver as a source of amino acids and protein for cellular metabolism. In addition, it aids in transport of fatty acids and other molecules and plays an important role in maintaining the osmotic pressure of blood. Albumin is one of the blood proteins that is rapidly adsorbed to surfaces and may modify the blood clotting activity of biomaterials.

Lipids present in blood include

- cholesterol and its esters
- phospholipids

- glycerides and
- free fatty acids.

They are attached to proteins to form lipoproteins and are transported throughout the body in this form. These lipoproteins include chylomicrons, very low density lipoproteins, low density lipoprotein, and high density lipoproteins. Lipid adsorption to biomaterial surfaces can modify both the chemistry and mechanical properties of a surface as well as mediate calcification.

Other proteins, involved in the immune system, stimulate plasma cell synthesis of antibodies that react with foreign surfaces, especially if they are protein in nature. The immune system is involved in the body's defence against infection, tumor formation and 'foreign' (not self) substances. B lymphocytes on exposure to an 'antigen' present on a foreign surface, differentiate into plasma cells and begin synthesizing immunoglobins, a class of proteins given the names IgA, IgD, IgE, IgG and IgM. The binding of antibodies to antigens present in blood lead to destruction of foreign matter via monocyte and T cell mediated mechanisms. In addition, antibody–antigen complexes present further stimulate antibody and T cell production. Antibodies to implant surfaces can result in implant destruction, prolonged inflammation and tissue necrosis.

Proteins involved in the complement pathway function in parallel with the immune system to defend against foreign cells and matter. Activation of the complement pathway can lead to direct foreign cell death as well as mediate inflammation. Materials that activate complement may cause prolonged inflammation and compromise implant function as well as lead to unacceptable side effects in humans. A more detailed presentation of the complement pathways is presented by Silver and Doillon (1989) in reference to the biocompatibility of materials.

Coagulation of blood prevents small leaks in the cardiovascular system from leading to excessive blood loss. Blood coagulation is a complex process as summarized in Table 5.8. Biomaterials that activate the contact factors initiate the formation of fibrin and are not likely to be good materials for replacement of vascular surface components except in high shear, high flow rate situations such as for replacing sections of large arteries including the aorta. Blood clotting also involves platelets and their surface components further confusing effective evaluation of the tendency of surfaces to clot blood and cause platelet adhesion and aggregation. Tests used to evaluate blood compatibility of surfaces include whole blood clotting time, platelet adhesion and aggregation, thrombin time, prothrombin time and other in vitro and in vivo (Table 5.9) evaluations discussed by Silver and Doillon (1989).

Activation of the contact factors for blood coagulation also trigger activation of the kinin system. The kinin system in blood involves conversion of prekallilrein to kallikrein which triggers conversion of high-molecular-

Table 5.8 Summary of events leading to blood clotting*

Activation of intrinsic cascade via surface
                or
Activation of extrinsic cascade via tissue damage
Complex formation between blood proteins and platelet surface
Activation of prothrombin and formation thrombin
Activation of fibrinogen and formation of fibrin clot

---

* Silver and Doillon, 1989

weight kininogen to bradykinin. Bradykinin induces leakage of fluid from the vascular system into the surrounding tissues and is associated with the inflammatory response.

Once a blood clot forms to limit bleeding, a process is set into motion that lyses it so that blood flow is not interrupted peripherally. The fibrinolytic system is activated via release of cellular components and fragments of blood proteins and results in degradation of fibrin networks that make up the clot. Plasminogen is an enzyme found in blood and its conversion to plasmin initiates fibrinolysis. Degraded fibrin networks are digested by inflammatory cells in the wound area.

5.4 Mechanical properties of aorta and valve

Although the aortic wall and cardiac valves do not experience the high loads that are transmitted by tendons and ligaments, they do undergo mechanical fatigue because these tissues are cycled through billions of repeated loadings. The loads are both normal (perpendicular to aortic wall and valve surface) and shear (parallel to surface) and change in intensity as the heart goes from systole to diastole. This loading profile results in the development

Table 5.9 Tests used to evaluate blood compatibility*

Test	Purpose
Platelet adhesion	Adhesion to surface
Platelet aggregation	Aggregation of platelets
Prothrombin time	Determine rate of conversion of prothrombin to thrombin and fibrinogen to fibrin
Thrombin time	Determine rate of conversion of fibrinogen into fibrin
Whole blood clotting time	Determine effect of a surface on clotting

* Silver and Doillon, 1989

of tears or points of stress concentration that ultimately lead to aortic aneurysms or abnormal valvular calcification. Therefore any candidate material for replacement of these tissues must be able to duplicate the properties of the material that has been developed by evolution over millions of years.

5.4.1 Mechanical properties of aortic valve

Fluid flow in the cardiovascular system is a wonder of natural science. Cardiac valves open and close with such precision that blood is pumped from the vena cava, at a pressure of 70 mm to the aorta, at a pressure of 120 mm with repeated reproducibility. During the systolic-diastolic cycle, the valve components experience stress variations as well as changes in the direction of curvature. The total stress on the valve becomes a sum of the normal, shear and bending stresses. Analysis of these stresses has been attempted based on in vitro and in vivo studies. Chapter 5 of Thubrikar's (1990) recent book gives a detailed analysis of the important considerations and only an overview will be given here.

Mechanical stresses experienced by the aortic valve are a consequence of the bending and reversal in curvature that occurs from diastole to systole, and increases in valve dimensions that occur in the circumferential (across the valve in the anatomical position) and radial (in the valve height) positions. The mechanical properties of valve components have been determined from in vitro measurements of the load-deformation properties of excised valve leaflet material and from in vivo measurements of circumferential and radial dimensions of valves at known pressure gradients.

In vitro, the stress (load per unit cross-sectional area)–strain (change in length/original length) curve for human leaflets is similar to that of other soft connective tissues since it consists of an initial linear region followed by non-linear and a second linear region. In the circumferential direction the stress–strain curve is characterized by a fairly early (strain about 10%) transition into the high strain region. In the radial direction, the slope of the stress–strain curve (modulus) is much lower in the two linear regions; however, the valve can undergo higher strains prior to failure. The moduli of the two linear regions are 1.99 and 599 g/mm^2 (1 g/mm^2 equals 104 N/m^2) in the circumferential 1.13 and 174 g/mm^2 in the radial direction. The transition strains are 12.8% and 23.9% in the circumferential and radial directions (Thubrikar, 1990). These values are consistent with the microscopic anatomy which shows that the collagen fibrils are orientated in the circumferential direction and offer resistance to stretching in that direction while in the radial direction the extracellular matrix between the collagen fibrils provides the resistance. In the circumferential direction the low modulus region is believed to be associated with the uncrimping of the collagen fibrils similar to what happens in tendons and ligaments. Whether the crimp can be observed under normal physiological conditions remains unclear.

Although the stress–strain properties of valve leaflets do not appear to be altered by storage at low temperature or room temperature up to 120 days they are altered by freezing particularly in the radial direction. For this reason the behaviour of valve replacements such as allografts (human grafts implanted in a genetically different individual) are biomechanically altered during preservation by freezing.

In vivo, the mechanical properties have been estimated by placing radiopaque markers on the leaflets and then determining the position of the markers as a function of pressure gradient (Thubrikar et al., 1980). Length decreases of 10.6% from diastole to systole did not appear to change with normal systemic pressure and calculated values of systolic and diastolic moduli of 2×10^6 and 6.7×10^7 dynes/cm^2 were observed (10 dynes/cm^2 equal N/m^2) which are similar to values reported in vitro. Although the leaflet is more deformable in the radial direction in vitro (40%); in vivo, very little deformation is measured beyond a strain of 18% (Thubrikar et al., 1986) probably because deformation in the circumferential direction limits that in the radial direction (Thubrikar, 1990). Since the stiffness in the radial direction is less than that in the circumferential one, deformation in the radial direction does not significantly affect the behaviour of the leaflet in the circumferemtial direction (Thubrikar, 1990).

Using an average modulus of 350 g/mm^2, stress analysis was carried out for a pressure load of 1 g/mm^2 (diastolic pressure of 73.6 mm Hg) assuming linear elasticity and a finite element approach representing curved, triangular, thin shell elements. Maximum principle stress was in the range of 15–27 g/mm^2 and was found to be along the circumferential direction and the minimum principle stress in the radial direction. Thubrikar (1990) concluded that all elements in the leaflet were under tension, some bi-axial while others uniaxial.

Considering that the leaflet is cycled through tension and then flexed, fatigue and flexion stresses contribute to failure of the valve. Total stresses in the circumferential direction is the sum of the tensile stress in the membrane and the flexion stress which can be tensile or compressive depending on the location of the neutral axis. Thubrikar et al., (1986) determined that the membrane stress in the circumferential direction was 1.7 g/mm^2 in systole and 24.5 g/mm^2 in diastole. In addition, they found that the total stress on the aortic surface was 4–9 g/mm^2 during systole and 9–15 g/mm^2 during diastole while on the ventricular surface it was 0.3–0.8 g/mm^2 during systole and 36–75 g/mm^2 during diastole. In the radial direction the total stresses were 0.85 g/mm^2 during systole and 12.1 g/mm^2 during diastole. In the area of leaflet attachment, tensile stresses of 76–95 g/mm^2 in the circumferential and 37–44 g/mm^2 in the radial direction occurred during diastole (Table 5.10). Deck et al. (1988) concluded that excessive wear and tear would likely occur in the region of leaflet attachment.

170 Cardiovascular implants

Due to the movement of the sinuses during the cardiac cycle, Deck *et al.* (1988) evaluated the stress sharing between the leaflet and the sinuses. They noted that the decrease in the circumferential radius of curvature in the circumferential direction of the sinus from systole to diastole suggests that the high stress in the circumferential direction on the leaflet is shared between the leaflet and the sinus. Histological examination indicates that principle stress bearing element in the leaflet is a collagenous layer of fibres termed the lamina fibrosa in which the collagen fibres are aligned with the free edge of the leaflet.

5.4.2 Mechanical properties of aortic wall

The mechanical status of the aorta has been evaluated using the parameters seen in Table 5.11. These include characteristic impedance (Z_o), pulse wave velocity (C), circumferential elastic modulus (E_o), pressure-strain elastic modulus (E_p), percentage of variation in diameter (PVD), and Young's modulus (E).

In order to determine the physiological variables that can be used to define mechanical properties, two general approaches have been developed. The first measures pressure and volume in various segments of the arterial tree. However, the limitations associated with this approach include low sensitivity, inadequate dynamic response of volume-measuring methods, and site-to-site geometric variation of arteries. It is difficult to interpret pressure and volume measurements found for a length of vessel because of geometric differences.

The second approach used in the evaluation of mechanical properties is based on measurements using segments of vessels isolated from the vascular

Table 5.10 Stresses on the surface of aortic valve leaflets*

Direction of surface	Stress systole gm/cm^2	Stress diastole gm/cm^2
Aortic surface	4–9	9–15
Circumferential	1.7	24.5
Leaflet attachment circumferential radial	76–95 37–44	
Radial	0.85	12.1
Ventricular surface	0.3–0.8	36–75

* Thubrikar *et al.*, 1986

Table 5.11 Evaluation of aortic mechanical parameters

Parameter	Equation
Percentage variation in diameter, PVD	$\text{PVD} = \dfrac{\Delta d}{d} \times 100$
Pressure-strain elastic modulus, E_p	$E_p = \dfrac{\Delta P(d)}{\Delta d}$
Circumferential elastic modulus, E_o	$E_o = \dfrac{(\Delta P) r d}{h(\Delta d)}$
Pulse wave velocity, C	$C = \dfrac{\sqrt{E_p}}{2\varrho}$
Young's modulus, E	$E = \dfrac{C^2 \varrho d}{h}$
Characteristic impedence, Z_o	$Z_o = \dfrac{\varrho C}{\pi r^2}$

Note: D, end-diastolic diameter; Δd, maximum change in diameter (end-systolic dia. − end-diastolic dia.); h, end-diastolic wall thickness; ΔP, pulse pressure (systolic pressure − diastolic pressure); ϱ, density of blood; r, average radius.
From Silver *et al.*, 1989

tree. Information gathered in this manner does not yield dynamic mechanical properties in the intact animal (Peterson *et al.*, 1960).

Invasive and noninvasive methods for evaluating aortic mechanical properties are examined below.

Invasive measurements using strain gauges
Patel *et al.*, (1960) and others (Greenfield and Patel, 1962; Barnett *et al.*, 1961; Patel and Fry, 1964) conducted in vivo studies that involved the use of low-mass calipers with a strain wire-sensing element attached to two limbs of the calipers. The calipers were sutured to the surface of the arterial wall and changes in the vessel circumference were detected by the relative displacement of the calipers. Pressure in the vessel was recorded simultaneously.

Other researchers have used the same technique in their studies; however, different animal models were used. Peterson *et al.*, (1960) extended the study by Patel and co-workers to include a wider range of vessel sizes using

172 Cardiovascular implants

additional animal models. They applied acetycholine or norepinephrine directly to the wall of the test vessel to induce relaxation and contraction, respectively, of the smooth muscle. Acetylcholine was found to increase the circumferential strain from 1.03–1.24% in the femoral artery, while norepinephrine was used to decrease the circumferential strain in the carotid artery from 1.87–0.71%. These observations examine the effects of smooth muscle activity.

Feigl et al., (1963) performed a series of studies using dogs to evaluate the mechanical properties of the femoral artery before and after chronic hypertension was induced. Substantial differences were noted and the change was related to the electrolyte and water composition of the wall.

Values of circumferential strain and pressure-strain elastic modulus found using the strain gauge technique are relatively similar for the studies reported by Patel et al., (1960) and Peterson et al., (1960). Differences were attributed to the animal model used and the subject age and weight.

Measurements on isolated vessel segments

Bergel (1960a, b; 1961) conducted in vitro studies on isolated human aortic segments connected to the ends of two metal tubes. The tubes were adjusted to the in vivo length of the aorta segment. Bergel used a beam of light in conjunction with a photo cell to measure changes in relative diameter in such a way that the aortic wall intersected the collimated beam of light so that changes in diameter resulted in changes in output of the photo cell.

Limitations to this approach include the removal of connective tissue that normally tethers the aorta and severing the vaso-vasorum, which supplies blood and nutrients to the aortic wall.

When pressure-strain elastic modulus, measured on isolated vessel segments, is compared with measurements made using the strain gauge technique, significant differences are observed. Results of strain gauge studies (Peterson et al., 1960; Patel et al., 1960) yielded higher values of modulus than the results based on measurements on excised vessels. Pulse wave velocity, based on measurements using isolated vessel segments, is closer to values obtained based on multiple-point pressure measurements (Bergel, 1961a, b).

Angiographic measurements on intact vessels

In the late 1960s and early 1970s angiography was introduced to assess aortic mechanical properties. Angiography is a procedure commonly utilized to visualize vessels after injection of radiopaque dye in the vascular system (Whitley and Whitley, 1971). Arndt et al., (1971), Gozna et al., (1973), and others (Olson et al., 1971; Arndt et al., 1970) measured the internal diameter using fluoroscopy and performed studies to determine the mechanical properties of the aorta.

Arndt et al., (1971) reported noninvasive measurements on the hydraulic properties of five unexposed thoracic cat aortas. Measurements of pressure and diameter were made at various locations along the aorta. Pressure measurements were performed using a catheter attached to a strain gauge monometer. The catheter was positioned at the junction of the aorta and the brachiocephalic artery. Approximately 25 ml of Thorotrast®, a radiopaque dye, was injected intravenously to visualize the aorta. Measurements were made from exposures taken at midsystole and late diastole.

Results of these studies indicated that the percentage of variation in diameter of the aorta in situ was found to be two times higher than that of the isolated aorta in vitro. Distensibility and diameter decreased as a function of distance from the root and it was observed that there was a pronounced tapering of the aorta from the ascending to the descending region.

Variation in diameter with increased pressure also decreased as a function of distance from the aortic root as reported by Arndt et al., (1971). The distance between diameter vs. pressure curves decreased with pressure, which suggested that distensibility decreased with increased pressure.

Gozna et al., (1973) used cineangiography to determine the relationship between aortic diameter and intravascular pressure in humans. They reported that the major arteries were two to three times more distensible then reported by Bergel (1960a, b; 1961).

From the observed relationships, Gozna et al., (1973) computed values for modulus of elasticity and pulse wave velocity. The mechanical parameters they computed included pressure-strain elastic modulus, E_p, circumferential elastic modulus, E_o, and pulse wave velocity, C, along the ascending aorta.

Gozna et al., (1973) used 25 human subjects with normal blood pressures in his study. Of these subjects, two demonstrated no cardiac disease, three had cardiomyopathy, four had coronary artery disease, 11 had mitral valve disease, and five had mild aortic valve disease with normal aortic pressure.

Ascending and descending thoracic aortas were studied in all patients. Patients were examined in the supine position to assure that the aortas were orientated in a plane orthogonal to the x-ray beam using routine anteroposterior projections. Observations were made at data rates of 30–60 frames per second for high resolution. Changes in the diameter were detectable down to 2% and intravascular pressure was monitored using a catheter coupled to a pressure transducer.

Approximately 15 ml of the contrast media, Renovist®, was injected per exposure. The pressure measurements were made during the first three to five cardiac cycles in order to avoid errors in measurements due to contrast media effects. All diameter measurements were made during the same time period at end-systole or end-diastole when the rate of pressure and diameter change was minimized.

Gozna et al., (1973) found that the mean values for PVD, E_p, E_o, and C were $10.3 \pm 3.26\%$, 711 ± 309 g/cm², $3.6 \pm 1.5 \times 10^6$ dyn/cm², and 5.6 ± 1.28 m/s respectively. E_o, E_p, and C were found to be about 20% smaller than those values found using the strain gauge technique.

Merillon et al., (1978) performed experiments similar to those of Gozna et al. (1973) using 30 human subjects. The patients were divided into three groups. Group I consisted of 18 people free from any valvular or aortic disease. Of these patients, five showed signs of congestive heart failure. The remaining 13 patients were considered normal for this study. Group II consisted of nine patients having arterial hypertension (diastolic pressure above 100 mm Hg) and group III consisted of three patients with aortic insufficiency.

Aortic diameters were measured from cineangiograms taken at a speed of 50 frames per second. Radioselecta 76 was injected into the pulmonary artery or into the right atrium at a dosage of 1 cm³/kg. Diameters were measured frame by frame 2–3 cm above the sinuses. As in the study reported by Gozna et al., (1973) only extreme values for pressure and diameter were utilized for evaluating elastic moduli. This study also determined values of characteristic impedance, Z_o, a determinant of left ventricular performance that represents the contribution of the aorta to afterload as discussed by McDonald (1968) and Milnor (1975).

In 15 patients, a synchronized ventricular extrasystole was set off every four beats as early in the cardiac cycle as possible using a right ventricle electrical stimulus. This allowed the measurement of an additional level of diastolic pressure and diameter to be used for the calculations. Two points for pressure and diameter were obtained for 15 patients (diastolic and systolic) and three points were determined in the remaining 15 patients (two diastolic points and one systolic). The new systolic point corresponding to the second diastolic value was not used. For all the postextrasystolic beats, Z_o was calculated for extreme values of pressure and diameter. Z_o was also compared to systemic arterial resistance.

In 18 patients, of whom eight were subjected to postextrasystolic stimulation, aortic elasticity and Z_o measurements were supplemented by simultaneous recording of blood flow in the aorta and left ventricular pressure (LVP).

The pressure-diameter relationship in the ascending aorta was found to be nonlinear for the 15 patients where three points were obtained. In addition, a wide variation in values among individuals was observed.

E_p observed in normal patients (group I) was found to increase significantly with age when compared with age-matched subjects (Kalath et al., 1986). E_p was also observed to increase with diastolic pressure and radius. Group II hypertensive patients exhibited increased values of E_p with increased diastolic pressure; however, no correlation was found with age or radius. Observations on group II patients indicated that E_p was significantly higher.

The average value of E_p reported by Merillon et al., (1978) was close to that reported by McDonald (1960) for the ascending aorta, $0.46 \times 106 \, \mathrm{Nm^{-2}}$.

The value found for pulse wave velocity in the ascending aorta is 400 cm/s. This value is close to that reported by King (1950) and McDonald (1960).

Merillon et al., (1978) found a significant correlation between characteristic impedance, Z_o, and age, but not between Z_o and diastolic pressure in group I patients (normals). In group II patients, a significant correlation was observed between Z_o and diastolic pressure. A comparison between the values of Z_o for patients in groups I and II indicates that Z_o is not significantly higher among hypertensives (group II) relative to normal subjects (group I) despite higher values of E_p. Merillon et al., (1978) suggested that this phenomena is related to an increase in aorta radius in the case of hypertensive patients.

Z_o has been observed to be related to systemic arterial resistance (SAR), age, and aortic pressure. In group I, no correlation was observed between Z_o and SAR. However, a significant correlation was found between Z_o and age, but not with diastolic pressure. Group II had a significant correlation between Z_o and diastolic pressure, but none with age. Z_o has been noted to decrease for all individuals in group III. Finally, Merillon et al., (1978) noted that blood flow acceleration and outflow resistance are inversely related. A comparison of mechanical properties reported by Merillon et al., (1978) and other investigators using different techniques is shown in Table 5.12.

Based on Table 5.12, it is obvious that the elastic moduli (E_p, E_o), measured using the strain gauge technique, are higher than those measured in intact animals using angiography. The use of a strain gauge device requires a thoracotomy and extensive dissection of the connective tissue bed surrounding the artery. Pressure-diameter relationships in the aorta are thought to be influenced by connective tissue and intercostal arteries (Hughes et al., 1979). This may account for the wide discrepancies in the literature on the mechanical properties of major arteries.

Using angiography, PVD is seen to be two to three times greater for all age groups compared with those values found using the strain gauge device. The mean value for PVD found using angiography is seen to be between 12 and 18.5%, compared with values between 3.0 and 5.4% found using the strain gauge technique. Values for elastic moduli and pulse wave velocity are significantly less using angiography compared with those using the strain gauge technique. These observations suggest that the aorta appears stiffer based on the strain gauge technique as compared with angiography.

Several factors affect these measurements, including:

1. the strain gauge technique involves surgical invasion, affecting vasomotor tone;
2. drying of the exposed vessel may alter the observed properties;
3. excessive strain gauge stiffness may affect the wall motion of the vessel; and
4. angiography makes use of the inside diameter, whereas the strain gauge technique uses the outside diameter. Use of the inside diameter

Table 5.12 Comparison of aortic mechanical properties obtained using various techniques

Method and subject	p^b	PVD %	E_p (g cm^{-2})	E_o (dyn cm$^{-2} \times 10^{-6}$)	C (m/s)
Strain gauge					
Human	52–206	5.2	960	4.8	6.9
Dog	105		600	0.30	4.9
Dog^c	118	3.0	1320	0.66	7.9
Dog	99	5.4	665	0.33	5.6
Angiography					
Cat^c	100	15.5	401	0.20	4.3
Cat	100	18.5	402	0.20	4.3
Human	65–115	10.3	711	3.6	5.6
Human		12.0	337	0.33	3.9
Transit time					
Dog^c	120		488	0.24	4.8
Dog	120		339	0.17	4.0
Echograph – Human		7.9	741	3.41	

^{a} Number next to subject indicates number tested.
^{b} P = mmHg.
^{c} Indicates descending aorta.
From Silver et al., 1989

increases PVD about 25%, assuming a wall thickness to radius ratio of 0.10 (Marble et al., 1973).

Greenfield and Patel (1962) reported, based on strain-gauge measurements, that changes in aortic diameter were limited to only a few per cent and would not be measurable based on angiography. However, angiographic studies clearly illustrate diameter changes greater than a few per cent (Gozna et al., 1973).

Ultrasonic methods for assessing aorta mechanical properties
The ability to noninvasively image organs and tissues of the body became possible with the advent of ultrasound technology. Several techniques have been developed to assess the mechanical properties of the aorta and other vessels using ultrasound. These techniques include transit-time measurements, intra-aortic ultrasonic catheterization, and echocardiographic measurements.

Transit-time measurements Bertram (1977) describes an ultrasonic transit-time system that was developed to measure pulsatile changes in arterial diameter. This technique involves the placement of ultrasonic transducers on the external wall of the test artery, and is able to resolve changes in distance smaller than 1μm. The transducers are implanted on the outside of the artery walls for the determination of diameter.

In this system a piezoelectric crystal transducer produces an ultrasound burst that is transmitted through the wall of the vessel, across the lumen, through the opposite wall, and is received by a second crystal that converts the sound waves to an electrical signal. The distance between the transducers can be computed at a given instant in time if the velocity of ultrasound through the vessel and the time-of-flight is known (Hughes et al., 1985).

The ultrasonic transit-time technique has been shown to accurately measure arterial diameter. Bertram showed pressure and diameter traces that closely paralleled each other for the femoral artery of a greyhound in vivo and found a 4% change in diameter associated with a cardiac cycle. The vessel is loaded minimally by the transducer, and, since the system measures only the shortest path between the two transducers, the output is independent of transducer orientation. Calibration measurements in vivo have been made using rubber tubes of known diameters.

Values for E_p, E_o, and C were recorded using the transit-time technique by McDonald (1968) and Nichols and McDonald (1972). Values found using this technique were very close to those determined using angiography (Table 5.13).

Measurements using an intra-aortic ultrasonic catheter Another method used by Hughes et al., (1979; 1979a) to study the mechanical parameters of the aorta involves the use of a catheter containing three 10-MHz piezoelectric crystals spaced equiangularly (120°) around the tip of a catheter (Hughes et al., 1979; Hughes et al., 1979a). The crystals were mounted in the catheter so that the ultrasound beams would be perpendicular to the long axis of the catheter. The pulse-echo technique was used to obtain time-of-flight distances from the transducer and the position of the inner and outer walls of the aorta to determine radius and wall thickness. Corrections were made to account for the catheter diameter. A detailed mathematical description is reported by Hughes et al., (1979).

Hughes et al., (1979) initially used this technique to obtain a simultaneous record of dynamic wall motion and aortic pressure. They found that there was a striking similarity between the vessel radius waveform and the pressure waveform. These findings were very similar to the wave traces observed by Bertram (1977) using the transit-time technique for studies on the femoral artery in the dog. Hughes et al., (1979) were able to observe an 8% change in the inner and outer radii of the aorta.

Hughes et al., (1979) extended this study and used the values found for diameter and wall thickness to compute Young's modulus for the ascending and descending aorta. They then performed inflation tests on isolated aortic tissue in vitro to compute Young's modulus for the ascending and descending aorta and found that the two moduli measured in vitro increased exponentially with mean distending pressure. Hughes *et al.*, (1979) also noted that the two moduli were not significantly different; however, the value of the modulus of the descending thoracic aorta determined in vivo exceeds that for the descending thoracic aorta determined in vitro. This result is consistent with the increased stiffness observed in vivo using the ultrasound technique and was suggested to be due to the tethering of the aorta to the spine. Comparison of the ultrasound and strain gauge results are shown in Table 5.13.

Echocardiographic technique Kalath *et al.*, (1986) used an echocardiograph of the aortic root to evaluate mechanical properties of 50 normal human subjects. The patients were divided into young, middle-aged, and old groups. Kalath measured diameter and wall thickness changes based on M-mode echographs of these individuals taken using a 3-MHz transducer. All measurements were made at systole and diastole.

Pressure measurements were made using a sphygomanometer and elastic moduli were calculated using blood pressure in phase with strain. Dynamic evaluation of the pressure and diameter relationship was made by approximating blood pressure at any time using a triangular relationship based on in vivo measurements reported by Greenfield and Patel (1962). A triangular pressure pulse was constructed and divided into 16 (0–15) equal time intervals. It was assumed that minimum pressure occurred at intervals 0 and 15 and maximum blood pressured occurred at interval 6. Diameter measurements were made at intervals 0 and 15 corresponding to minimum diameter (end-diastolic diameter) and at interval 6 for maximum diameter (end-systolic diameter). Electrocardiographic tracings were simultaneously recorded. Mechanical parameters were computed for each subject. All computations were made using values of anterior wall thickness during diastole and using inside diameter measurements. The results indicated that the elastic aortic stiffness in the circumferential direction increases with age.

The increase in aortic elastic stiffness in the circumferential direction was also found to be associated with decreased aortic auxiliary pumping efficiency. The pumping efficiency of the aorta was found to decrease to 56% in older individuals compared with the young group.

Mechanical parameters computed by Kalath *et al.*, (1986) using the echocardiographic technique are shown in Table 5.12 to be very close to those observed based on angiography. There is a significant difference between the results of Kalath *et al.*, (1986) and those of Greenfield and Patel (1962). The difference could be attributed to surgical invasion, the use of outside diameter for strain gauge measurements, and the use of inside diameter for calculations based on echocardiographs.

Kalath et al., (1987) used this echocardiographic procedure to evaluate the mechanical status of the aortas of individuals with the connective tissue disorder, osteogenesis imperfecta. In the majority of the patients studied, the computed elastic moduli were significantly elevated compared with age-matched controls, indicating an acceleration of ageing.

Buntin and Silver (1988) studied the use of ultrasound to noninvasively determine the value of wall thickness of the rabbit aorta. A comparison was made between wall thickness determined using ultrasound and that obtained from direct measurement on fixed aortic preparations. The wall thickness values found for the fixed aortas, after correction for shrinkage effects occurring during histologic processing, were within 10% of those found based on measurements using ultrasound. The results indicated that echocardiographic examination is a viable method of obtaining accurate wall thickness measurements.

Tables 5.12 and 5.13 compare values found for mechanical parameters computed based on the various techniques presented above. Based on these tables, it is seen that the mechanical properties depend on the type of technique used for data collection. Invasive techniques tend to generate higher values of elastic moduli and lower values of relative change in diameter. It is likely that measurements made noninvasively reflect the specific properties of the aorta in vivo.

5.5 Repair of cardiovascular tissue

Aortic wall and heart valves normally do not repair themselves if mechanical injury occurs; instead they undergo a process of wound healing that leads to the formation of a scar tissue very similar to that seen in skin. Normal aorta and valve contain collagen fibres, elastic fibres, proteoglycans and cells in

Table 5.13 Compliance values determined using ultrasound and other techniques

Method	Subject[a]	P diastolic (mmHg)	PVD %
Ultrasonic catheter	Dog (7)[b]	80	18.8
Transesophageal	Dog[b]	100	6.0
Strain gauge (excised aorta)	Dog	100	7.6
Echocardiograph	Human (50)		7.85
Angiography	Human (18)	66	12.0

[a] Figure in parentheses indicates number of subjects studied.
[b] Indicates descending aorta studied.
From Silver et al., 1989

the appropriate layered structures. Aorta wall is a tri-laminar structure while heart valve is bi-layered. However, injury beyond loss of a few endothelial cells that line the blood contact surface, is followed by deposition of aligned collagen fibres and removal of denatured macromolecules. The problem with this wound healing response is that the mechanical properties of the new collagenous tissue are more like that of tendon than that of normally compliant cardiovascular tissue.

One model of the cardiovascular wound healing response that has been studied in great deal, is the tissue ingrowth into porous textile prostheses. The morphology of the formation of a new cellular lining as well as tissue to replace the media and adventitia has been reported. Hertzer (1981) summarized four theories of endothelialization/ingrowth of vascular grafts (Jerusalem et al., 1987).

1. Cells derived from both vascular stumps invade the prosthesis by crossing the points of anatomoses (suture lines).
2. seeding of the inner surface by circulating white blood cells and endothelial transformation;
3. Immigration of fibroblasts from the adventitia into the inner layer of the graft and transformation into endothelial like cells;
4. migration and transformation of smooth muscle cells from the media.

A report by Jerusalem et al. (1987), followed the formation of neo-intima in textile prostheses by means of light and scanning electron microscopy. They reported that two independent cellular layers (intimal and adventitial) developed on the free surface at the blood interface under the fibrin clot, replacing the fibrin clot from the outer free surface. The inner layer of tissue invades the prosthesis from the aortic stumps (proximal and distal) and extends over the fibrin clot, or replaces it. This layer consists of smooth muscle cells covered by endothelial like cells. The ingrowth layer at the outer free surface contains fibroblasts, myofibroblasts (contractile type of fibroblast) and smooth muscle cells that invade the outer pores of the prosthesis.

Endothelial cell proliferation is promoted by binding to specific cell receptors including fibronectin (Hynes, 1987; Ruoslahti, and Pierschbacker, 1987), heparin and acidic fibroblast growth factor. Extracellular matrix macromolecules have been postulated to alter endothelial cell growth based on their ability to mediate attachment and thus alter cell shape. During initiation of capillary development, endothelial cells respond to angiogenic mitogens by remodelling underlying extracellular matrix, extending long processes, and increasing their proliferative rates (Folkman, 1982). Ingber (1990) recently reported that fibronectin controls capillary endothelial cell proliferation based on its ability to support tension-dependent alterations of cell shape, i.e., both by binding to cell-surface integrins and by resisting mechanical loads that are applied to these receptors.

5.6 Pathophysiology of aortic and valvular diseases

Although aortic and valvular tissue undergo billions of cycles in many individuals without any evidence of tears or deposition of calcium, others suffer each year from these problems. Tears (dissections) occur in the aorta as well as areas where the aortic wall abnormally balloons out (aneurysm) or is narrowed due to atherosclerosis. Valvular leakage (stenosis) is associated with abnormal calcification at points of stress concentration and eventual stiffening resulting in ineffective valve closure. Below the pathophysiology of each of these cardiovascular tissues is analyzed in more detail.

5.6.1 Aneurysm formation and atherosclerosis

Atherosclerosis is characterized by formation of plaques composed of fatty deposits and fibrous tissue (collagen and extracellular matrix components) on the intimal side of the vessel lumen (Buja, 1987). Deposition of plaque narrows the vascular lumen and is associated with degenerative changes in the media and adventitia. Aortic atherosclerosis leads to the formation of aneurysms most commonly in the abdominal area of the aorta with involvement of the iliac, femoral and popliteal arteries. Aneurysm is the term used to describe an abnormal dilatation of artery and vein walls and frequently occurs in the aorta (Buja, 1987). The causes of aneurysm formation include

- congenital defects,
- traumatic injury

or systemic disease including

- atherosclerosis,
- syphilis and
- medionecrosis.

Aneurysms that form as a result of these conditions can grow to a diameter of up to 15 or 20 cm triggering blood clotting and can potentially lead to dissections (tears in the aortic wall), bursting of the vessel wall and subsequent death.

Atherosclerotic aneurysms are the most frequently observed sub-type and are prevalent in males after the age of 50. These lesions occur most commonly in the abdominal area of the aorta, usually below the renal arteries. They take the form of sack like swellings in which the media of the aortic wall is destroyed by atherosclerosis and filled with blood clots. Occlusion to the iliac, renal, and mesenteric arteries may result from pressure exerted on these vessel walls by the aortic wall swelling. In addition the blood clot may be released into the cardiovascular system (embolize) and block a vessel down stream causing a variety of complications. Rupture occurs most frequently when the aneurysm is larger than six cm in diameter.

Aneurysms are most commonly found below the renal arteries and can be replaced with a prosthesis.

Cystic medial necrosis is a disease of unknown origin that is characterized by loss of the elastic and muscular tissue that makes up the media of the aortic wall. Dissecting aneurysm is a relatively frequent complication of this disease and is associated with formation of a longitudinal tear through the media of the aorta or artery until it reaches the outside or inside walls. In the case where the tear exits from the adventitia, blood exits into the body cavities. When the the tear re-enters the lumen of the vessel, the blood that exits into the wall now re-enters the system. In the latter case the aorta becomes a double bored vessel with two almost parallel vessel openings present for blood to follow.

Dissections in the ascending portion of the aorta extend both towards the heart and the abdominal aortic region. More commonly, the tear begins in the descending aorta past the subclavian artery and proceeds away from the heart.

A consequence of aneurysm formation and rupture in the arterial system is the abnormal feeding of arterial blood into the venous system. The process of abnormal transfer of blood between arteries and veins as a result of rupture of an arterial aneurysm is termed arteriovenous fistula.

Valvular diseases
Isolated aortic valve disease was once considered a consequence of rheumatic fever associated with inflammatory injury resulting from bacterial infection. It is now more widely accepted that isolated aortic valve disease usually has a non-rheumatic origin and is caused most commonly by degenerative calcification of malformed valves as well as valves in the elderly (Schoen and Sutton, 1987). Malformed aortic valves are found in uni-, bi-, and tetra-leaflet forms that are present at birth. In addition, mitral valve prolapse, a condition where the valves are 'floppy', leads to improper valve closure.

There are a variety of ways that aortic valves become diseased; however, all diseased valves either block blood flow and cause **stenosis** or cause inefficient blood transfer by not closing completely. This is clinically referred to as **regurgitation or incompetency** (Thubrikar, 1990). Valvular incompetency is evaluated by injecting radiopaque dye into the aortic root and observing under x-ray if the dye flows back into the left ventricle when the valve is closed.

Aortic stenosis is commonly caused by

- calcification of bicuspid valves
- commissural fusion
- degenerative calcification of tri-leaflet valves
- leaflet fibrosis and

Aorta and heart valve replacements   183

- post-inflammatory calcification of valves from patients with rheumatic disease (Subramanian *et al.*, 1984; Passik *et al.*, 1987).

Aortic insufficiency has been observed by itself or in combination with aortic stenosis. The origin of pure aortic insufficiency include (Olson *et al.*, 1984):

- post-inflammatory disease of rheumatic origin
- aortic root dilatation
- incomplete closure of bicuspid valves
- heart wall infection (infective endocarditis), and
- valves with four leaflets.

Aortic calcification and stenosis are thought to be secondary to mechanical wear and tear that result from cycling the valve through tensile and bending deformations. This applies to both bi-leaflet and tri-leaflet valves (Sell and Scully, 1965). In tri-leaflet valves changes to the leaflets with age include fibrous thickening of the leaflet with associated calcification within the fibrosa and annulus. Changes in the aortic valve appear to be similar to those described for atherosclerosis; however, some morphological differences exist (Thubrikar, 1990). The earliest calcification deposits are found at the site of leaflet attachment and along the lines of contact between the leaflets.

5.7 Aorta and heart valve replacements

A variety of natural and synthetic materials have been used to replace both vessels and valves that leak or do not perform the normal physiologic functions. In some cases, such as aortic replacement, patient survival requires the use of synthetic materials since no other vessel of the size of the aorta can be used to replace large portions of the major elastic artery in the body. In other cases, such as for replacement of small diameter vessels such as the coronary arteries, no synthetic material currently available today meets the design criteria for replacement. Therefore, clinical use of both natural and synthetic materials has led to trial-and-error adoption of approaches that most commonly lead to patient survival. Below we will discuss some of the accepted clinical approaches to replacement of vessels and valves.

5.7.1 Aortic and small diameter vessel replacements

Vascular prostheses can be classified based on the materials of construction, method of construction and according to the diameter (Silver and Doillon, 1989). The distinction between large and small diameter vessel replacements is arbitrarily based on the degree of blood compatibility. Large diameter (12–38 mm in diameter) vascular replacement with poly(ethylene terephthalate), commercial products containing Dacron™, is the accepted clinical practice (Table 5.14). Medium diameter vessel replacement with poly(tetrafluoroethylene), tradenamed Gore-Tex™, in addition to Dacron™ and biologicals dominate the market (5–10 mm in diameter). In small diameter applications (less than 4 mm) biologicals and materials currently under development are the hope for replacement of cerebral and coronary arteries.

The commercial market is split almost evenly between large and medium diameter vascular prostheses. The companies involved include Meadox Medical, Bard, W.L. Gore & Associates, Pacesetters, Impra and Golaski as listed in Table 5.15. Nearly all large diameter vascular prostheses are made of Dacron™; Bard and Meadox are the leaders in this area. Three-quarters of these prostheses are bifurcated while one fourth are straight. The bifurcated prostheses are used to repace the lower part of the aorta where it branches. About 70% of the medium diameter market is held by Gore-Tex™ while Dacron™ and biologicals account for 25% and 5%, respectively. Currently only 1% of the small diameter market is held by synthetic grafts due to lack of blood compatible materials.

5.7.2 Construction of large and medium diameter vascular prostheses

According to Sauvage *et al.* (1986), the modern era of effective reconstructive arterial surgery began in 1952 when Voorhees, Jaretski and Blakemore introduced fabric prostheses for replacement of the abdominal aorta. High rates of success are reported for tightly woven, crimped, non-supported Dacron™ fabric prostheses in the thoracic aorta; for knitted, crimped, non-supported Dacron™ in the abdominal aortoiliac area; and for knitted, noncrimped, supported Dacron™ prostheses for axillofemoral and femoropopliteal bypass (Sauvage *et al.*, 1986).

Graft preparation

Vascular grafts composed of Dacron™ are made using a variety of processes including fibre extrusion and fabric formation using knitting and weaving techniques (Silver and Doillon, 1989). Fabrics composed of woven and non-woven yarns are made using standard textile manufacturing processes.

Table 5.14 Vessel replacement using synthetics*

Graft size	Type used
Large diameter (12–38 mm)	PET
Medium diameter (5–10 mm)	PET, PTFE
Small diameter (<4mm)	Vessel autografts

PET = Poly(ethylene terephthalate); PTFE = poly(tetrafluoroethylene)
* Silver and Doillon, 1989

Aorta and heart valve replacements 185

Table 5.15 Manufacturers of vascular grafts

Company	Products
Bard/USCI	Dacron™ and Dacron™/Albumin Grafts
Golaski	Dacron™
Impra	Poly (tetrafluoroethylene)
Intervascular	Dacron™
Meadox Medicals Inc.	Diameter Dacron™, Dacron™/Collagen and Umbilical Cord Graft
Pacesetters	Dacron™

Large diameter vascular grafts are supplied in both porous and non-porous forms. The porosity of these fabrics is related to the number of fibres present, their diameter and the presence of a type I collagen or albumin coating to seal the pores between the fibres.

On a microscopic level the pores between the fibres in vascular grafts promote tissue ingrowth from the tissue–implant interface which leads to adhesion to the surrounding tissue (Silver and Doillon, 1989). Fabrics with pores 10–45 µm in diameter promote optimal tissue ingrowth and rapid wound healing. The liquid permeability of vascular grafts is expressed in ml/cm^2 per minute and relates the rate of water movement through a fabric at a pressure of 120 mm Hg. Porosity is typically measured by pressurizing tubes of the material to be tested. Most prostheses display porosities of 2300–5300 ml/cm^2; however, with the recent introduction of coated grafts the rate of liquid penetration through the graft is significantly decreased without adversely affecting tissue ingrowth. Traditionally, a balance of blood loss due to the porous nature of grafts was required to support rapid tissue ingrowth. Other parameters of critical importance are biocompatibility, blood compatibility, graft stiffness, fatigue lifetime and handling characteristics. All of these properties depend on the type of fibre used and the geometry of fibres in the finished textile product.

The properties of the textile product reflect the individual yarns used to make a fabric. Yarn properties in turn reflect the number and twist of individual fibres as well as the material properties of the polymer used. Continuous fibre is termed monofilament, which differs in physical properties from yarn composed of similar polymeric materials. Physical properties of a fabric are also influenced by the presence of crimp, degree of twist in the yarn, the direction of the fibre axis, and the yarn diameter.

Fibres can be heat processed to form a regular zig-zag (crimp) that results in a low modulus region to the stress–strain curve. In addition, they can be twisted together to form yarns that resist deformation in proportion to the twist. Yarn can be processed into fabrics by either weaving or knitting. The direction of the fibre with respect to the axis of the prosthesis can be either parallel (warp direction), circumferential (weft) or wrapped at an angle (bias) to the axis. Increased degrees of extension can be obtained along the prosthesis axis when the yarn is incorporated in the bias direction.

Woven structures are constructed by criss-crossing layers of fibres that are orthogonal to each other. The yarns pass over and under each other creating interfibre friction which increases the bending stiffness of a fabric. The ability of a fabric to drape or lie smoothly over a surface is related to the diameter or denier and the fibre stiffness. In contrast, knitted structures are prepared by looping the yarn with a moving needle and then interconnecting the loops to form a continuous structure. As a result knitted fabrics tend to be highly porous and have lower ultimate tensile strengths compared to woven ones.

During surgery, porous vascular grafts are pre-clotted with the patient's own blood to decrease the leakage, once the graft is sutured in place. During pre-clotting, proteins such as albumin and fibrin are integrated along with blood cells into the wall of the prosthesis. The material is replaced by connective tissue.

Types of Dacron™ prostheses

Tightly woven, crimped prostheses are used without preclotting in large diameter, high flow arteries. The porosity has been lowered by coating the prosthesis pores. Commercial grafts include USCI® Debakey® woven Dacron® prosthesis and Meadox® Cooley Veri-Soft® woven Dacron Graft. The difficulty of suturing these grafts led to the design of knitted grafts which have preferred handling properties.

Knitted, crimped Dacron® prostheses both bifurcated and straight are flexible, easily sutured because of their greater porosity, and exhibit good tissue ingrowth. Pre-clotting is used to lower the graft porosity. These grafts have long term stability in large and medium calibre arteries. Weft knit grafts which were produced in the 1950s (Edwards, 1959) were improved in the mid-1960s by imparting a filamentous texture in the form of a velour surface (Hall et al., 1967; Sauvage et al., 1971). Commercially warp knit Microvel™ by Meadox has filamentous internal and external surfaces and Bionit by Bard is filamentous only on the external surface. These prostheses dominate usage in the large diameter market including abdominal aorta and iliac arteries. A ten year patency of 95% is reported for these grafts (Sauvage et al., 1986). An infection rate of 2–5% is common with Dacron® grafts.

Graft infection may occur several years post-surgery and is diagnosed by either localized wound infection accompanied by fever, elevated leukocyte count, pseudoaneurysms, graft thrombosis, emboli containing bacteria, suture line haemorrhage or systemic infection (Szilagyi et al., 1972). A recent report concluded that 50 cases of patients with infected vascular grafts, among 212 vascular explants evaluated, indicates that infection may be associated with a high risk of graft failure (Vinard et al., 1991).

5.7.3 Medium and small diameter arterial replacement

In contrast with the success that has been achieved using knitted, crimped unsupported (external support) Dacron® prostheses for abdominal aorta and iliac artery replacement, reduced success rates have been measured for these grafts as bypasses for axillofemoral and above-knee femoral popliteal, below-knee femoropopliteal and below-knee femorotibial sites (less than 50% patent). These grafts were modified to reduce kinking by adding external support to non-crimped, knitted Dacron prostheses. Increased numbers of patent grafts were reported after these modifications; however, today about three-quarters of the grafts used to repair diseased arteries in the leg are made of expanded poly(tetrafluoroethylene), PTFE.

Microporous expanded PTFE is currently the most successful graft material for small diameter arterial reconstruction (White, 1987). After evaluating various modifications of expanded porous PTFE, it was determined that a pore size of 20–30 µm was optimal (Campbell et al., 1974) with external support. This provided the best handling and clinical success rates (White, 1987). Above the knee these grafts were as effective as autografts up to 30 months (Bergan et al., 1982); below the knee, they were less effective (Hobson et al., 1980).

5.7.4 Vein and artery autografts

Host arteries and veins are commonly used in vascular surgery to replace or bypass diseased small diameter arteries. Cells in these grafts remain viable after transplantation and divide and synthesize connective tissue components. In children they increase in size in proportion to the normal bodily growth rate. The flexibility and other physical properties compare with that of the normal vessel. Blood compatibility is better than that of synthetic materials. For these reasons autografts are used to bypass obstructions in the coronary and other small diameter arteries.

The saphenous vein, a major external vein in the lower leg, is widely used to bypass blocked regions of the coronary artery, femoropopliteal and for patch angioplasties. Because of its external location it is surgically accessible and the remaining ends can be tied off without any short or long-term complications. Implantation of this vein has several long term disadvantages including:

- proliferation of intimal fibroblasts
- aneurysm formation
- atherosclerotic build up in the vessel lumen
- disappearance of the endothelial cell lining, and
- lumenal narrowing due to deposition of collagen

As a substitute for the saphenous vein, the mammary artery is used in coronary bypass procedures. Other autografts used in vascular surgery include (Silver and Doillon, 1989):

- Common internal and external arteries
- Human umbilical cord
- Mammary artery
- Superficial femoral artery
- Xenografts

Human umbilical cord vein grafts have been used for replacement of small-diameter vessels (Dardik and Dardik, 1975; Dardik et al., 1975a). Biograft® is a glutaraldehyde treated human umbilical cord vein graft supported with a polyester mesh and is reported to be an acceptable alternative to use of the saphenous vein. Complications include (Dardik, 1986):

- aneurysm formation
- foreign-body reactions
- infection
- thrombosis

Arteries from animals (xenografts) have been used after glutaraldehyde treatment for replacement of human arteries. These materials become calcified and brittle over time and the use of xenografts for replacement of the aorta or femoral arteries is questionable based on the low five year patency rates.

Endothelial cell seeded vascular grafts
Research and clinical studies have led to the conclusion that saphenous vein autografts are preferred blood vessel substitutes for peripheral vascular reconstructions. However, because this graft is a biological product, person-to-person variation in length and varying availability due to the presence of diseased segments or prior surgical intervention, limit its use in patients. Small diameter vascular prostheses composed of synthetic materials have had limited success not only because of the problem of blood compatibility but also because of the technical problems encountered during graft insertion into vessels with low flow rates. Several research groups have reported improved small diameter vascular graft performance as a result of seeding protheses of Dacron® (Schmidt et al., 1984) and PTFE (Graham et al., 1982; Shepard et al., 1986) with autologous endothelial cells. A recent report on PTFE grafts with pore sizes between 28–52 µm, seeded with autologous endothelial cells, showed higher mean flow rates than did non-seeded grafts. The study also concluded that endothelial cell seeding of small diameter PTFE vascular grafts improved patency and the amount of thrombus-free surface areas were greatest when the pores were 40 µm in

diameter; however, neither endothelial cell seeding nor pore size affected the performance of PTFE grafts under conditions of reduced flow.

Another approach to fabrication of small diameter vascular replacements involves use of a variety of polyurethanes (Lyman *et al.*, 1977; Lelah and Cooper, 1986) consisting of a fibrous conduit spun on a rotating mandril (Annis *et al.*, 1978). However, animal and clinical results have been disappointing and a recent report indicates that occlusion of polyurethane grafts is a result of a hyperplastic response (Teijeira *et al.*, 1989).

5.8 Cardiac valve replacements

The most commonly used valve replacements are mechanical devices involving a ball or disc in a housing, and bioprosthetic valves that are derivatives of natural valves. Mechanical valves are made totally of synthetic materials while bioprosthetic valves are pig or human valves that are chemically perserved and attached to a sewing ring for stabilization during surgery. A disadvantage of mechanical valves is that patients receiving this prosthesis must be maintained on anticoagulants to prevent systemic clotting while patients receiving bioprosthetic valves do not require anticoagulant therapy, but these valves fail by calcification and degeneration.

5.8.1 Mechanical valves

Mechanical valves come in several basic designs consisting of various modifications of the ball-in-cage, caged disc and tilting disc concepts (Schoen, 1987; Williams, 1987; Thubrikar, 1990) (Table 5.16).

Early prototypes of the Starr-Edwards (Starr, 1960) valve had a ball composed of silicone rubber, a cage of stellite (cobalt-chromium-molybdenum alloy) and silicone rubber sewing ring. These designs left the valve struts (supports holding ball in the cage) uncovered while later designs employed covered valves to limit clotting and embolism formation. Problems with the ball composition were encountered and modifications to the silicone rubber as well as substitution of stellite resulted in variable results. Later models of the Starr-Edwards valve utilized ultrathin

Table 5.16 Types of mechanical valves*

Valve type	Examples
Ball-in-cage	Starr-Edwards, Smeloff-Cutter, Debakey-Surgitool
Caged disc	Kay-Shiley, Beall-Surgitool, Starr Edwards
Tilting disc	Bork-Shiley, St. Jude Medical, Medtronic Hall, Omniscience, Lillehei-Kaster

* Schoen, 1987; Williams 1987; Thubrikar, 1990

polypropylene cloth on the stellite cage with a part of the strut on the inside left bare and a sewing ring composed Dacron® (Bonchek and Starr, 1975). Valves were introduced for the mitral and aortic positions in 1972 (Williams, 1987). A success rate of 90% after four years is expected in the mitral position. The disadvantages of this valve include the need for continued anticoagulation of the blood of the patient and red cell lysis. Other designs including the Smeloff-Cutter and Debakey-Surgitool valves were similar in design to the Starr-Edwards; however, they never were as widely used because of technical problems.

Caged-disc valves were associated with several problems that stemmed from the large size of the cage required to hold the disc in place. Low cardiac output as well as outflow obstruction has led to the development of disc valves. Among the designs were the Kay-Shiley, Beall-Surgitool, and Starr-Edwards as summarized by Williams (1987).

Tilting disc valves solved some of the problems encountered in caged-disc valves. In the Bork-Shiley tilting disc valve, pyrolite coated graphite is used for the disc and Haynes 25 for the housing. Problems with clot formation on the metal components of the orifice and disc have plagued these valves.

The St. Jude Medical valve contains two semi-circular leaflets of pyrolitic carbon. In the Medtronic Hall and Omniscience tilting disc valve, pyrolitic carbon is used for the disc and titanium for the housing. Most of these valves have sewing rings composed of either poly(ethylene terephthalate) or poly(tetrafluoroethylene). The Lillehei-Kaster valve consists of a pivoting disc suspended in a titanium housing. Pyrolytic carbon coats the disc. Clot formation in this valve can result in occlusion.

Several design criteria have been used to evaluate the effectiveness of mechanical valves. These include the pressure drop resulting from forward flow through the valve, and reverse flow required for valve closure should not cause incompetence. In the mitral position, a maximum pressure drop of 2 mm Hg at 5 l/min and a diameter of at least 23 mm is required to result in clinically acceptable stenosis (Williams, 1987). The pressure drop in the aortic position should be 20 mm Hg (Table 5.17).

5.8.2 Bioprosthetic valves
These valves are preferred over mechanical valves primarily because the patient does not have to be maintained indefinitely on anticoagulant

Table 5.17 Acceptable pressure drop criteria for valve design*

Mitral position	2 mm Hg at a flow of 5 l/min
Aortic position	20 mm Hg

* Williams, 1987

therapy. Bioprosthetic valves are made by chemically treating porcine aortic valves or bovine pericardium (sac that surrounds heart) with glutaraldehyde. Glutaraldehyde treatment cross-links the collagen fibrils increasing resistance to enzyme degradation, mechanical wear and transplant rejection. Most biological valves have additional components such as metallic or plastic stents and polymeric sewing rings.

The types of bioprosthetic valves include the Carpentier-Edwards, Agell-Shiley, Liotta, and Hancock porcine valves and Ionescu-Shiley and Mitral Medical pericardial valves. The Carpentier's-Edwards design involves treatment of aortic valves from young pigs with a 0.625% solution of phosphate buffered pH 7.4, glutaraldehyde and sewing them into a metal frame covered with PTFE (Table 5.18). The sewing ring has a silicone rubber insert covered with porous PTFE (Carpentier et al., 1982). The Angel-Shiley valve is similar to the Carpentier's-Edwards valve except that fixation is achieved using 0.5% glutaraldehyde and Dacron® covered Delrin stents are used (Angell et al., 1977). Hancock valves are treated with 0.2% glutaraldehyde and mounted on a stent consisting of a polypropylene frame and a Stellite ring (Reis et al., 1971). Liotta's valve (Liotta et al., 1977) was a low profile valve for implantation in small hearts.

The Ionescu-Shiley valve is obtained by mechanical cleaning and trimming pericardium from calves 6–18 months old. It is placed in a sterile physiological solution for three to six hours and then stored in 0.5% glutaraldehyde in phosphate buffered saline for two weeks or more. The tissue is attached to a titanium stent post covered with Dacron®. Valves are stored in 40% formaldehyde buffered with acetate (Williams, 1987).

None of the commercially available bioprosthetic valves have similar values of design parameters. Thubrikar (1990) notes that the Carpentier's-Edwards, Hancock and Ionescu-Shiley valves have values of α, ϕ, Rb/Rc

Table 5.18 Types of bioprosthetic valves*

Angel-Shiley	Pig aortic valve treated with glutaraldehyde
Carpentier's-Edwards	Pig aortic valve treated with glutaraldehyde attached to PTFE metal frame attached to Dacron® covered Delrin®
Hancock	Pig aortic valve treated with glutaraldehyde mounted on poly(propylene) frame and a Stellite ring
Ionescu-Shiley	Cleaned, trimmed pericardium from calf treated with glutaraldehyde and attached to titanium stent covered with Dacron®

* Thubrikar, 1990

and H/Rc that differ significantly from the values found for canine aortic valve. He goes on to note that in the Carpentier's-Edwards valve the large value of the angle φ makes the leaflet edge too long resulting in fold formation during systole. In the Hancock valve, the large angle φ and the small distance between the stent posts make the valve orifice appear triangular. The small angle φ in the Ionescu-Shiley valve and the spherical shape make the flow profile uneven and somewhat obstructive. Therefore use of all of the bioprostheses is somewhat of a compromise compared to the normal valve.

5.8.3 Failure of heart valves

Despite the availablility of a large number of prosthetic valves, according to Schoen (1987a), the long-term survival of patients following valve surgery is not particularly sensitive to the type of device used. Five year survival is about 70–80%, while ten-year survival is about 55–70% (Cohn, 1984; Cobanoglu et al., 1985). The thromboembolism rate for patients with mechanical valves, who are on anticoagulant therapy, is about the same as that of patients receiving bioprosthetic ones. The advantage of bioprosthetic valves is that patients do not need to be on anticoagulant therapy continually. Bioprosthesis failure rate during the first five years is 1%, and 2% per year thereafter, and therefore appears more favourable in the first ten years (Oyer et al., 1984); however, this advantage does not occur after ten years (Cobanoglu et al., 1985).

Prosthesis associated deaths include local occlusion of the prosthesis or thromboembolism from the prosthesis. Causes of failure requiring re-operation include:

- endocarditis
- mechanical dysfunction
- thrombosis
- tissue degeneration
- tissue overgrowth
- valvular leakage

Bioprostheses fail by degeneration and subsequent calcification at points of maximum stress.

5.9 Summary

Replacement of components of the cardiovascular system includes use of tissues as well as synthetic materials to achieve normal blood distribution systemically. Synthetic polymeric materials are fashioned into straight and bifurcated tubes for replacement of large diameter vessels including the aorta and its branches. Composites of metals, polymeric materials and allografts are used to replace valves that fail to close normally. Glutaraldehyde treated valves and pericardium are fashioned into valve replacements in humans. Veins and arteries are used to bypass sections of small diameter vessels to restore normal blood flow to the coronaries.

Research in the area of biomaterials used to replace cardiovascular tissues continues to focus on use of both synthetic and natural materials to replace biological tissues. These different materials are needed since no one material has properties that are sufficient to replaced all cardiovascular tissues.

6.
Facial Implants

6.1 Introduction

Use of autografts, homografts and synthetic polymers was, up to the 1990s, sufficient to generate acceptable cosmetic results in facial surgery (Glasgold and Silver, 1991). However, during the last ten years advances in surgical techniques, appreciation of the consequences of homograft resorption and decreased use of homografts because of the increased risk of viral contamination, have led to the need for more available implant materials.

The development of implant materials, both biological and synthetic has previously occurred via two almost independent pathways. Surgeons have pioneered the development of biological graft materials while scientists and engineers have largely been responsible for introduction of synthetic polymers in a variety of medical applications.

Increased sophistication of facial plastic surgeons has led to increased numbers of procedures to correct genetic, traumatic, and cosmetic deformities as well as an increased expectation for positive results by the patient. As our population ages so does the demand for procedures that minimize cosmetic changes associated with ageing. The growing awareness of cosmetic procedures as well as the patient's expectation for ideal results have led to a need for improved techniques and implants for each procedure discussed in this chapter. Cosmetic procedures that were the gold standard of the 1980s are unacceptable by present standards.

6.1.1 Anatomy and physiology of facial structures

Facial implants are used in over twenty areas of the face as diagrammed in Figure 6.1, which includes (Glasgold and Silver, 1991):

- alar cartilages in the nostrils
- cheek
- chin
- creases above eye
- dorsum of the nose
- earlobe
- forehead
- glabella frown lines
- infra-orbital groove
- labial groove

Introduction 195

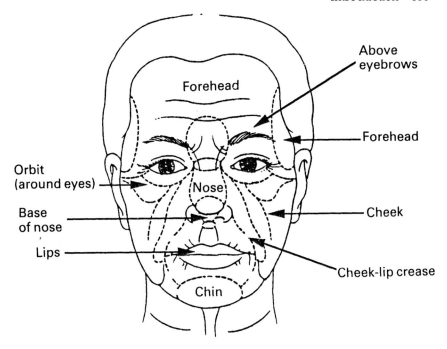

Figure 6.1 Areas of the face where biomaterials are used. Reprinted with permission from Orentreich and Orentreich (1991) copyright CRC Press, Boca Raton, FL.

- lips
- malar area
- nasolabial crease
- periorbital groove
- radix furrows
- temple
- tip of the nose

Facial structures that are replaced or that interface with implants include skin, cartilage and bone. The microscopic structure of skin has been reviewed in section 2.1.1 and therefore the reader is referred to this section for a description. In the case of cartilage, it comprises the septum that separates the two nostrils internally as well as comprises the walls of the nose and ear. Bones of the face make up the upper and lower mandibles, orbits, chin and other structures that are repaired or interface with biomaterials.

6.1.2 Types of cartilage

There are three different types of cartilage (Wasserman and Dunn, 1991, for a review) including hyaline, fibrocartilage and elastic cartilage. Hyaline cartilage is the predominant form and contains structural components including territorial matrix, interterritorial matrix, matrix vesicles, lacuna, proteoglycans, chondrocytes and collagen fibrils (Table 6.1). Hyaline cartilage has a glossy translucent appearance due to the high water content and small diameter of the collagen fibrils that make up the interfibrillar material.

Hyaline cartilage contains chondrocytes, proteoglycans and narrow diameter collagen fibrils of type II collagen. Chondrocytes synthesize several different types of collagen (primarily type II) and proteoglycans and

Table 6.1 Structural components of cartilage: their location and function

Structure	Location	Function
Territorial matrix (TM)	Surrounds the lacuna; forms a capsule around the chondrocyte	Fine CF and small PB form a fibril basket that provides support for C; provides an ideal chemical environment for C
Interterritorial matrix (ITM)	Area between chondrocytes; begins outside of the TM	Coarse CF and PG aggregates provide compressive stiffness to cartilage
Matrix vesicles (MV)	Form clusters in the TM and ITM; bud off of C cell membrane	Provide a seeding site for mineralization
Lacuna	The cavity which contains a chondrocyte	Provides a compartment and ideal environment
Proteoglycan (PG)	Exist as monomers and aggregates; distributed throughout cartilage	Holds CF together and to C cell membrane; cements all components of cartilage together
Chondrocyte (C)	Cells of cartilage; sit within a lacuna; are surrounded by the territorial matrix	Produce CF, PG, and MV; maintain cartilage viability
Collagen fibrils (CF)	Compose the TM and ITM; fibrils are held together by PG	Forms a basket which holds C; forms cartilage suprastructure

Note: Listed are the components of cartilage. The location and function of these components are described.
From Wasserman and Dunn, 1991

eventually are surrounded by extracellular matrix. Chondrocytes are found in compartments termed lacunae that are surrounded by a ring of extracellular matrix (Figure 6.2 from Wasserman and Dunn, 1991).

Cartilage ultrastructure has been reviewed in detail by Sheldon (1983) and the reader is referred to this reference for additional information.

Proteoglycans found in cartilage are composed of

- chondroitin sulphate,
- dermatan sulphate, and
- keratin sulphate glycosaminoglycans

(Mayne and von der Mark, 1983; Mayne and Irwin, 1986). Proteoglycans are found in the form of monomers, and aggregates attached to hyaluronic acid via link proteins forming proteoglycan aggregates or matrix granules (Heinegard and Paulsson, 1984; Rosenberg and Buckwalter, 1986).

The collagenous material surrounding the chondrocyte forms a region referred to as the territorial matrix (Clark, 1974). Several chondrocytes may be found within this matrix as well as cytoplasmic processes. Small vesicles bud off from the ends of these processes and remain situated in the matrix around the cells.

Matrix vesicles may play a role in mineralization of cartilage. Outside the territorial matrix fewer vesicles are found and collagen fibrils are coarser and more widely spaced. The latter region is termed the interterritorial matrix.

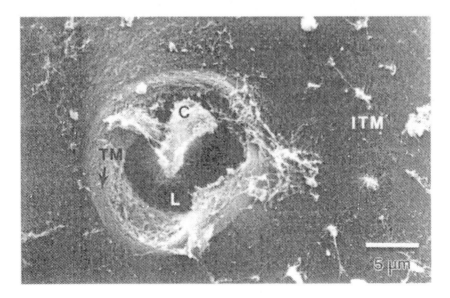

Figure 6.2 scanning electron micrograph of nasal septum. Reprinted with permission from Wasserman and Dunn (1991) copyright CRC Press, Boca Raton, FL.

Large proteoglycan aggregates are found in the interterritorial matrix and smaller ones in the territorial and pericellular areas.

Cartilage found in the face is primarily hyaline; this includes:

- nasal septum
- lower lateral cartilage
- upper lateral cartilage

Attachment of cartilage to the bones of the face is described in a review by Morris (1988).

Elastic cartilage is also found in facial or associated structures including

- auricle of external ear
- larynx
- epiglottis and
- external auditory canal

It differs from hyaline cartilage principally by the presence of elastic fibres in its matrix (di Fiore, 1981). Large chondrocytes are seen in lacunae in the interior and smaller ones towards the periphery that make a transition towards fibroblasts in the surrounding layer of perichondrium. Elastic fibres enter the cartilaginous matrix from the perichondrium and branch into a network of fibres in the interior.

Fibrocartilage is only a minor component of the face. It is composed of extracellular matrix and type I collagen, fibroblasts, hyaline cartilage and chondrocytes. It acts as a capsular membrane that surrounds many organs, transition zone between tendon and bone as well as a tough linkage between the bone found in the vertebral bodies.

6.1.3 Types of bone

There are two types of bones, flat or membranous bones and long bones. Membranous bones and long bones differ in the way in which the extracellular matrix is mineralized. Membranous bones mineralize in a cartilage independent manner while in long bones deposition of cartilage is followed by subsequent mineralization.

Flat bones compose the clavicle, bones of the face and skull vault. Membranous bones mineralize by mesenchymal cell deposition of collagen fibres and differentiation into osteoblasts producing and secreting organic matrix of bone, osteoid (Bouvier, 1989). Osteoid then undergoes calcification by deposition of calcium-phosphate salts becoming bone matrix. At the point when the original collagen matrix is surrounded by bone, a series of long thin pieces of bone, trabeculae, are observed (Figure 6.3 from Wasserman and Dunn, 1991). At the same time the primary centre of ossification is vascularized, trabeculae fuse forming porous (cancellous) bone and the trabeculae become filled with blood elements.

Biochemistry of facial tissues 199

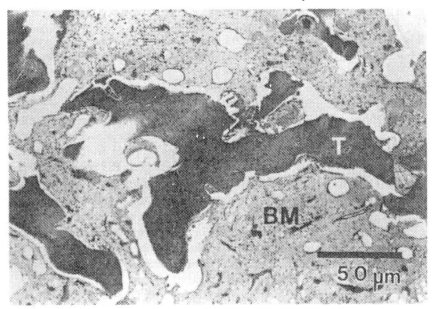

Figure 6.3 Light micrograph of cancellous bone. Reprinted with permission from Wasserman and Dunn (1991) copyright (1991) CRC Press, Boca Raton, FL.

Cancellous bone that forms the developing bones of the skull incease their size by appositional growth and conversion of cancellous bone into compact or cortical bone. Appositional growth involves osteogenic cells covering the trabeculae, differentiation into osteoblasts and deposition of bone mineral over the trabeculae.

The structure of long bones was reviewed in Chapter 4 and the reader is referred there for details.

6.2 Biochemistry of facial tissues

Biochemistry of skin, cartilage and bone is an important consideration of the differences that exist between these tissues. Details of the biochemistry of skin are presented in section 2.2.0 and therefore the reader is referred there.

Cartilage is a specialized extracellular matrix containing cells, collagens, proteoglycans, glycoproteins, elastin and other elastic fibre components, hyaluronic acid, a cell attachment factor (anchorin), and water (Geesin and Berg, 1991).

Cartilage contains six types of collagen including types II, V, VI, IX, X, and XI, three of which, II, IX and XI, are specific to this tissue (Miller and

Gay, 1987). Recent evidence suggests that collagen fibrils found in cartilage are heterotypically assembled from all three of these collagen types (Mendler *et al.*, 1989). Types IX and XI collagens may have a role in limiting fibril diameter of type II collagen fibrils.

Cartilage contains large chondroitin sulphate monomer (molecular weight of about 2×10^6) as well as two small proteoglycans (PG I, biglycan and PG II, decorin) (Table 6.2). Large chondroitin sulphate proteoglycans (PGs) form aggregates with hyaluronic acid and are stabilized by link protein. Each monomer consists of a protein core to which numerous glycosaminoglycan (GAG) side chains are attached. PG monomers and aggregates contain numerous fixed negative charges that associate with water molecules and ions which maintain the swelling of cartilage.

Small proteoglycans (PG I and PG II) from cartilage have molecular weights less than 100 000. PG I and PG II have core proteins of similar size (40 000) with PG I having two GAG chains while PG II has only one. Differences in the core proteins and self association of these PGs have been reported (Choi *et al.*, 1989; Neame *et al.*, 1989).

A variety of other matrix proteins have been identified and play a role in the normal physiology of this tissue (Geesin and Berg, 1991). These molecules include fibromodulin, anchorin, chondrocalcin, collagen-binding protein, cartilage matrix protein and CH 21. Fibromodulin and anchorin bind to type II collagen.

Bone contains collagens, proteoglycans, mineral and other matrix proteins (Table 6.3). The collagens found in bone include types I, V and X, although type I collagen predominates. Biglycan and decorin are the PGs present in bone as well as bone sialoproteins, gamma carboxyglutamic acid containing (Gla) protein, SPARC (osteonectin), thrombospondin and BP2.

6.3 Mechanical properties of facial tissues

The physical properties of skin, cartilage and bone are important considerations in the design of biomaterials. Skin is highly extensible and can absorb impact loads without permanent deformation. The mechanical properties of

Table 6.2 Proteoglycans found in cartilage*

Type	Molecular weight
Large chondroitin sulphate	2×10^6

Small proteoglycans
  PG I, biglycan
  PG II, decorin
	$<1 \times 10^5$

* Choi *et al.*, 1989; Neame *et al.*, 1989

Table 6.3 Bone specific proteins

	Function
Collagens	
Type I collagen	Fibril formation, matrix structure
Type V collagen	Fibril organization
Type X collagen	Mineralization?
Proteoglycans	
Glycosaminoglycans	
Bone small proteoglycan I, biglycan	Matrix organization
Bone small proteoglycan II, decorin	Matrix organization, collagen binding
Other matrix proteins	
Bone acidic glycoprotein	Cell attachment, mineralization
Osteonectin, SPARC, BM-40	Regulation of mineralization
Osteopontin, bone sialoprotein I (BSP)	Cell adhesion (RGD) binds hydroxyapatite
Bone sialoprotein II	Matrix organization
Osteocalcin, bone Gla protein	Regulation of mineralization Ca homeostasis
Matrix Gla protein	Regulation of mineralization Ca homeostasis
Chondrocalcin, carboxy-terminal propeptide	Mineralization
Phosphoproteins	Mineralization
Phosphoryn (dentin only)	Mineralization
BP2	Mineralization
BMP	Differentiation
Osteogenin	Differentiation
Thrombospondin	Cell adhesion (RGD)

from Geesin and Berg, 1991

this tissue are presented in section 2.3. Although highly hydrated, cartilage to some degree behaves similar to skin in terms of its stress–strain behaviour; both of these tissues can undergo almost 100% tensile deformations prior to failing. Initial loads applied to hyaline cartilage are dissipated by rapid elastic deformation; however, with inceasing time the load is dissipated by displacement of water molecules from the spaces between the collagen fibres. Cartilage shows increased modulus as the strain is increased. Bone in contrast to skin and cartilage, initially exhibits an almost linear stress–strain curve which plateaus at strains of about 1% depending on the strain rate.

6.3.1 Mechanical properties of cartilage

Cartilage is a multi-layered connective tissue containing an aligned network of collagen fibres in the superficial zone (surface), a bracing network of fibres orientated at +/- 45° in the intermediate zone and a system of fibres perpendicular to the bone that is found beneath it. The factors influencing the mechanical properties of cartilage to a first approximation (Silver *et al.*, 1992) are:

- collagen cross-link density
- collagen fibre diameter
- orientation of collagen fibres
- number of zones or layers
- proteoglycan content
- rate of deformation
- source of tissue

The extracellular matrix of cartilaginous tissue is generally composed of 60%–80% water, collagen fibres and proteoglycans. The latter two components compose 60% and 40 % of the dry weight, respectively. Proteoglycans contribute to the mechanical properties due to the high negative surface charge that is surrounded by a layer of counterions that increases the charge density of the collagen matrix. This high concentration of charges results in osmotic pressure within the collagen matrix. In the unloaded state, the Donnan osmotic pressure, which tends to expand the tissue, is balanced by the tensile stiffness of the swollen collagen network. When a compressive load is applied to cartilage, fluid is expressed increasing the effective swelling pressure. When the load is removed the tissue swells until the pre-loaded state is achieved. The large bottle brush configuration of PGs and the large volume of water bound to the charged side chains prevents free diffusion of all water molecules. The large 'excluded' volume of water bound to PGS attached to collagen fibres laterally stiffens these structural units.

Craniofacial cartilages do not support large mechanical loads and therefore the modulus and not the failure properties are physiologically important. Glasgold *et al.* (1988) have reported the stress-strain behaviour for human nasal septum. Their results indicated that this behaviour was non-linear and characterized by lower and upper stiffnesses of 0.41 and 19.3 MPa and ultimate strength and strain of 3 MPa and 70%, respectively (Figure 6.4). In comparison, Yamaguchi and Katake (1960) report a strength and ultimate strain of 3 MPa and 30%, respectively.

6.3.2 Mechanical properties of bone

Bone is a hard connective tissue consisting of about 67% hydroxyapatite and 30% collagen (dry weight basis) designed to provide mechanical support for skeletal motion and to protect non-mineralized structures (Wasserman and

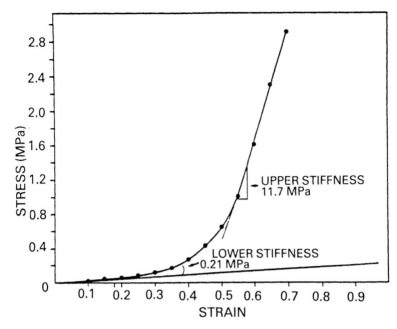

Figure 6.4 Typical stress-strain curve for nasal septum.

Dunn, 1991). Its properties are a consequence of mineralized collagenous tissue structures that are continually remodelled in response to applied stress. Therefore, the mechanical properties of bone are dependent on the type of loading, and mineral content.

Collagen fibres in osteon units are unable to withstand compressive forces in the absence of hydroxyapatite that is deposited within the hole region and between the fibres. The mineral composition of bony tissues varies from 5–50% for compact (cortical) bone and 30–90% for spongy (cancellous or also trabecular) bone. Tissue mechanical properties are influenced by the amount of bone present as well as the geometry of the macrostructure.

Katz *et al.* (1984) identified four levels of structure that are important in determining cortical bone mechanical properties which include:

- collagen-hydroxyapatite interactions
- macroscopic size and shape
- microstructural effects including woven versus flexiform versus Haversian bone
- molecular properties of collagen and proteoglycans

Based on ultrasound measurements they reported that the modulus of cortical bone was between 30 GPa in the longitudinal direction and 17 GPa in the radial direction (Table 6.3). Ultimate strengths range from 60 MPa

204 Facial implants

Table 6.3 Mechanical properties of bone*

Type	Ultimate tensile strength (MPa)	Modulus (GPa)
Compact (cortical)	60 (shear) 200 (compression)	30 (longitudinal) 17 (radial)
Cancellous (spongy)	51–237	6–22

* Cowin, 1989

under shear loads to 200 MPa in compression. As pointed out by Cowin (1989), the mechanical properties are strain rate dependent. This dependence can change the ultimate properties by a factor of two. The modulus is inversely dependent on the porosity and increases with calcium content and mineral volume fraction.

In cancellous bone, the variation in mechanical properties reflects anatomic location, type of loading, bone density, and species of donor. Measured moduli range from 6–22 GPa and strengths between 51 and 237 MPa have been reported (Cowin, 1989). The properties of cancellous bones are listed in Table 6.3.

The bones of the skull are composed of inner and outer layers of cortical bones separated by a layer of porous bone. Mechanical properties of bones of the skull reported in the literature were recently reviewed by Wasserman and Dunn (1991). Values for the modulus, tensile strength and compressive strength for bones of the skull are less than $\frac{1}{2}$ of the values reported for long bones (Table 6.4).

6.4 Repair of facial structures

Repair of skin, cartilage and bone are all wound healing responses as discussed in detail in a recent review by Silver and Parsons (1991). Repair of skin defects involving the dermis occurs exclusively by the deposition of scar tissue through the wound healing process as described in section 2.4. Healing of skin occurs via a series of events including

Table 6.4 Mechanical properties of long bone and skull*

Site	Test direction	Modulus of elasticity (GPa)	Strength (MPa) Tensile	Compressive
Long bone	Longitudinal	18	136	150
Skull	Tangential	5.6	48	96
	Radial	2.4	37	74

* adapted from Wasserman and Dunn, 1991

inflammation, proliferation of cells and granulation tissue deposition, and remodelling of granulation tissue. Activation of biological systems and release of cellular and other regulatory factors restores normal turnover of connective tissues.

In contrast to skin, the repair of cartilage is somewhat more complex. Much of the literature is focused on repair of articular cartilage that lines the joint surfaces. Repair of hyaline cartilage found in joints has been studied in order to optimize surgical reconstruction of these structures after injury associated with trauma, contact sports and osteoarthritis.

The degree to which articular cartilage can repair itself (Silver and Parsons, 1991) is a function of the following.

- Age
- Protection against abrasion
- Proximity to blood vessels
- Wound depth and location

In general, the extent of restoration of the joint surface is incomplete making this a significant clinical problem.

Loss of the superficial layer of articular cartilage results in little or no loss of blood and therefore blood clotting and inflammation are not triggered. Repair under these conditions occurs by division of chondrocytes adjacent to the wound (Table 6.5). The edges of the wound are not closed by cells as is the case in dermal healing. Microscopic evaluation of superficial cartilage wounds shows a thin layer of fine collagen that is deposited by chondrocytes local to the wound.

In contrast, deep lacerations that penetrate subchondral bone damage blood vessels intiating blood clotting and the repair response. Repair tissue consists of fibrocartilage containing type I collagen (compared to type II found in normal cartilage). Repair proceeds in a pattern that follows that seen in the dermis (section 2.4).

Bone repair is a regenerative process that differs from skin healing in that scar tissue is normally not formed. Regeneration occurs either through formation of membranous bone or through mineralization of cartilage. Membranous bone growth involves calcification of osteoid tissue (endochondral bone formation). This process occurs in facial bones, clavicle, mandible and subperiosteal bone.

Table 6.5 Mechanisms of cartilage repair*

Depth of injury	Repair mechanism
Superficial	Division of chondrocytes at edge of wound
Deep	Deposition of fibrocartilage

* Silver and Parsons, 1991

Because of the structural complexity of long bones, regeneration involves both membranous and endochondral bone formation. The stages of repair include

- induction
- inflammation
- soft callus formation
- callus calcification
- remodelling

During induction, cells in the region of disruption divide and begin to form new bone. These cells may derive from the periosteum or endosteum, or may be activated osteocytes. Other cells include fibroblasts, endothelial cells, muscle cells, and various mesenchymal cells which may differentiate into cartilage and bone forming cells under the appropriate stimulus. A variety of osteoinductive proteins have been identified and are believed to be involved in promoting differentiation of cells to form bone (Toriumi and Larrabee, 1991) including:

- bone morphogeneic protein
- demineralized bone matrix
- osteoinductive factor
- transforming growth factor β

Inflammation occurs during induction and normally lasts until significant cartilage and bone formation occurs. Blood clots that formed during trauma begin to lyse and macrophages remove necrotic tissue. Callus is formed by a combination of membranous bone formation from the periosteal surface and cartilage formation at the site of the fracture. Soft callus converts into hard callus and osteoclasts continue the remodelling process. Hard callus is converted into woven bone which is eventually remodelled into lamellar bone.

6.5 Types of procedures performed in facial plastic surgery

A considerable number of procedures in facial plastic surgery involve the use of either biological or synthetic materials. The ideal implant in the face must be permanent and must not stimulate a chronic inflammatory response since any change in implant position and or size will negatively affect the long-term outcome of a procedure. Both biological and synthetic implants have significant merits in a variety of applications. The long-term success of any implantation requires careful selection of the appropriate material.

Biomaterials are used to correct depressions in the face, recontour the nose, lips, cheeks, chin and forehead (Glasgold and Silver, 1991) (Table 6.6). The exact materials chosen may be both of synthetic and natural origin; however, the exact mode of introduction and method of insertion is carefully worked out in the clinic.

Table 6.6 Locations where biomaterials are used in the face*

Site	Correction
Cheek	Malar augmentation – create high cheek bones
	Submalar augmentation – fill in depressed areas
Chin	Mentoplasty – extend chin forward
Forehead	Augmentation
Nose	
Nasal dorsum	Augmentation
Nasal contour	Defects
Nasal base	Project nose
Premaxilla	Increase angle between nose and lips
Skin	
Scars	Elevation
Furrows	Elevation
Contouring	Elevation

* Glasgold and Silver, 1991

6.5.1 Use of biological grafts in the face

A wide variety of tissues are harvested and used to augment, re-contour and replace defective structures found in the face. These include

- bone
- bone-muscle grafts
- cartilage autografts
- cartilage transplants
- dura
- fascia
- pericranium

All of these materials require extensive surgical procedures to procure and may require a second surgical site. Below, each of these materials and its uses are examined in detail.

Cartilage autografts

Cartilage autografts are perhaps the most widely used implants in the face (Glasgold and Glasgold, 1991). Although synthetics are used in most areas of the face, their use in the nose is not recommended because of several complicating factors including:

- extrusion of polymeric implants
- thinness of the nasal skin

- susceptibility of the nose to trauma and infections
- tissue scarring

Cartilage autografts remain viable after transplantation, continue to grow when implanted into young hosts and do not appear to resorb over periods of time as long as 12 years. Factors that appear to be important in graft survival include the absence of dead space or blood in the surgical field, graft smoothness, and curvature of the implant (Table 6.7). Rib autografts appear to warp especially when placed over the bridge (nasal dorsum). Contact with adjacent cartilage and adequate coverage with soft tissue are also required for long-term survival when used on the nasal dorsum.

The major sources of cartilage autografts include nasal (septal or lateral) cartilage, lobe of the ear (chonchal cartilage) and the rib (costal cartilage) (Table 6.8). Of these sources the septum, a cartilage that separates the left and right nostril below the dorsum, is easily accessible during nasal surgery. It is easy to contour and elicits no host reaction; however, it may be missing or defective due to trauma. Septal cartilage is removed from inside the nose (endonasal approach) or externally by separating the medial crura that separates the nostrils at their base.

Table 6.7 Factors important in survival of cartilage grafts*

Factor	Outcome
Blood	Graft resorption
Dead space	Infection
Rough surface	Graft resorption
Curved implant	Warping or shape change
No cartilage interface	Graft resorption
Thin skin covering	Extrusion of implant

* Glasgold and Glasgold, 1991

Table 6.8 Sources of cartilage autografts*

Autograft	Source
Nasal septum	Nose
Lateral cartilage	Nostril base
Chonchal cartilage	Auricle of ear
Costal cartilage	Rib

* Glasgold and Glasgold, 1991

The lower lateral cartilage, which is often removed in nasal tip surgery, is often used to fill in a defect in another part of the nose. When asymmetry exists, lateral cartilage can be remove from one side of the nostril and inserted into the other.

Chonchal cartilage from the auricle of the ear is another source of cartilage autografts. Removal of this material does not result in scarring or deformity of the ear. It can be sutured together to form a multi-layered material, rolled to form a tube and used in conjuction with perichondrium.

Large segments of costal cartilage can be obtained from the sixth and seventh rib. The long operating time leads to an increased morbidity associated with this procedure. It remains viable when stored at 4°C for days and must be carved carefully to counteract its tendency to warp. It is used to reconstruct malar and mandibular contour defects and for reconstruction of auricular defects.

Clinically, cartilage grafts are used to augment a variety of areas in the face, but primarily in nasal reconstruction (Table 6.9). They are used for augmentation of the dorsum in patients with congenital abnormalities, traumatic injury or defects that arise from previous surgery. Normally septal cartilage is used in a layered graft; however, auricular and rib cartilage can also be employed.

Nasal contour and base defects can be corrected using cartilage from the nasal septum or auricle of the ear. Grafts are inserted to correct depressions and to assist tip projection, rotation, and correction of the angle between line drawn from the top of the nose to the tip and the line from the upper lip to the tip (nasolabial angle).

Cartilage homografts

Fresh cartilage autografts are the material of choice for facial reconstruction in the area of the nose; however, this material is not always available in large amounts or a second surgical procedure is not warranted. An alternative is to use preserved cartilage as a graft material. The down side of this approach is that the preservation technique must be shown to kill all viruses and infectious agents that may be transmitted via transplantation. Donald and Brodie (1991) have recently reviewed the use of human cartilage (homo)grafts and the reader is referred there for additional details.

Table 6.9 Use of cartilage autografts in nasal reconstruction*

Nasal dorsum (bridge)	Septal cartilage
	Auricular (chonchal) cartilage
	Rib (costal) cartilage
Nasal base augmentation	Septal, lateral or chonchal cartilage
Nasal tip projection	Septal or chonchal cartilage

* Glasgold and Glagold, 1991

In order for a cartilage homograft to be useful, it must be preserved between the time it is harvested and the time it is ready to be used. Preservation is accomplished by:

- cold storage in saline, antiseptic or antibiotic solutions
- freeze drying, and
- irradiation

Exposure to these treatments is designed to maintain sterility of the graft, destroy any viral contaminants and reduce absorption. Homografts are not matched for histocompatibility antigens since graft rejection is not observed. The lack of a rejection reaction is possibly due to the avascularity of cartilage.

Resorption of cartilage homografts has been reported in the literature to be somewhat variable. Gibson (1977) reported that a dead homograft undergoes resorption over a prolonged period of time and reviewed the results of studies that indicated that live chondrocytes were necessary to maintain the integrity of the cartilage matrix. Observations based on human clinical studies using Merthiolate® treated homografts suggested that fibrous tissue encapsulation around the implant slowed resorption (Gibson and Davis, 1959).

Dingman and Crabb (1960) and Schuller et al. (1977) described the use of irradiated cartilage homografts to repair facial defects. In follow-up studies that lasted as long as three years, there was no evidence of resorption. Donald (1986) recently showed a high rate of resorption of irradiated cartilage grafts in animals (85.7%) and a lower rate of resorption of Merthiolate®-treated grafts (43.6%) over a two to six-year period. From these studies it is apparent that the rate of homograft resorption depends on the preservation technique.

Irradiated homografts are obtained from the costochondral junction of ribs four or five to rib number seven of cadaver donors under the age of 35. Grafts are not accepted from donors who died of cancer or infection or were HIV or hepatitis virus positive. Cartilage is stored in sterile lactated Ringer's solution or normal saline with an air tight lid and kept refrigerated (Donald and Brodie, 1991). Grafts are exposed to a dose of 2.5 Mrad of gamma-irradiation. The shelf life of the irradiated specimen is two years.

Lyophilized cartilage grafting has been reported on extensively by Sailer (1983). Cartilage is harvested from the costochondral junction, stripped of muscle and other soft tissue taking care to preserve the perichodrium (Donald and Brodie, 1991). Sterilization is achieved by immersion in a 1% solution of beta-propiolactone solution at 37°C for two to three hours. Cartilage pieces are then rinsed twice for two hours in a buffered solution. Alternatively, cartilage can be sterilized with ethylene oxide gas; however, tissue reactivity and inflammatory diseases have been linked to ethylene oxide sterilization of some biomaterials.

Sterilized cartilage is then placed in sterile saline, frozen at −70°C for 30 minutes and then freeze-dried at −40°C for 36 hours. Freeze-dried materials are stored in vacuum packed containers prior to utilization. Prior to surgery, the freeze-dried material is rehydrated.

Bone grafts

The use of bone grafts in facial plastic surgery has been recently reviewed by Marentette (1991). Although the use of cadaver and allogeneic bone grafts has received increasing attention during the 1980s, bone autografts are still the material of choice in facial reconstructive procedures. Bone grafts either free or in combination with their vascular supply are used. Free grafts are used to repair facial defects and bone grafts (including their blood supply) are used in facial plastic surgery (Table 6.10). Also, grafts including arterial and venous vascular tissue are harvested and then connected to vascular tissue at donor sites. These are referred to as microvascular free bone grafts.

Illiac crest is used in the head and neck to fill in mandibular defects greater than 1 mm in size. Non-union of the mandible is associated with movement of the ends of the bone at the fracture site. Removal of any scar tissue in the non-union is required for fracture healing with a bone graft. Particulate spongy bone from the iliac is used to pack the defect and is stabilized with a plate or other fixation device.

Split rib grafts are taken from the fourth, fifth or sixth rib. They can then be used to reconstruct midfacial deformities, mandible, and alveolar ridge. In contrast to rib, calvarium is harvested as a partial thickness graft by removing only part (inner table or outer table) of skull and avoiding a full thickness defect.

All free bone grafts resorb which is a disadvantage of their use. The rate of resorption depends on the mobility of graft, the degree of vascularization and the site of implantation. Transferred cells die prior to adequate blood

Table 6.10 Tissues used in bone grafting*

Free grafts
    iliac crest (outer surface of iliac bone in pelvic area)
    split rib
    calvaria (skull)

Muscle-bone grafts
    pectoralis major osteocutaneous flap (rib-chest muscle-skin graft for intraoral defect correction)
    trapesius osteomyocutaneous flap (skull-neck muscle-bone graft for mandibular reconstruction)
    temporal composite calvaria graft (skull-muscle on side of head to augment malar areas)

* Marentette, 1991

supply and therefore grafts that transfer both bone and its blood supply are preferred over those that involve only bone.

Grafts involving connective tissue

Connective tissue grafts including fascia, pericranium and dura mater have found increasing use in head and neck surgery (Brodie and Donald, 1991). In general these grafts are composed primarily of fibrous connective tissue that result in strong easily handled materials. Anatomically, fascia is the connective tissue that forms bands that hold together the tissues and organs that make up the body. Pericranium is the connective tissue layer that covers the bones of the skull. Dura mater is another connective tissue membrane that prevents mechanical attachment and damage to brain tissue.

Facial grafts are obtained from either the deep fascia of the thigh or gluteal region and from the fascia near the temporalis muscle in the side of the head. In the thigh, the graft is obtained using a device that forces a razor blade over the fascia and produces a strip of tissue. Pericranial grafts are obtained either through an incision or via dissection during other procedures involving the skull. Dura, in comparison, has been obtained from cadavers and used after chemical treatment as a graft material.

Grafts of fascia (Brodie and Donald, 1991) have been used in

- facial contour augmentation, to fill defects and cover bone irregularities – overcorrection by about 20% is recommended to account for shrinkage
- correction of contour irregularities in the forehead or nose, depressions or humps in bone after removing irregular areas or depressions
- correction for defects in the auricle of ear or eyelid
- creation of a bed for skin grafting, and
- grafting in the oral cavity can be achieved using fascial grafts.

Pericranial grafts are used to

- augment temples, nasolabial folds, frown lines, lips and around orbits
- coat bone grafts and metallic plates
- repair of ear, cleft palate and skull wounds
- repair scalp defects

Other uses include repair of ear and cleft palate as well as complex scalp wounds.

Dural grafts from cadavers are processed and sterilized by a variety of procedures. Processing includes freeze-drying (lyophilization) and sterilization by gamma irradiation or exposure to ethylene oxide. Another form of dura is treated with enzymes, dehydrated with an organic solvent and then gamma irradiated.

Histologically, dura is composed of dense parallel sheets of collagen fibres which are interconnected by elastic fibres. The outer layer is more cellular containing fibroblasts and osteoblasts while the inner layer is thinner and contains collagen fibres that are perpendicular to those of the outer layer.

The inner layer is lined by flattened mesothelial cells. Following implantation of processed dura, it is replaced by endogenous connective tissue from the outside edges towards the centre. The graft serves as template for deposition of new dural tissue.

Dural grafts have been used to correct defects that lead to leakage of cerebrospinal fluid and surgical defects. In most applications dural grafts have been successfully used to repair these defects with a 1–2% rate of infection. However, isolated cases of Creutzfeldt-Jacob disease, a rare neurodegenerative disorder, have been reported following implantation of processed cadaveric dural grafts, which has resulted in concern of continued use of this material.

Dural grafts have been used to reconstruct periodontal, esophageal, mucogingival and oral tissues. It is used as a filler over which epithelial flaps can be placed and eventually become attached to.

6.6 Synthetic implant materials

Synthetic implants offer a number of advantages over tissue grafts. These include eliminating the time required to secure the graft as well as the pain and risk of infection or sickness associated with a second surgical site. In addition, implants for standard procedures such as chin and cheek augmenation come in a variety of sizes and shapes. Some materials like silicone rubber and Teflon can be easily carved by the surgeon to modify an existing implant shape or size. A number of materials are used in facial applications including:

- collagen
- poly(dimethyl siloxane)/Silicone
- poly(terafluoroethylene)/Teflon
- poly(ethylene)
- poly(ethylene terephthalate)/Dacron
- poly(glycolic acid)

The host reaction to synthetic implants varies widely depending on the degradation rate and porosity of the materials. Porous mesh implants allow extensive ingrowth and are effectively fixed to the tissue by fibrous tissue. Solid implants have minimal porosity and therefore are held in place by fibrous tissue that forms a capsule surrounding the implant. Polyglycolic acid and collagen are rapidly replaced by fibrous tissue; however, even by overcorrection using a large implant, the defect may not be permanently removed.

Systemic antibiotics are recommended to be used before and after all procedures performed using implants. Many implants are soaked in antibiotic solutions or the antibiotic solution is forced into the pores within an implant by freeze-drying or exposing the implant to an antibiotic solution under vacuum.

Implants used in the face can be arbitrarily classified by their physical form. Using this approach the classifications include liquids (injectables), solids and meshes. Below, the materials that fall into these categories are described.

6.6.1 Injectable implant materials

A number of injectable polymers are used to augment tissues of the face. They include poly(dimethyl siloxane) also known as silicone and collagen. Although silicone is not approved by the FDA for use as an injectable material in the face, it is use in many facial plastic techniques as a 'touch-up' procedure to remove any small depressions or wrinkles. Collagen is used in an injectable form to remove depressions and wrinkles and mask acne scars.

Injectable silicone

Orentreich and Orentreich (1991) have recently reviewed the use of silicone for soft tissue augmentation. They outline the requirements for an ideal augmentation material as given in Table 6.11. Although no material exists that meets these requirements, silicone oils have been tested for facial augmentation.

Silicone is a term used to refer to polymers that contain the element silicon. The chemical name poly(dimethyl siloxane) includes an acronym derived from **sil**icon, **ox**ygen and meth**ane** (siloxane). A medical grade silicone oil is manufactured by Dow Corning and has viscosity of 350 cSt. This material has an average molecular weight from several thousand to ten thousand and is used for: lubricating suture materials, disposable hypodermic needles and syringes, coatings for containers and in protective skin preparations.

The uses of injectable silicone in the face include treatment of scars and defects in the following.

Table 6.11 Requirements for an ideal augmentation material*

Availability at a low cost
Capable of repeated sterilization to avoid wastage
Long shelf-life at room temperature
Ease of implantation
Chemically inert; does not initiate inflammation or foreign body response
Nontoxic, noncarcinogenic, nonallergenic and nonteratogenic
Mechanical properties similar to host tissue
Persistent over long periods of time; does not calcify or degenerate
Corrects defect in one session

* adapted based on Orentreich and Orentreich (1991)

- Chin
- Crow's feet
- Earlobes
- Eyelids
- Mouth
- Neck
- Nose
- Rhytides (age-associated furrows)

Three principal methods have been used for injection of silicone beneath the skin:

- the microdroplet serial puncture technique,
- the fanning procedure and
- the tattooing method.

These techniques differ in the angle at which the needle is inserted into the skin and the amount of materials injected in a droplet. The microdroplet technique inserts the needle at an angle to the surface of the skin and multiple droplets are injected with a separation distance between droplets of several mms. In the fanning technique the needle is inserted parallel to the surface of the skin and the material is injected forming a droplet that parallels the skin–air interface. Tattooing involves stabbing the needle into the skin at multiple sites maintaining a constant plunger pressure.

Using the microinjection technique, 50–150 needle punctures are needed to treat a typical patient. Treatments are repeated monthly until the desired effect is observed. The material is deposited within the epidermis and dermis if they are less than normal thickess or is placed subdermally when the skin thickness is normal.

Adverse reactions including pain, swelling, redness, skin discolouration, embolism, granuloma formation, silicone migration and connective tissue disease. Silicone is unsuitable for use in eyelids, fibrocystic lesions, inflamed or infected sites and patients with allergic reactions to silicone.

Injectable collagen

Injectable collagen dates back to 1977 (Knapp *et al.*, 1977) when the first report of use of this material in humans was made. Since then, its use has been quite controversial because of the temporary nature of the material and reports of hypersensitivity to the material (Kamer and Churukian, 1984). These events have evoked concern related to this procedure.

Churukian *et al.* (1991) recently reviewed the use of injectable collagen implants including Zyderm I (35 mg/ml), Zyderm II (65 mg/ml) and Zyplast (glutaraldehyde cross-linked Zyderm). Correction with these materials requires continuous maintenance due to the limited persistence of the implant (six to nine months). Patients must be carefully selected and a skin test conducted prior to injection in the face to minimize the possibility of adverse reactions.

New patients undergo two skin tests a month apart prior to treatment. A dermal injection of 0.05–0.1 cc in the forearm is used to raise a bump that can be easily visually identified. If the test site shows any response at 48 and 72 hours, the patient returns for examination. A second injection in the opposite forearm is conducted and the patient is instructed to report any redness, swelling or colour change. About 3.5% show a positive reaction at the initial test site while 1.3% show delayed hypersensitivity (Kamer and Churukian, 1984).

The amount of collagen to be injected into sites chosen for tissue augmentation is judged based on the degree of resorption at the test site. The skin is washed with alcohol prior to and after injection of collagen. After implantation, the skin is treated with steroid cream and massaged. Ice is applied for 20 to 30 minutes following treatment. Topical or oral drugs are used to relieve pain in patients with low thresholds.

Of patients having adverse clinical responses to injectable Zyderm, 56% occurred following the first treatment, 28% after the second, 10% after the third and 6% following subsequent exposures (DeLustro et al., 1987). Patients responding to the first treatment were further broken down to 45% having symptoms within ten days, 22% at more than 30 days (DeLustro et al., 1987).

Differences in collagen implants include concentration of collagen and the introduction of cross-links to decrease the resorption time. Correction with concentrated solutions of collagen resulted in correction with decreased volumes of material. Cross-linked materials were formulated to reduce the antigenicity and increase the persistence time. Cross-linked collagen implants exhibited slower fibroblast colonization and increased collagen deposition in comparison to uncross-linked materials (Stegman et al., 1987).

6.7 Solid facial implants

Although autograft materials are the gold standard for augmenation or reconstruction of facial defects, due to the need of a second surgical site and because of limited amounts of graft tissues, synthetic materials have been developed. The properties of an ideal implant are well defined. In the case of synthetic materials in the form of solid implants, the problem of extrusion of the implant must be considered. This effect has been termed 'rejection'; since there is no evidence that it involves either cell mediated or antibody dependent mechanisms, it is unlikely to be equivalent to classical tissue or organ rejection.

Adams (1991) recently reviewed the use of solid implants for facial augmentation. She concluded that there are four surgical factors that influence implant extrusion. These factors include:

- depth of soft tissue coverage
- implant movement
- infection associated with use of an implant
- introduction of tension in the skin

Coverage of the implant with poorly vascularize thin skin, movement of the implant, infection and closure of the wound containing the implant under tension frequently lead to implant extrusion.

Four polymers including poly(dimethyl siloxane), poly(tetra fluoroethylene), poly(ethylene) and poly(acrylates) are used in facial implants. The first two polymers, poly(dimethyl siloxane) and poly(tetra fluoroethylene) are most widely used; however, the other materials are employed for facial augmentation.

6.7.1 Poly(dimethyl siloxane) solid implants

Poly(dimethyl siloxane), Silastic™ is widely used in areas of the face including the chin and cheek. It is available as a gel-filled implant for augmenation of soft areas and in rubber form for areas of the face that are stiffer. Implants are inserted after soaking in an antibiotic solution and patients are given prophylactic antibiotics before and after surgery.

Chin augmentation with Silastic™ is a successful procedure as a result of a thick layer of soft tissue that is present over the implant and the relatively little motion that the implant experiences. It is easily inserted since it will deform and makes a good fit over the mandible. The wide variety of sizes available as well as the ability of this material to be carved by the surgeon allows on site custom implant design.

The size implant is determined by dropping a vertical line from the chin and by measuring the distance between the chin and vertical line. Implants are available to increase the projection of the chin 4–14 mm. Implants are normally inserted through an incision in the mouth (intraoral route), although insertion is also achieved by an extraoral route by making an incision in the crease between the lower lips and chin.

Infrequent complications include:

- bone erosion
- bleeding
- implant extrusion
- improper positioning
- infection

Patients experiencing tenderness, swelling and redness around the implant are treated with antibiotics for three weeks. In some cases the infection will re-occur and re-treatment with antibiotics is recommended. If the infection does not clear after treatment with antibiotics, then the implant must be removed.

Cheek (malar) and augmentation to areas below the cheek (submalar) are procedures commonly used to improve the appearance of high cheek bones and maintain a young appearance, respectively. Although the complication rate observed with malar implants is low, a complication rate as high as 12.6% is reported for submalar implants (Binder *et al.*, 1981).

Augmentation of other areas of the face including the forehead have been reported with Silastic™. The nose, because of its high flexibility and mobility and thin soft tissue covering, is the only part of the face that is avoided when using this material. High extrusion rates have been reported when it is used as a nasal implant.

6.7.2 Poly(tetra fluoroethylene) solid implants

Poly(tetra fluoroethylene) implants contain either carbon fibres or aluminium oxide as reinforcing materials. Both of these soft tissue implants are manufactured as sponges with pores occupying about 70% of the volume. Pore sizes are in the hundreds of micrometres making these implants easy to 'carve' into custom shapes and sizes.

Initially this polymer initiates a significant inflammatory response that eventually subsides in a period of months (Arem *et al.*, 1972). It is used for augmentation of (Adams, 1991):

- alveolar ridge
- cheek
- chin
- forehead
- mandible reconstruction
- middle ear
- nasal dorsum
- orbital floor
- temple
- tibiomandibular joint

6.7.3 Poly(ethylene) solid implants

Porous high density polyethylene is used in facial tissue augmentation, and as an ossicular implant. Rubin *et al.*, (1981) reported use of poly(ethylene) implants as malar and skull grafts. Berghaus (1985) reported correction of frontal, orbital rim and external ear defects in four patients with this material.

6.7.4 Acrylic solid implants

These materials are either polymers of acrylic acid or of methacrylic acid. They are formed just prior to implantation using polymer powdered granules that are mixed with liquid monomer at room temperature. Any residual monomer remaining unreacted will contribute to adverse reactions to this material. For this reason the mixing time of this material is very critical. Mixing times of 2.5–3 minutes are optimal with frequent beating required to ensure monomer reaction. A total of seven minutes is required for mixing and fitting the implant into the desired space. An additional seven minutes is then required for hardening.

The exothermic nature of the reaction results in the generation of heat thus requiring constant irrigation to avoid death to the surrounding tissues. Although orthopaedic surgeons have reported several adverse effects of methacrylate monomer including allergic reactions, none have been reported for facial or skull augmentation (Adams, 1991). These materials have been used for chin and forehead augmentation.

6.8 Mesh materials

A number of synthetic polymers are used in the form of an open mesh work of fibres including poly(glycolic) acid and poly(lactic acid) copolymer, tradenamed Vicryl™, poly(amide) tradenamed Supramid™ and poly(ethylene terephthalate) tradenamed Mersilene™.

Mesh materials are used for any site requiring augmenation where small defects or contour defects exist such as the bridge of the nose, the chin, and the cheeks. Vicryl™ has been used to smooth out irregularities on the nose where the skin is thin (Beekhuis and Colton, 1991). Mesh products have been used for chin augmentation, mandible angle, forehead and jawline recontouring.

6.9 Summary

Both biological and synthetic polymeric materials are used in facial plastic surgery. Tissue grafts include cartilage, connective tissue, bone, bone-muscle, rib, and ear lobe. Synthetic implants include injectables, solid implants and meshed products. Each of these materials works well in specific applications.

In the nose, tissue grafts are superior to synthetics. Use of synthetics in the nose can result in implant extrusion. Injectable implants are used to correct small defects and scars. These materials include silicone, collagen and other products that are injected sub-dermally. Solid implants are used to make large corrections of defects. The later classification includes chin and cheek implants that are produced in a variety of sizes.

The increasing desire for plastic surgery is creating a demand for new implants. The increasing concern over the long-term effects of medical implants will result in the continued controversy over use of permanent polymeric materials.

7.
Dental Implants

7.1 Introduction

A number of materials are used in the practice of dentistry including impression materials to copy the contours of the gum, appliances and dentures to replace or correct deficiency of the grinding surfaces, and restorative materials to correct defects in natural surfaces (Table 7.1).

According to *Skinners Science of Dental Materials* (Phillips, 1991), there are a number of considerations to development of materials to be used in the mouth and specifically as restorative materials. These include

- consideration of thermal changes
- minimization of contact between dissimilar materials, and
- prevention of microleakage

Microleakage of oral fluids through restorative materials leads to penetration of acids and micro-organisms into the pulp of the tooth. This problem arises as a result of less than adequate adhesion of dental filing materials to the tooth surface especially in areas where the contour changes are discontinuous. Thermal conductivity and coefficient of thermal expansion are two material properties that determine whether excessive pressure will be exerted on the dental pulp as a result of changes in temperature. Temperatures as high as 65°C are associated with eating hot and cold foods. Finally, when two dissimilar metals contact each other in the presence of a conductive environment, a half-cell current is produced that leads to

Table 7.1 Types of materials used in dentistry

Material	Use
Impression materials	formation of negative and positive replicas of gum surface
Dentures and appliances	replacement and correction of grinding surface defects
Restorative materials	correction of defects in natural grinding surface

corrosion and dissolution of restorative materials. This is a very important concept that should be considered early in the implant design phase.

As with implants designed to be used internally within the body, dental materials are first subjected to standard safety tests to determine if they are sterile, non-pyrogenic, non-cytotoxic, non-mutagenic, non-carcinogenic or induce an allergic reaction (Table 7.2). Once safety tests (level I testing) are completed successfully, other tests (level II testing) in primates or other species are initiated to evaluate pulp reactions, repair and inflammation in comparison to positive (silicate cement) and negative (zinc oxide) controls. If the results of these tests are positive (i.e., no reactions are observed), then human testing (level III testing) is initiated.

7.2 Impression materials

Impression materials are used to make a reproduction of the gum surface as a mould for 'casting' replacement materials and dentures. They are used for corrective lining in a preliminary impression. In addition, to these impression materials, colloids and elastomeric materials are used in some part of the fabrication of an impression (Table 7.3).

The steps used in formulation of primary and secondary impression materials are

1. place primary impression material in contact with gum (plaster);
2. using primary impression made above, make a cast using dental stone;
3. using acrylic or other polymer, a tray is fabricated over the stone cast; and then
4. a secondary impression is made in the tray using zinc oxide-eugenol paste.

7.2.1 Gypsum and plaster of Paris

Gypsum is the common name given to the compound calcium sulphate dihydrate (Table 7.4). When gypsum is heated to temperatures between 110° and 130°C it is converted to calcium sulphate hemihydrate also known

Table 7.2 Safety and efficacy testing of dental materials

Type of test	Tests conducted
Level I	Sterility, pyrogenicity, cytotoxicity, mutagenicity, carcinogenicity and allergic reaction induction
Level II	Evaluation of pulp reactions, repair and inflammation
Level III	Human studies

Table 7.3 Types of impression materials

Type	Use	Advantage or (disadvantage)
Plaster of Paris	Primary impression	Inexpensive
Dental stone cast	Formation over primary impression	Rigid cast material
Zinc-eugenol	Secondary impression	Some distortion when used to take impression over teeth
Hydrocolloid	Primary impression	Gels at room temperature
Elastomeric	Primary impression	Reproduces impression of teeth

Table 7.4 Formation of plaster of Paris and dental stone

Gypsum + elevated temperature =
  calcium sulphate hemihydrate (plaster of Paris)
  Plaster of Paris used to make impression of surface

Gypsum + calcined under steam = alpha-hemihydrate (dental stone)
  Dental Stone used to make a cast by pouring over impression material and then it is allowed to harden

as beta hemihydrate or plaster of Paris. This is a loose crystalline form of calcium sulphate in contrast to alpha-hemihydrate (dental stone), a more highly crystalline form. Alpha-hemihydrate is calcined under steam pressure at temperatures between 120° and 150°C. Plaster of Paris is used to make impression materials (negative model of surface) while dental stone is used to form a cast (positive model of surface) by pouring it into dental impression materials.

Gypsum materials are characterized by setting times, or the time required to form crystalline materials from a water suspension.

7.2.2 Zinc-eugenol impression materials

Zinc oxide-eugenol materials are used as impression materials, cements, and filling materials. They are formulated from zinc oxide paste that is mixed with eugenol (an alkyl phenyl) to form zinc eugenolate. Accelerators include water, acetic acid, zinc acetate, and calcium chloride (Table 7.5). Initial setting times of between three and six minutes and final setting times of between 10 and 15 minutes are frequently observed.

Zinc-oxide eugenol pastes are used to aid in retention of medications on the surface of wounds and in wound healing. They are also used as

Table 7.5 Formation of zinc-oxide eugenol materials

$$\text{Zinc oxide paste} + \text{eugenol} \xrightarrow{\text{accelerators}} \text{zinc eugenolate}$$

Accelerators = water, acetic acid, zinc acetate, calcium chloride

---

temporary crown and bridge cements. Their use is somewhat limited by the stinging and burning sensation that occurs when they are applied to soft tissues as well as the gastric disturbance that occurs with free eugenol digestion.

Paste impression materials often result in distortion when used to take an impression of teeth. The distortion is introduced when the impression is removed from the locations that contact the gum–tooth interface. To overcome this problem, elastic impression materials have been developed.

7.2.3 Hydrocolloid impression materials

Hydrocolloid impression materials used in dentistry include reversible and irreversible materials. Hydrocolloids are materials containing large amounts of water and large particles. At high temperatures the material will flow like a liquid while if the colloid gels (particles clump together) as the temperature is lowered a solid forms. Normally the material is placed in an impression tray in the solution state and impressed against the mouth tissues to be reproduced. The tray is held in place and water circulating through the cooling tubes causes the hydrocolloid to solidify. When the material has gelled the tray is removed and it is prepared for pouring dental stone on top of the impression. In order for a colloid to be useful as an impression material it must be liquid at a temperature tolerated by dental tissues and must gel at or above oral temperature.

Reversible hydrocolloid impression materials include agar, a linear polysaccharide containing galactose and sulphuric acid esters, which is derived from seaweed. These materials gel by cooling below the gelation temperature and can be liquified by reheating. The gelation temperature for agar is 37°C which is in the range (36–42°C) typically found for dental materials (Table 7.6). Typically the composition of the hydrocolloid includes agar (8–15%) and Borax (0.2–0.5%) which strengthens the gel. Specifications set by the American Dental Association for the mechanical properties of these materials include compressive strength above 0.245 MPa and permanent set after a 10 % linear strain applied for 30 seconds not to exceed 1.5%.

Irreversible hydrocolloids do not liquify after reheating above the gelation temperature. They include brown seaweed which is a polymer of anhydro-beta-D-mannuronic acid trivially known as alginic acid (Table 7.7). Several salts including the sodium, potassium and triethanol amine are used in

Table 7.6 Formation of impression materials from reversible hydrocolloids

Agar (liquid at temp > 42°C) + additives $\xrightarrow{\text{cool to 37°C}}$ Gelation

Composition: Agar (8–15%), Borax (0.2–0.5%), water

Specifications: Compressive strength >0.245 MPa, permanent set after a 10% linear strain for 30 seconds <1.5%

Table 7.7 Formulation of irreversible impression materials

Alginate + calcium sulfate $\longrightarrow$ insoluble calcium alginate

Composition: 15% alginate, 16% calcium sulphate, 60% diatomaceous earth, 2% sodium fluoride, 4% zinc oxide and 3% fluoride

Properties: Geling times of 3 to 4 minutes give compressive strengths >0.343 MPa

dental impression materials. Gelation is achieved by mixing soluble alginate with a solution of calcium sulphate which causes the complex, calcium alginate to precipitate into an insoluble complex. The composition of the final mixture is about 15% alginate, 16% calcium sulphate, 60% diatomaceous earth, 2% sodium phosphate, 4% zinc oxide and 3% fluoride. The diatomaceous earth, fluoride and zinc oxide act as fillers to firm the gel. Insolubility is believed to occur as a result of divalent calcium cations bridging two adjacent polysaccharide chains. Optimal gelling times of three to four minutes at 20°C give compressive strengths greater than 0.343 MPa.

7.2.4 Elastomeric impression materials
Included in this classification are synthetic polymers used in the production of impressions. They include

- poly(sulfides)
- silicones
- Poly(ethers)

These impression materials can undergo large deformations reversibly without failing or loss of dimensions and are therefore used over areas where the impression material must come in contact with existing teeth.

Poly(sulfides) are polymers that contain sulphur atoms linked together into long chains. They are cross-linked from a pre-polymer via sulfhydryl groups (SH) that react in the presence of lead oxide and peroxides. This material is mixed on a sheet of plastic lined paper or glass prior to use.

Two types of silicone impression materials are used including condensation products which yield by-products of polymerization and addition type products that react without generating additional chemical species. Condensation products derive from a hydroxyl terminated poly(dimethyl siloxane) which has a backbone of repeating silicon atoms separated by oxygen atoms. Two methyl side chains are attached to each silicon atom. In the presence of tri- and tetrafunctional alkyl silicates, cross-links are formed releasing an alcohol as a byproduct. To these products are added silica or metal oxide particles to stiffen the polymer chain backbone.

Addition type silicone polymers are derivatives of dimethyl siloxane with vinyl ($-CH=CH_2$) end groups. Cross-linking is achieved using a silane coupling agent. The polymer is formed by mixing the pre-polymer which is contained in one tube with the cross-linking agent contained in a second tube.

7.3 Denture base resins

Dentures consist of a base in which artificial teeth are embedded.
The formation of dentures is as follows.

1. Prepare primary impression of gum
2. Form stone cast over primary impression
3. Place the base constructed from sheets of polystyrene on top of stone cast
4. Position artificial teeth on base using wax
5. Set cast, base plate and positioned teeth in freshly made dental stone or plaster in a denture flask
6. Separate the flasks and remove dental base and wax
7. Place material in mould with denture resin material
8. After denture formed and cured, remove from flask and finish

Poly(methyl methacrylate) is the principal polymer used in formation of the dental base material. It is employed in the form of a powder containing small spherical beads and dispersed by mixing with a solution containing monomer. The solubility of the polymer in the monomer is increased by addition of 5% or less of a co-polymer of methyl methacrylate and ethyl acrylate or by adding 8–10% of a plasticizer such as dibutyl phthalate. The plasticizer must be soluble in the polymer causing it to swell. An initiator is added such as benzoyl peroxide as well as 1–2% of a cross-linking agent such as glycol dimethyacrylate into the solvent. A pigment is added to colour the base to match the gum.

7.4 Restorative resins

A number of materials are used to repair defects in teeth involving either the filling in of cavities or the replacement of the grinding surface. Cavities are filled in using what are termed resin materials either by directly pressing a viscous material that later sets in place or by constructing a mould for casting

Table 7.8 Definitions of terms referred to in restoration of grinding surfaces

Word	Definition
Resin	Polymer containing mixture
Inlay	Cast material used to fill in cavity
Unfilled resin	Does not contain particulates for mechanical reinforcement
Filled resin	Contains particulates for mechanical reinforcement
Conventional	Contains 70–80% particulate material $> 1\mu m$
Microfilled	Contains 30–50% of particles 0.04–0.06 μm

a piece of material that will fit into the defect (inlay) (Table 7.8). Resins are classified as unfilled or composites. Composite resins are further broken into the categories of conventional and microfilled resins.

7.4.1 Unfilled and composite resins

Unfilled resins consist of a two component system such as an acrylic polymer in powder form that is mixed with monomer containing about 5% methyl methacrylate prior to use (Table 7.9). The mixture initially is a viscous liquid that reacts with cross-linking agents to polymerize in the cavity into a hard material. The powdered polymer normally contains an initiator such as a peroxide (0.3–3% benzoyl peroxide) to initiate cross-linking while the liquid contains an amine to complete the reaction. Resins prepared using this approach have compressive strengths of about 69 MPa, moduli of about 2.4 GPa, water absorption of about 2% (after one week at 37°C) and 7% polymerization shrinkage.

Table 7.9 Composition and properties of unfilled resins

Acrylic polymer	+ Monomer	+ 5% methyl methacrylate
(powder)	(liquid)	(liquid)

+ cross-linking initiator (peroxide)

Physical properties: Compressive strength = 69 MPa, modulus = 2.4 GPa, water absorption = 2%

Conventional composite resins consist of a resin binder, a filler and a coupling agent (Table 7.10). The resin, normally contains a polymer such as BIS-GMA, which is a derivative of methyl methacrylate. The polymer in paste form is mixed with peroxide to initiate cross-linking after mixing with another liquid or paste which is composed of dimethacrylate monomer and amine which is also required to complete the cross-linking reaction. In addition, UV and visible light curing systems are also available for resin cross-linking.

Composite systems contain 70–80% of filler material such as crystalline quartz and/or lithium glass ceramics, calcium silicate, glass beads, glass fibres and calcium fluoride. Particle sizes between 1 and 100μm are commonly used in the formulation of the system. A coupling agent such as vinyl silane or gamma-methacryloxy propyl silane is used to bond the filler particles to the polymer chains. The resulting resin mechanical properties include compressive strength of 235 MPa, modulus of 13.7 GPa, water absorption of 0.6% and polymerization shrinkage 1.4%. Glazing agents are used to coat the resin surface to eliminate roughness and minimize wear of the restorative material.

Microfilled composites are similar to conventional composites except that the filler is composed of very fine particles (0.06–0.04). The use of fine particles improves surface smoothness and wear. Optimum mechanical properties are obtained when filler particles make up 35–50% by weight of the resin. Mechanical properties of these resins include compressive strength of 276 MPa, modulus of 4.5 GPa, water absorption of 1.4% and polymer shrinkage of 1.7% (Table 7.11).

7.4.2 Alloys used as restorative materials

A variety of metal alloys are used in the mouth for repair of cavities as well as for preparation of crowns and bridges. Among the best known

Table 7.10 Composition and mechanical properties of conventional composite resins

---

Resin Binder
    BIS-GMA, initiator, cross-linking agent

Filler (70–80%)
    crystalline quartz, lithium glass ceramics, calcium silicate, glass beads, glass fibres, calcium fluoride

Coupling agent
    vinyl silane or gamma-methacryloxy propyl silane

Properties: Compressive strength = 235 MPa, Modulus = 13.7 GPa, water absorption = 0.6%, shrinkage = 1.4%

Table 7.11 Comparison of mechanical properties of unfilled and filled resins

Type	Compressive strength (MPa)	Modulus (GPa)	Water absorption (%)
Unfilled	69	2.4	2
Conventional composite	235	13.7	0.6
Microfilled composite	276	4.5	1.4

materials include dental amalgums used to repair cavities as well as alloys of gold used for construction of dental appliances. Other uses for alloys include wires used for clasps with partial dentures in addition to metal-ceramic composites.

Amalgams are metal alloys that contain mercury. An amalgam is made by taking a metal alloy powder and mixing it with liquid mercury. The mixture is a paste that hardens as the mercury dissolves away the surface of the alloy particles. The hardening reaction is a result of formation of a precipitate at the grain boundary interfaces. It has been estimated that over 160 million amalgam restorations are conducted each year. Failure of dental amalgams is a result of excessive expansion leading to interfacial separation between the enamel and the alloy.

Amalgam systems used include low and high copper systems. Low copper amalgams typically contain 6% copper, 65% silver and 29% tin while high copper amalgams contain anywhere from 6–30% copper. Silver-tin amalgams are brittle unless a small amount of copper is used to replace silver atoms. Inclusion of zinc increases ductility and acts as an oxygen scavenger to prevent oxide formation.

High copper amalgams include admixed and single composition alloys. Admixed alloys are formed by mixing low copper alloy particles with spherical silver-copper alloy particles. Single composition alloys involve silver, copper and tin atoms contained in the same particle. The advantage of single composition and admixed alloys is the improvement in compressive strengths and decrease in creep rates (see Table 7.12).

7.4.3 Direct filling gold

Gold is used in various forms as a filling material. It is supplied free of surface contaminants (cohesive gold) or with non-volatile agents adsorbed to the surface (noncohesive gold). Available forms include foil, electrolytic precipitate, powder and in alloys with calcium.

Table 7.12 Mechanical properties of amalgums

Amalgam	Compressive strength (MPa)	Creep* (%)	Tensile strength (MPa)
Low copper	343	2.0	60
Admix	431	0.4	48
Single composition	510	0.13	64

*Creep is measured as change in length divided by original length between one and four hours after a compressive load of 36 MPa is applied at 37°C to a cylinder 8 mm long and 4 mm in diameter that was aged for one week.

Noble metal alloys are also used in dental appliance construction (crowns, bridges and partials). They contain gold, silver, copper, palladium, platinum, and zinc atoms. One per cent of palladium atoms is required for every 3% silver to offset the tarnishing propensity of silver.

Inlays or crowns are made directly or indirectly. Using a die or the indirect method, a wax pattern is made of the tooth using paraffin. The wax is surrounded by a gypsum containing material (investment material) and the alloy is cast in the investment material after removal of the wax.

7.5 Cements for restorations

Cements are used in dentistry for restorations to correct temporary, intermediate or aesthetic problems:

- silicates
- glass ionomer
- zinc phosphate
- zinc-eugenol
- polycarboxylate

The major cements used include silicates and glass ionomer.

Silicate cements consist of a powder and liquid system that are mixed prior to use. The powder consists of finely ground ceramic termed acid soluble glass that contains about 40% silica (SiO_2), 30% alumina (Al_2O_3), 19% calcium phosphate with lime (CaO), sodium fluoride (NaF), calcium fluoride (CaF_2) and cryolite (Na_3AlF_6) (Table 7.13). The liquid component is similar to that used in zinc phosphate cements and contains phosphoric acid, zinc, aluminium and magnesium phosphate.

When the powder and liquid are mixed an acid-base reaction occurs with hydrogen ions of the phosphoric acid attacking the glass and displacing aluminium, sodium and calcium positively charged ions. Displaced ions collect in the semi-liquid phase and as the pH rises, metal ions precipitate as

Table 7.13 Composition of powder and liquid components of silicate cements

---
Powder-acid soluble glass
   40% silica, 30% alumina, 19% calcium phosphate, sodium fluoride, calcium fluoride, and cryolite

Liquid
   phosphoric acid, zinc, aluminium and magnesium phosphate
---

phosphates and fluorides. The physical properties of silicate cements are given in Table 7.14.

Although silicate cements have higher strengths as compared to glass ionomer base material, they will generate a severe tissue response when placed in contact with pulp. Therefore, silicates are applied after a base coating has been used consisting of zinc oxide-eugenol or calcium hydroxide cements.

Glass ionomer cements are used for cosmetic corrections and for restoration of lesions (Table 7.15). They involve a system consisting of a liquid and a powder that are activated by mixing. The liquid contains polyacrylic acid (a co-polymer of acrylic and itaconic acid) and 5% tartaric acid. The powder contains aluminosilicate glass prepared using fluoride fluxes. Once the powder and liquid are mixed, a paste is formed in which the glass surface is

Table 7.14 Physical properties of cements

Property	Silicate cement	Glass ionomer
Compressive strength (MPa)	180	140
Tensile strength (MPa)	3.5	2.7
Solubility at 24 hours	0.7%	0.4%
Pulp response	severe*	mild

* Generates pulp response due to acidic pH; normally pulp protected by covering with a layer of zinc oxide-eugenol or calcium hydroxide cement prior to silicate use.

Table 7.15 Components of glass ionomer cements

Powder
   aluminosilicate glass

Liquid
   poly(acrylic acid), 5% tartaric acid
---

attacked by the acid, and aluminium, calcium and sodium ions are liberated. The polyanion chains are cross-linked by calcium and aluminium polysalts that form during the reaction.

7.6 Dental porcelains

Porcelain used are given in Table 7.16. Dental porcelains consist of crystalline materials in a glass matrix. The glass phase is made from finely divided powders, sintered or compacted together at high temperatures. Materials can be classified as high (1288–1371°C), medium (1093–1260°C) and low (871–1066°C) temperature fusing materials. Artificial teeth contain high temperature fusing materials and consist of 75–85% feldspar which contains potassium aluminium silicate ($K_2O\ Al_2O_3\ 6SiO_2$) and albite ($Na_2O\ Al_2O_3\ 6SiO_2$). Feldspar melts at 1250–1500°C and when cooled fuses to become a glass containing free crystalline silica.

7.7 Base metal alloys for dental castings

Removable prosthetics used in the mouth are composed largely of chromium-cobalt-nickel alloys. They are used in the fabrication of partial dental frameworks. The cobalt is the base element of these alloys and can be present at levels up to 70%. Nickel or chromium is added at levels up to 30% to protect against corrosion. Other alloys including combinations of cobalt and nickel or cobalt and chromium and iron and chromium are used. Mechanical properties of these alloys are given in Table 7.17.

Table 7.16 Use of porcelains in dentistry

Artificial teeth
Inlays
Jacket crowns
Veneers over cast crowns

Table 7.17 Mechanical properties of partial denture alloys*

Alloy	Tensile strength (MPa)	Failure elongation (%)	Modulus (GPa)
Co-Cr	870	1.6	223.5
Ni-Cr	800	3.8	182
Co-Cr-Ni	685	8	198
Fe-Cr	841	9	202

* adapted from Phillips (1991)

The ductility of Co-Cr-Ni alloys is better than that of either Co-Cr and Co-Ni alloys while the tensile strength and modulus are only somewhat lower than that of these other alloys. Therefore Co-Cr-Ni alloys give optimum overall mechanical properties.

7.8 Other materials, collagen

The materials discussed above are widely used in dentistry. A number of new materials such as collagen are beginning to find applications including promotion of ingrowth into synthetic implants, prevention of oral bleeding, support of regeneration of periodontal tissues, encouragement of new bone growth, promotion of healing of mucosal lining and prevention of migration of epithelial cells. Below, in Table 7.18, the development of these materials is discussed.

Dressing materials containing collagen are needed to promote healing of defects in oral mucous membranes. Mitchell (1983) reported the use of a porcine collagen graft as a dressing for denuded mucous membrane. In this study, lyophilized sterilized porcine collagen from the dermis was immersed in saline, cut into the desired shape and sutured into place over mucosal defects. The mucosal defects were created by removal of a variety of pathological lesions. The material acted as a biological dressing and the denuded areas quickly became covered by normal mucous membrane.

Collagen has also been used to promote attachment to implant materials. Yaffee et al. (1982) reported the treatment of acrylic dental roots with collagen. The implantation of acrylic teeth normally is associated with less than desirable attachment between the implant and the host tissue. This ultimately leads to rejection of the implant. Native soluble dog-skin collagen was reconstituted and acrylic roots were immersed in collagen solutions. The coated root replicas were then inserted into extraction sockets. The results of these studies indicate that collagen treated roots were retained and accepted, leading to connective tissue proliferation and new bone formation around the implants.

The use of collagen as an agent to control bleeding in general surgery has led to its use in the oral cavity. Stein and co-workers (Stein et al., 1985) reported the use of collagen absorbable haemostatic sponges to control bleeding at a mucosal graft donor site. The procedure used evaluated control of bleeding of a mucosal graft bed taken from the lateral-posterior surface of the palate using a collagen sponge material. After removal of the donor tissue, a sterile collagen sponge was cut to the size of the donor site and directly applied to the wound. After completion of the graft procedure, the collagen sponge was left in place and covered with a periodontal dressing. One week later, any remaining collagen sponge was removed from the wound. At this time the wound showed no evidence of infection, necrosis or tissue reaction. Well formed granulation tissue was observed in the palatal donor area and wound healing proceeded normally.

Table 7.18 Uses of collagen in dentistry

Material	Observation	Reference
Collagen	Collagen sponges decreased seepage of blood during periodontal mucogingival surgery	Stein et al., 1984
Collagen	Collagen membranes have capacity to support regeneration of periodontal tissues	Pitaru et al., 1988
Collagen-allogeneic bone	Collagen gel-allogeneic bone implant encouraged ingrowth of regenerative tissue and new bone	Blumenthal and Steinberg, 1990
Collagen-tricalcium phosphate	Collagen-tricalcium phosphate grafts resulted in less soft tissue recession	Blumenthal et al., 1986
Collagen coated root implants	Long lasting retention of collagen coated acrylic root implants	Yaffee et al., 1982
Collagen solution	Collagen solution applied to root surface suppressed epithelial migration and new tissue formation	Minabe et al., 1988
Collagen graft	Collagen graft promoted formation of normal mucous membrane	Mitchell, 1983
Collagen-allogeneic bone	Bone collagen grafts reduced probing depths and gained new attachment	Blumenthal and Steinberg, 1990
Collagen solution	Application of collagen solution to root surface suppressed epithelial migration and promoted new cementum formation	Minabe et al., 1988
Collagen film + tetracycline	Topical administration of tetracycline on a collagen film remains active for two to three weeks	Minabe et al., 1989

Periodontal flap surgery is conducted to re-establish a stable healthy periodontal environment by reducing pocket depth and the associated propensity for infection. Repair of gingival or bony pockets using flap surgery results in less recession and some new soft tissue attachment; however, some associated bone loss remains a problem. Both hydroxyapatite and tricalcium phosphate are synthetic ceramic materials that have been used to fill periodontal defects (Meffert et al., 1985; Baldock et al., 1985).

Blumenthal et al. (1986) and Blumenthal and Steinberg (1990) reported the use of collagen membrane barriers in conjunction with combined demineralized bone-collagen gel implants in dog and human bony defects. Their goal was to promote bony defect healing since many of these defects fail to heal after surgical treatment. Other studies indicated that epithelium that migrate between the tooth and adjacent tissues prevents regeneration (Canton and Zander, 1976; Polson and Heijl, 1978) and attachment of gum to bone.

Blumenthal et al. (1986) studied a combination of autolysed antigen-extracted allogeneic (AAA) bone and collagen gel on gaining new attachment in surgically created defects in dogs over 24 weeks. Results reported in this study include that the collagen gel encouraged ingrowth of regenerative tissue-fibroblasts in the early stages of wound healing while allogeneic bone induced new bone formation. In a later study, Blumenthal and Steinberg (1990) compared debrided controls at one year with autolysed antigen-extracted allogeneic (AAA) bone grafts alone, combined AAA bone-microfibrillar collagen grafts, and debrided grafts covered with a collagen membrane. Results of these studies indicated that the best bone fill and defect morphology was observed in wounds treated with AAA-microfibrillar collagen and covered by a collagen membrane.

Blumenthal et al., (1986) used tricalcium phosphate ceramic (TCP) in conjunction with microfibrillar collagen as a space filler in pocket elimination surgery. Using this approach 16.74% less soft tissue recession was observed compared to control sites. It was concluded that this treatment modality may have value in reducing aesthetic deformities, food impaction areas, and root exposure that often occurs following periodontal surgery.

Pitaru et al. (1988) used collagen membranes to prevent migration of epithelium during periodontal wound healing. The use of a Millipore filter as a barrier between root surfaces and periodontal flaps has been shown to prevent apical migration of epithelial cells during the initial stages of wound healing. They showed that the treated root surface allowed colonization of gingival or periodontal ligament fibroblasts that may lead to connective tissue attachment to bone (Melcher, 1976).

Results of this group (Pitaru et al., 1988) indicate that

1. collagen membranes have the capacity to support regeneration of periodontal tissues;

2. collagen membranes are either incorporated within the healing tissues or degraded by these during the healing process.

Exposure of dentin collagen resulting from demineralization of the root surface provides a collagen fibre scaffold as a matrix for cellular attachment (Boyko et al., 1980; Polson and Proyne, 1983). Minabe et al. (1988) evaluated the effects of application of collagen solution after periodontal flap surgery and demineralization of the root surface. In their studies the root surface was washed with saline followed by citric acid pH=1.0 and then a 2% collagen solution. The experimental results indicated that application of the collagen solution after acid conditioning in flap surgery promoted suppression of epithelial migration and new cementum formation. They hypothesized that in the presence of collagen increased cementum formation occurred via proliferation of periodontal ligament cells.

Collagen has also been used as a carrier substance for immobilization of various active substances used in dentistry. The amount of tetracycline released from a cross-linked collagen film in the liquid pool within the periodontal pocket exceeded the minimal inhibitory concentration (8 µg/ml) even ten days after insertion (Minabe et al., 1989a). In a later study Minabe et al. (1989) evaluated the therapeutic effect after administration of the collagen film with immobilized tetracycline. The collagen film immobilized tetracycline patient group showed significantly lower values for bleeding upon probing the pocket depth for three to four weeks. In addition, the density of micro-organisms and proportion of motile rods and spirochetes were also significantly decreased three weeks after administration.

7.9 Summary

Polymers, alloys, and ceramics are used in different phases of dentistry. Polymeric materials are used as impression materials, denture base and restorative resins, cements and materials that promote repair of periodontal and muscosal defects. Metal alloys are used for preparation of crowns and bridges, inlays and repair of cavities. Ceramics are used as impression materials, in cements and in artificial teeth.

The safety and efficacy of dental materials is evaluated based on standard biocompatibility testing (Level I) evaluation of pulp reactions, repair and inflammation (Level II) and human studies (Level III). Although the biocompatibility is an essential component of the evaluation, other mechanical and chemical factors are important in the usefulness of a material in a particular application. Factors such as setting time, ultimate tensile strength, modulus, percent shrinkage and dimensional stability are all important design parameters.

8.
Breast implants

8.1 Introduction

An estimated 150 000 women undergo breast augmentation each year (Sprague Zones, 1992). About 80% of these women have the surgery to increase the size of their breasts for cosmetic reasons, the remainder have implants that are inserted for reconstruction after removal of breast tissue for health related reasons. The US market alone for these implants is about $100 million annually which is about three times the European market. Major commercial suppliers include Aesthetech, Cox-Uphoff, Dow Corning Wright, McGhan, Mentor and Surgitek. Implant classifications include smooth gel-filled, textured gel-filled, polyurethane covered, saline-filled, double lumen and permanent expander (Table 8.1). The smooth gel-filled implant is most commonly used based on published estimates (Sprague Zones, 1992). The total breast implant market has been estimated to be 300 000 units per year in 1986.

Breast augmentation as a surgical procedure began over 90 years ago with the transplantation of autograft material. Unsatisfactory results due to tissue resorption and donor site scarring led to the search for the ideal polymeric material. Prior to 1976, the year of the Medical Device Amendment to the Federal Food, Drug, and Cosmetic Act of 1938, the FDA did not regulate the distribution and sales of breast implants on the market. After 1976,

Table 8.1 Percentage of breast implants used for augmentation and reconstruction*

Type of implant	Augmentation	Reconstruction
Smooth gel-filled	37.0	25.2
Textured gel-filled	26.4	23.8
Polyurethane covered	18.8	22.2
Saline-filled	5.5	3.1
Double lumen	12.4	11.2
Permanent expander		14.5

* adapted from Sprague Zones, 1992

manufacturers were required only to show safety and efficacy data if their device was not substantially equivalent to a pre-1976 implant. For this reason most breast implants on the market were developed based on substantial equivalence to pre-1976 devices.

In November 1988, the General and Plastic Surgical Devices Advisory Panel reviewed confidential information from Dow Corning, indicating that silicone gel leakage was associated with development of cancerous tumours in animal models. The panel recommended that the FDA provide educational materials describing the benefits and risks of breast implants for consumers.

In a recent release (February, 1991), the FDA provided background information on 'The Possible Health Risks of Silicone Breast Implants' as a result of the growing concern about their safety. The FDA has required all manufacturers of these implants to provide scientific evidence for the safety of their products by the summer of 1991.

In April 1991, the FDA announced that the manufacturers of silicone gel-filled breast implants must file PMAs within 90 days or stop distributing their implants. Later in 1992, the FDA limited the use of these implants to breast reconstruction following cancer excision.

The risks as described by the FDA related to silicone breast implants are two-fold. The first relates to difficulty imaging the breast for abnormalities in the presence of an implant while the second involves deposition and contraction of fibrous tissue that surrounds the implant causing pain. In some cases leakage of fluid from the implant and migration of the released material requires a second surgical procedure to remove as much of the material as possible.

8.2 Anatomy and physiology of the breast

The breast is a superficial organ consisting of the nipple, areolar glands, lobes containing a duct system, lobules of glandular tissue, supporting connective tissue and surrounding fat (see Figure 8.1 and Table 8.2). It extends over the superficial layer of abdominal muscles and up to the pectoral muscles (Hall-Craggs, 1990). A single lactiferous duct from each lobe opens onto the nipple by combining with other ducts to form lactiferous sinuses. Milk is produced in the lobules of the glandular tissue and flows through the duct into the sinuses. The nipple is lubricated through areolar glands contained in the circular pigmented area (areola).

Microscopically, dense connective tissue is observed between the lobes that make up breast tissue. Lobes are in turn made up of lobules containing small groups of tubules, interlobular ducts and intralobular connective tissue (Figure 8.2). Contained in the intralobular connective tissue are fibroblasts, some lymphocytes, plasma cells and eosinophils. Surrounding the lobule is dense interlobular connective tissue and fat (diFiore, 1981). During pregnancy lactiferous ducts appear as well as alveoli that form from

238 Breast implants

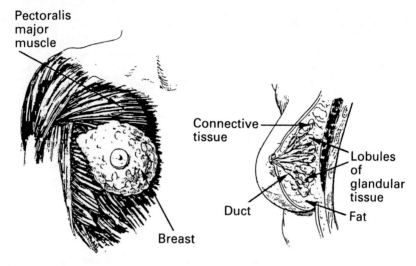

Figure 8.1 Diagram of gross anatomy of breast showing pectoralis major muscle and components including the lobules, ducts, connective tissue and fat.

the ends of the smallest ducts. Each lactiferous duct collects the secretions of a lobe and transports them to the nipple. As pregnancy proceeds secretion into the alveolar lumen occurs.

Table 8.2 Anatomical components of breast tissue*

Component	Function
Nipple	Collection point for milk from lobes that make up breast
Areolar glands	Lubricate nipple during nursing
Lobes	Individual units (15–20 in number) that make up a breast
Lobules	Contains groups of small tubules lined with cuboidal or low columnar epithelium
Tubules	Epithelial cell-lined channels through which milk flows into ducts
Connective tissue	Fills in space between lobules
Fat	Found in spaces between lobules

* Hall-Craggs, 1990

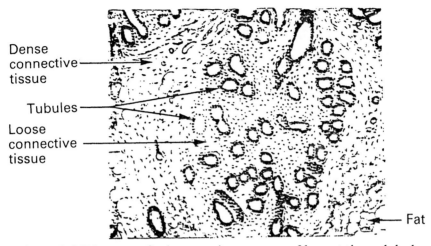

Figure 8.2 Diagram of microscopic anatomy of breast tissue lobule showing tubules, loose and dense connective tissue and fat.

8.3 Psychology of breast augmentation

Since most breast augmentation procedures are done for primarily psychological reasons, it is important for the biomaterials scientist to understand the motivating factors. Although the results of studies reported in the literature provide conflicting impressions, since the parameters considered are not readily measured objectively and patient self-evaluation may lack credibility, most women who have undergone surgery to have breast implants would undergo the procedure again.

Early studies reported that many women undergo breast augmentation because of strong feelings of self-consciousness and sexual inadequacy since adolescence (Baker et al., 1974). The implants enhance self-image, attractiveness and sensuality (Grossman, 1976) and patients seeking implants are as stable psychologically as other women (Shipley et al., 1977). In one study 96% of the patients stated that they would have the operation again while only 1% would not (Hetter, 1979). In other studies, 85–89% of patients receiving prostheses are pleased with the results while only 3–4% have regrets (Hetter, 1979; Meyer and Ringberg, 1987).

Patients seek consultation with a plastic surgeon regarding breast surgery for one of three primary reasons. Small breasted women may wish to have breast enlargement for personal and/or social reasons. In this case surgery corrects developmentally small breasts or hypoplastic breasts by augmenting size and shape. Another group of women have had breast tissue removed during cancer surgery. The creation of a breast in these women is more complicated and may require multiple surgical procedures. The final group of patients have had surgery to remove subcutaneous tissue (subcutaneous mastectomy) leaving the skin and nipple intact. This group is at risk for the development of cancer.

8.4 Types of breast implants

Several types of implants have been evaluated for use in breast augmentation (Batich and DePalma, 1992):

- Liquid injectable silicone
- Sponge
- Gel-filled
- Inflatables
- Double lumen
- Poly(urethane) covered gel-filled

All of these designs have advantages and disadvantages which are discussed further below. Implant surgery costs between $2 000 and $6 000 depending on the geographic location, physician, type of procedure and medical requirements of the patient (Sprague Zones, 1992).

Before 1964, liquid silicone was promoted and used in the form of serial injections to augment breast tissue (Berkowitz and Elam, 1985). Reactions to this material were mainly noted when it was mixed with other additives including peanut oil. Reactions to this mixture ranged from some minor swelling to a anaphylactic response. The main disadvantage was the time required to perform repeated injections as well as the use of a vibrator to disburse the injected droplets.

The next generation of implants were composed of porous sponges, some treated with antibiotics while others were covered to limit ingrowth. Materials with open pores as opposed to solid silicone implants were reported to become hard and/or extrude regardless of the material used in fabrication (Broadbent and Woolf, 1967). In some cases pain and distortion were noted and believed to be a result of formation of a fibrous capsule that surrounded the implant. Antibiotics were used to prevent infection associated with the implantation procedure (Edwards, 1963).

Sponge implants are no longer considered a viable prototype for breast implants since the fibrous tissue response was similar regardless of the material used. Problems with peripheral contracture around the implant are still experienced with other implants.

Gel-filled implants consisted of liquid silicone encased in a silicone 'bag' to which Dacron® patches were applied to provide attachment to muscle (Berkowitz and Elam, 1985). Subsequent studies indicated that silicone gel leaked from the bag into surrounding tissue spaces and was felt to be responsible for fibrosis and capsular contraction around the implant (Barker et al., 1978). Results of other studies indicate that silicone bleeds from all types of implants. It is passed through the implant shell and can be detected in capsules surrounding the implants in humans (Barker and Schultz, 1978; Barker et al., 1978).

Modifications of the gel-filled implants included the introduction of a silicone-gel implant covered by a thin layer of polyurethane. The polyurethane covering was designed to fix the implant to the chest wall. In addition, the Ashley (Ashley, 1970) implant had an internal septum (the Natural-Y) and was reported to be inert in animal tissues. In a follow-up study Ashley claimed reduced migration and contracture (Ashley, 1972); however, other studies reported marked foreign body reaction and inflammatory response to the polyurethane cover (Cocke et al., 1975; Smahel, 1978). A case report described the absorption of the cover after nine years in-vivo (Slade and Peterson, 1982) supporting previous evidence against the inertness of the implant. The Meme implant consists of an outer layer of polyurethane foam and an inner layer containing a low viscosity silicone gel (Herman, 1984). This implant lacked the internal septum that was present in the Natural-Y implant.

Molecular impact surface textured implants (MSTI) are textured silicone breast implants. These implants are fabricated by dipping a mandrel four or five times into a solution of silicone in toluene giving a final thickness of 10 to 15 thousandths of an inch. A final textured coating layer is applied on the surface before the material is cross-linked (Ersek, 1991). Capsular contraction with these implants was reduced based on the results of Ersek (1991). Table 8.3 gives the time sequence of formation of capsular contraction after implantation of smooth and MISTI implants.

Another type of implant was designed to be softer than the gel-filled implants and consisted of a thin-walled bag inflated with saline. Initial studies indicated problems with deflation while claiming a decreased incidence of capsular contraction (Cairns and de Villiers, 1980; McKinney and Tresley, 1983). Spontaneous deflation of these implants as late as seven years post-surgery was noted (Warton et al., 1980).

A double lumen prosthesis seeking to combine the best features of the silicone gel-filled implant and the inflatable prosthesis was proposed

Table 8.3 Capsular contraction around silicone implants*

Implant	Capsular contraction (%)	Time to contracture years (%)
Smooth	44.8%	one (30%) two (73%) seven (27%)
MISTI	0.262%	one and one-half (100%)

* From Ersek (1991)

(Hartley, 1976). It was hypothesized that at the time of capsular contracture, the outer saline filled lumen could be deflated by aspiration using a syringe and needle that is inserted through the skin into the implant. A beneficial feature of the implant is the semi-permeability of the outer saline-filled lumen which can be utilized to release antibiotics or steroids to surrounding tissues (Ellenberg and Braun, 1980).

8.4.1 Materials used in breast implants

Contemporary breast implants use only a limited number of materials for device construction. They include silicone polymers for fabrication of the shell or shells, silicone gel or saline for filling the inner sac, and polyurethane for covering the outer shell (Table 8.4). As a result of the recent review of silicone gel-filled implants, their use has been limited by the FDA.

Originally, the thin silicone layer that composes the elastomeric shell of an implant was about 0.010 inches in thickness (Batich and DePalma, 1992). Improvements in material processing and mechanical properties led to reduction in thickness of the shell to improve the implant softness.

Shell filling materials include silicone gel and saline. Silicone gel consists of a silicone network that contains silicone oil dispersed throughout the polymer. The amount of low molecular weight silicone controls the viscosity of the gel and influences the rate of migration of the gel across the shell. An ASTM standard for cohesion is used to evaluate the gel.

Saline-filled implants also have problems since fluid loss and deflation can occur even in the absence of tears in the shell (Batich and DePalma, 1992). However, saline loss into surrounding tissues does not pose the same risk that is presented by silicone gel. However, implant removal is required if deflation occurs as a result of loss of the filling material.

Other agents including silica in the form of SiO_2 are used in the shell to improve its mechanical properties. Amorphous particles of silica, 9–11 nm in diameter, are compounded with silicone rubber. The compounded rubber has superior strength and tear resistance compared with the pure polymer. Although crystalline forms of silica are believed to have adverse effects on some tissues, no evidence has been presented to indicate that amorphous

Table 8.4 Materials used for breast implants*

Material	Usage
Silicone polymers	Shell
Silicone gel or saline	Filling materials
Poly(urethane)	Shell cover

* Batich and DePalma, 1992

silica is released from breast implants and that it has an adverse effect on mammary tissues.

8.4.2 Polymer chemistry of implant materials

Silicone chemistry involves the synthesis of long chains of dimethylsiloxane that are subsequently cross-linked into a network. Synthesis involves heating a cyclo-tetramer (octamethylcyclotetra-siloxane) to 150°C with a small amount of sodium hydroxide to form a gum-like material. The gum is then cross-linked by mixing with an organic peroxide that gives rise to free radicals. The free radicals react with polymer chains and then combine to form cross-links between chains. Alternately, a vinyl compound is substituted into the siloxane chain. Vinyl groups within the chains are cross-linked with either peroxides or by a platinum catalyzed addition reaction. Residual platinum catalyst or peroxide derivative remain behind in the polymer.

Elastomer gums are reported to typically exhibit a molecular weight of 500 000 before cross-linking. After cross-linking the molecular weight increases. Low molecular weight gel material involves silicone with a molecular weight of approximately 1000 that increases in molecular weight during the cross-linking reaction (Batich and DePalma, 1992).

Poly(urethanes) containing the urethane linkage may contain other functional groups such as

- aromatic or aliphatic hydrocarbons
- epoxies
- poly(ethers)
- poly(esters)
- poly(olefins)
- silicones
- ureas

Batich et al. (1989) evaluated the composition of the polyurethane foams used to cover breast implants and reported the presence of a polyester linkage that was expected to be susceptible to hydrolysis. This suggested that commercial polyurethane covered silicone breast implants were likely to undergo hydrolysis during implantation.

8.5 Complications associated with use of breast implants

There are a number of complications associated with the use of breast implants including (McGrath and Burkhardt, 1984; Berkowitz and Elam, 1985):

- assymetry
- calcification of fibrous capsule
- capsular contraction

- excessive hardness
- extrusion
- implant deflation
- implant displacement
- infection
- numbness
- post-operative lactation
- leakage
- scarring
- sensitization
- interference with cancer detection
- potential for cancer formation
- visible and palpable prostheses.

In 1983, the FDA Advisory Panel on general and Plastic Surgery described the following risks of use of these devices: implant leakage, tissue or skin necrosis, haematoma, displacement of implant, calcification of fibrous capsule, post-operative lactation, and sensitization. In addition, connective tissue disease has been associated with reactions to breast implants. Connective tissue disease reported following augmentation mammoplasty includes:

- scleroderma
- rheumatoid arthritis, and
- systemic lupus erythematosus

(Fock *et al.*, 1984; Sergott *et al.*, 1986; Endo *et al.*, 1987; Spiera, 1988; Weisman *et al.*, 1988, Varga, 1989). Berkowitz and Elam (1985) indicate that post-operative bleeding is the most common factor precipitating early hardness. It usually is evident six to eight weeks post-operatively; however, it may take six to eight months to become symptomatic. Rigorous control of bleeding during surgery as well as post-operative exercises to eliminate any collected blood are reported to be valuable. Removal of the capsule surrounding the implant may ameliorate the problem.

8.5.1 Assymmetry
Proper breast symmetry is a result of proper dissection of a pocket into which the implant fits, choice of the implant size and volume, and displacement of the implant during encapsulation (Berkowitz and Elam, 1985).

8.5.2 Calcification of fibrous capsule
Calcification of the fibrous capsule surrounding the implant may result in cosmetic deformity and may require further surgical intervention or removal of implant (Redfern *et al.*, 1977).

8.5.3 Capsular contraction

Contracture of the fibrous tissue surrounding the implant may result in disfigurement, physical and psychological trauma, migration of the implant, or gross leakage of the contents.

Contraction around smooth walled silicone gel-filled prostheses is reported at variable rates between 0 and 75% in the clinical literature (Hetter, 1979; Williams, 1972; Rees *et al.*, 1973; Hipps *et al.*, 1978; Brandt *et al.*, 1984). Asplund (1984) reported a significantly higher rate of capsular contraction in silicone gel-filled implants (54%) when compared to saline-filled implants (20%). Free silicone around the implant may contribute to capsular contraction.

Lower contracture rates may be observed with poly(urethane) coated implants. Long-term clinical reports of contracture rates of 1–5% (Melmed, 1988) with poly(urethane) coated implants have been reported. The contracture rate increases for all types of implants in instances of breast reconstruction. Placement of the implant in a previously formed capsule is associated with increased incidence of capsular contraction indicating that an old capsule should be removed prior to implant introduction.

Burkhardt *et al.* (1986) reported that the use of a variety of local antibacterials in or around inflatable retromammary prosthetic devices reduced the early post-operative onset of certain types of capsular contraction by sevenfold and the final incidence by more than half. They hypothesized that capsular contraction in retromamary augmentation is due to bacterial contamination of the implant surface. This may occur during installation of the device through the surgical field.

8.5.4 Increased breast hardness

Increased breast hardness is also observed in the long-term and may be associated with estrogen therapy or other systematic conditions. The effects of estrogen on breast encapsulation and capsular contractures seem to be mediated through involvement of contractile cells.

8.5.5 Haematoma

The formation of a blood filled pocket (haematoma) is a significant complication of implant installation even using normal procedures to limit bleeding. Underlying coagulation defects induced by ingestion of aspirin or anti-inflammatory agents contribute to this problem. Haematoma due to small vessel rupture may require re-operation.

8.5.6 Implant deflation

Deflation of saline-filled implants is quite common (Berkowitz and Elam, 1985). Early deflations are due to valve failure while later ones are due to tears that develop where the material forms folds. When saline leakage and deflation does occur, it requires removal of both the failed and normal implant. If a gel implant fails, migration of the material away from the breast can be a problem.

8.5.7 Implant displacement
Migration of the implant below the skin may result in cosmetic deformity.

8.5.8 Infection
Infection rates of up to 4.2% are reported in the literature (McGrath and Burkhardt, 1984). Infection is believed to be caused by ill fitting prostheses and is limited by prophylactic use of antibiotics (Berkowitz and Elam, 1985). Organisms cultured from implants include predominantly Staphylococcus aureus and Staphlococcus epidermidis in a few instances. Extrusion is associated with infection or local use of steroids.

Clegg et al. (1983) reported periprosthetic infections due to Mycobacterium fortitum and Mycobacterium chelonei occurred in 17 women over a $3\frac{1}{2}$ year period, after implantation of mammary prostheses. Ransj'o et al., (1985) found mainly Staphyloccus epidermis and propionibacteria in female breast tissue. These bacteria were sensitive to penicillin G and/or isoxapenicillin. Use of poly(urethane)-covered implants leads to long-lasting complications including difficult removal of infected fragments of the coat and delayed foreign body reactions (Berrino et al., 1986). Ellenberger et al., (1986) found tissue-embedded poly(urethane) foam formed the focal point for persistent infection.

8.5.9 Numbness
Numbness of the nipple is a common phenomenon that is temporary. Sensation normally returns six to eight weeks post-implantation. Insertion of a large implant requires introduction of large pocket which may adversely affect the nerve supply or stretch nerves.

8.4.10 Post-operative lactation
There are a small percentage of patients taking oral contraceptives that experience lactation after surgical implantation of mammary prostheses (Hartley and Schatten, 1971).

In thin skin individuals visible or palpable prostheses can be encountered. This can be a problem with stiffer implants or implants with thicker shells.

8.5.11 Leakage
Implant rupture and leakage may result from intra– or post-surgical trauma; excessive stresses or manipulation in daily life; athletics and physical contact; mechanical damage before or during surgery and from other unknown causes. Manual compression of the breast tissue to limit capsular contraction may weaken the implant envelope and lead to rupture.

8.5.12 Sensitization and autoimmune reactions

Reports have been published of suspected immunological sensitization or hyperimmune responses to silicone mammary implants. Symptoms include localized inflammation and irritation at the implant area, fluid accumulation, rash, general malaise, severe joint pain, swelling of joints, weight loss, loss of appetite and breast implant rejection.

Human adjuvant disease, following silicone gel implant mammaplasty has been described by Baldwin and Kaplan (1983). The disorder was manifested by arthritis, arthalgias, skin lesions, malaise, pyrexia and weight loss. Byron *et al.*, (1984) reported a case of human adjuvant disease which occurred following the use of a saline filled silastic implant.

8.5.13 Interference with cancer detection

Breast cancer detection using mammography is reported to be impaired by the presence of implants (Hayes *et al.*, 1988; Dershaw and Chaglassian, 1989). Fibrous capsules that form around implants further obscure mammography readings. Women with implants who develop breast cancer generally have more advanced disease that may be associated with increased difficulty in diagnosis. There is no long term evidence associating implants with increased incidence of breast cancer (Silverstein *et al.*, 1985).

8.5.14 Potential for cancer formation

Silicone was recognized as having carcinogenic potential when Oppenheimer (1952) reported sarcomas induced in laboratory animals as a result of the implantation of solid plastic materials. Relatively inert smooth-surfaced materials have been shown to be the apparent cause of soft tissue sarcomas when implanted subcutaneously in rats (Turner, 1941; Oppenheimer, 1952). However, tumour formation in conjunction with breast implantation is relatively rare in humans (Fisher and Brody, 1992).

8.6 Complications with poly(urethane)-covered implants

The most common complications experienced with the poly(urethane)-covered implants include

- wrinkling
- rupture
- pseudopodic projections
- capsular contraction
- breast ptosis and
- silicone migration.

(Cohney *et al.*, 1992). Wrinkling of the implant occurs even with careful dissection to at least 1 cm in every direction past the proposed margin for the prosthesis. Rupture appeared due to the faulty connection between the anterior part of the prosthesis and the flat base, perhaps due to problems associated with adhesion. Pseodopodia are knuckle-like projections that occur at the periphery, or on the anterior surface of the prosthesis. Inflammation and the appearance of macrophages and lymphocytes occur in response to the poly(urethane) foam. It is this reaction that is thought to limit capsular contraction to 10% in the first five years and 30% over 15 years. Breast drooping (ptosis) of the overlying breast and subcutaneous tissue has been observed and may be reduced by skin reduction at the original augmentation. Silicone migration results in lymph node enlargement that is not necessarily a result of implant rupture.

8.7 Implant placement

Placement of the implant can either be beneath the glandular tissue (subglandular) where it can fill out the loss of breast tissue due to atrophy or it can be placed submuscularly. Subglandular placement is traditional according to Berkowitz and Elam (1985) and involves creation of a pocket within the breast tissue retaining the original breast shape. A disadvantage of this placement is that conditions of the breasts including fibrocystic disease, may affect the softness of the implant. In addition, the encapsulation rate may be higher than in the submuscular implant.

In patients with small breasts and thin chest walls, submuscular implantation may lower the encapsulation rate. It is difficult to insert a prosthesis larger than 300 ccs via this approach and the recipients generally have a flatness of appearance after surgery. Motion or exercise to the upper extremities may cause distortion of the breasts and therefore this approach is not recommended for athletic individuals.

8.8 Current concerns

The FDA and clinicians continue to be concerned about prevention of capsular contraction, breast neoplasia and detection of tumours in patients with these prostheses. Because of the widely varying reports of capsular contracture there is concern over how extensive these problems may be if all patients were followed more extensively. Although no tumour has been directly linked to implantation of synthetic polymers, there is continued fear that implants may somehow contribute to the rising incidence of breast cancer. At the very least, the implant makes detection of tumours more difficult especially if it is large.

All non-degradable and some biodegradable polymers will induce the formation of a collagenous sheath around the implant. This capsule is acellular and contains some vessels at its periphery. With time the fibroblasts in the sheath attempt to contract the capsule. Capsular contraction occurs with silicone, polyurethane and silicone-polycarbonate copolymers. It occurs in gel-filled, saline-filled and combination implants. Haematoma and infection contributes to capsular contraction. They can be prevented or ameliorated by submuscular placement of the implant, local use of steroids, local use of antibiotics, and by exercises that compress the implant. Capsular contraction is treated by surgical removal of the capsule and/or placement of the implant in another location.

While it is accepted in the field of biomaterials that no polymer has ever been directly linked to the formation of a tumour, there is evidence that monomer or biodegradation products of polymers can be tumourigenic. After insertion of large implants even the detection of tumours using mammography may be more difficult. Gel-filled implants may obscure the view of breast tissue more than ones that are saline filled.

8.9 Summary

A number of different types of breast implants have been developed for augmentation of mammary tissue. Due to risks associated with implant leakage, silicone gel-filled implants have been removed from the market except for use in patients who undergo reconstructive surgery after cancer. Saline-filled implants remain the only viable device for cosmetic augmentation of breast tissue.

Silicone implants are manufactured in smooth, textured and poly(urethane) coated varieties. Reports of reduced contracture with textured and poly(urethane) covered implants as compared with smooth implants have been made. However, careful controlled studies are needed to verify the exact rate and extent of contracture with each type of implant.

Although millions of breast implant procedures have been performed, the adverse effects of prolonged implant–host tissue interactions are still being evaluated. Infection, capsular contraction and implant leakage are among the most common problems associated with these devices. Continued concern over autoimmune diseases and cancer may have been expressed by researchers in the field to the point where the use of these implants is currently being carefully reviewed by the FDA.

9.
510 (k) and PMA Regulatory Filings in The US

9.1 Introduction

There are two primary pathways to gain approval to market a medical device in the US, 510 (k) notification and pre-market approval (PMA). These processes were introduced in chapter 1 (see section 1.6.1). 510 (k) notification involves marketing a device that is substantially equivalent to a device on the market prior to 1976.

Prior to 1976 the FDA was given little authority over medical devices. Although, the FDA by law had authority over medical devices that were shipped interstate, it was limited in its power and could only remove products from the market that were adulterated or misbranded. In 1976, Congress enacted the Medical Device Amendment to the Food, Drug, and Cosmetic Act that required the FDA to impose varying regulatory controls over medical devices, depending on the relative risks they present.

Pre-market approval required documentation of pre-clinical and clinical evaluation of the safety and effectiveness of a device. In addition, the FDA required review of package labelling and insert instructions for usage, as well as listing potential adverse reactions, as part of the regulatory approval process. The only devices that were not required to undergo pre-market approval were those that were considered 'substantially equivalent' in their design, materials and effective action to a device already on the market. In some cases it can effectively be argued that a new device is equivalent to more than one device marketed prior to 1976. The later devices may have more than one intended use. Regulation 510 (k) of the Medical Devices Amendment of 1976 provided a means to circumvent the PMA process by claiming that a device was substantially equivalent to one marketed prior to 1976. This approach eliminated the requirement for extensive pre-clinical and clinical testing. In addition, the 1976 Amendment required the FDA to establish and publish performance standards for Class II medical devices.

As a result of regulation 510 (k) and its broad interpretation by FDA, a great majority of the newly approved medical devices have been considered substantially equivalent to one or more devices marketed prior to 1976. Many of these devices were approved without extensive clinical testing that

Introduction 251

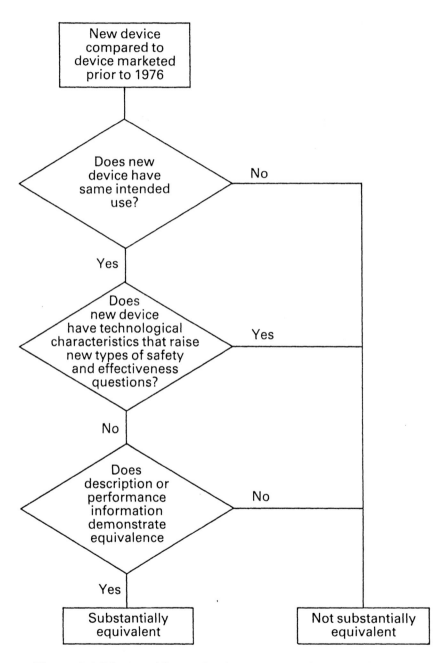

Figure 9.1 Diagram illustrating how 'substantial equivalence' is determined for a medical device.

is mandatory for devices requiring a PMA. Figure 9.1 shows a typical decision making diagram that is used to assess equivalency.

The strategic formulation of a regulatory approach requires analysis of the medical condition, the existence of marketed devices prior to 1976 and the desired product labelling claims. Below are given hypothetical examples of 510 (k) and PMA filings.

9.2 Components of a 510 (k) regulatory filing

The 510 (k) regulatory filing consists of sections including the following information:

- product name
- establishment name, address and registration number
- device classification
- labelling
- device description
- sterilization
- indications
- contraindications
- statement of substantial equivalence
- materials characterization and processing.

The purpose of the filing is to argue that the device is equivalent to a device or devices marketed prior to 1976. In addition, the sterilization of the device must be validated by an independent laboratory, the labelling must be identical to that of equivalent devices on the market and proper process controls and standard operating procedures must be established to prove that product production specifications exist. Other concerns of the FDA include whether the product be used properly and what precautions should be undertaken if the product is followed by an adverse reaction?

9.2.1 Product name
The product normally has a registered trade name and a common name. The product name is not a concern of the FDA unless it implies something about the usage of the product or composition that may not be true.

9.2.2 Establishment name, address and registration number
The FDA normally deals with companies and individuals. Registration of a Medical Device Establishment is obtained by filing form FD 2891. Once this form is filed, the FDA will subsequently assign an Establishment Registration Number.

9.2.3 Device classification

The device classification is given in the Federal Register and is listed in Table 1.26. The example used below will involve a wound dressing which is classified as a Class I medical device.

9.2.4 Labelling

The label contains the product name, manufacturer's name and address as well as the name and address of the distributor. Other information required includes product category, trade name, composition, description, action, indications, warning, contraindications, dosage and how product is supplied.

The composition should be listed by ingredients while the description lists the types of medical conditions (i.e. the types of wounds for a wound dressing) for which the product is used. For a wound dressing product, the labelling description is typically 'used in the management of' general conditions that are specified under indications. 'Action' describes how the product accomplishes its desired goal. For instance, a wound dressing prevents bacterial invasion into the wound by providing a physical barrier and therefore manages wound healing in this fashion. Indications include the exact medical usage of the product such as skin wounds, diabetic wounds, burns, cuts and scrapes, skin graft donor sites, pressure sores and other mechanical injuries to skin. Warning includes explicit instructions about how to use the product so that no injury occurs. In addition it states what is an inappropriate use of the product.

Contraindications include instructions on what events should lead to termination of product usage and what types of medical conditions do not warrant its usage. Dosage amount and frequency are given as well as instructions on how to properly use the product. Finally, the label contains information on how the product is supplied.

9.2.5 Device description

This portion is an expanded version of the description on the label detailing the components and amounts as well as the uses for the device. The components are always described by name, composition and manufacturer. Specifications are given for each component as well as for the packaging materials.

9.2.6 Sterilization

Devices can be sterilized in process or by end sterilization. End sterilization can be achieved by exposure to radiation, chemical treatment or high temperature. An outside testing lab must verify that the final product is sterile guaranteeing a sterility assurance level to or greater than 10^{-6}. This test must be conducted routinely on each batch manufactured.

9.2.7 Indications and contraindications
This information is identical to the information contained on the label.

9.2.8 Statement of substantial equivalence
The proposed product must be shown to be substantially equivalent to a product or products (i.e. wound dressing) that are marketed by one or more commercial organizations. There are numerous wound dressings on the market. By analysing the composition or properties of one or more of these commercial products, a comparison is made between the proposed and commercial products (Table 9.1). If the materials and the intended use are the same, then substantial equivalence is demonstrated. However, sometimes the materials are different but the use is the same and then substantial equivalence is shown by comparing the new product with two or more old products. One of the old products has the same composition and the other the same intended use.

9.2.9 Purity, identity, quality, safety and efficacy
This portion should establish the purity of the raw materials as well as standard procedures to evaluate the purity of each lot of raw material received from each supplier. Purity level specifications should be established for each material in order to demonstrate that device-to-device variation will be eliminated. The identity of the raw materials must also be established to enable a quick screening of all production batches. Most polymers have characteristic infrared spectra which can be used to identify the polymer.

Quality control procedures are next necessary to make sure that each processing step has a protocol and that specific quality control tests are conducted to maintain product specifications. Programs for quality control include chemical analysis for components, sterilization validation, and manufacturing parameter end points. If the product is a wound dressing then the chemical composition, purity, tensile strength, sterility and adhesion to surrounding healthy skin require quality control procedures.

Table 9.1 Comparison between proposed and commercial wound dressing

Characteristic	Proposed product	Duoderm flexible hydroactive dressing
Material	Polymeric materials	Carboxymethylcelluose other polymeric materials
Intended use	Manage healing of local skin wounds	Management of skin ulcers
Area of application	Skin	Skin

Safety testing normally involves pre-clinical tests that are described in Table 1.18. Typically for a wound dressing, acute systemic toxicity, agar overlay cytotoxicity, haemolysis, MEM elution cytotoxicity, primary skin irritation, USP rabbit pyrogen test, inhibition of cell growth, and LAL (endotoxin) testing are conducted (Table 9.2).

Efficacy portion of the application reviews the literature for data suggesting that the particular product (i.e. wound dressing) through some well defined mechanism solves a medical problem (i.e. promotes wound healing). The studies cited should include in vitro and in vivo results (animal and human data) so that a mechanism is established and that a correlation can be drawn between animal and human studies. It is not necessary to furnish clinical data on the proposed product usage in this section but only to infer from published studies that the product is effective in the claimed indications.

9.3 Premarket approval (PMA) application

Devices that are not equivalent to a device on the market before 1976 are automatically considered as class III if they are implantable. These devices

Table 9.2 Typical preclinical testing for a wound dressing

Test	Acceptable outcome
Acute systemic toxicity	No signs of respiratory, motor, convulsive, ocular, salivary, piloerectal, gastrointestinal or skin reactions
Agar overlay cytotoxity	No detectable zone of cell reactivity
Haemolysis	Less than 5% haemolysis
MEM cytotoxicity	No cytotoxicity of test material
Primary skin irritation	No primary skin irritation
USP rabbit pyrogen	No rabbit shows individual temperature rise of 0.6°C or for three rabbits the temperature rise is below 1.4°C
Inhibition of cell growth	No inhibition of cell growth at all extract concentrations
Limulus amebocyte lysate (LAL) testing	No LAL activity present

are approved based on the safety and clinical effectiveness demonstrated in a pre-marketing approval application.

As an example, the FDA (Division of Surgical and Rehabilitative Devices, Center for Devices and Radiological Health) provides a document entitled 'Guidelines For The Intraarticular Prosthetic Knee Ligament'. The guidelines state that the requirements for pre-clinical testing are influenced by the type of material, type of prosthesis, and history of previous use of the material in humans. If a material degrades, then the fate of the material in the joint must be tested as well as activation of the immune system.

Pre-clinical testing must be completed before an IDE (investigational device exemption) and clinical testing can be initiated. Pre-clinical testing recommended includes physical and chemical analyses, biological testing and animal implantation. 'If the device is claimed to be reasonably comparable to devices described in the literature, then these tests can be used to demonstrate that data from the literature can be extrapolated in support of the investigational device exemption'.

The objective of the physical and chemical analyses are to identify leachable materials in both polar and nonpolar solvents at body temperature for five days. Identification of the extracted material should be performed.

Biological testing includes standard pyrogenicity testing, haemolysis potential, acute toxicity testing, genetic testing (mutations), contact sensitization, sterility validation and mechanical testing. Mechanical tests to be reported include mean load–deformation curves, mean stress–strain curves, fatigue life, creep elongation, bending fatigue testing, fixation strength and abrasion testing. Tensile tests are conducted at a minimum of three different strain rates.

'Augmentation devices which are designed to degrade with time and which are not expected to retain any of their original properties in vivo may be excluded from long-term fatigue testing. For these devices, the intended function must be described in detail including the length of time the device is expected to carry a significant portion of the load imposed on the knee.'

Long-term animal studies should include up to one year of implantation in an animal stifle joint in a loaded configuration to characterize the type and time course of post-implantation biological and mechanical events. These data will be used to determine: the histological response to the device and particulate eminating from the device; immunological response to the device; device material degradation and loss of mechanical properties; device abrasion and damage; migration of particulate matter; and the fixation strength.

Animal models including sheep, goats and dogs are used in pre-clinical testing. A sham-operated procedure is used as a control two weeks prior to device implantation in the contralateral limb or in additional animals. Evaluations are recommended at three and 12 months post-implantation at a minimum. Histological studies are indicated on a minimum of three control and three device-treated animals and mechanical tests on six animals at each time point, bringing the minimum study to 24 animals.

At sacrifice, all joints should be examined and described in detail as well as surrounding joint components. The gross and microscopic pathology of tissue surrounding the device, the amount of ingrowth into the implant and various joint components should be analyzed. Abraded particles in the joint should be evaluated for amount, size and reaction. Gross examinations of systemic organs should be made for all animals. At least one slide per organ should be evaluated.

Mechanical testing should be conducted on the entire device with the fixation system intact and on the intra-articular material in order to test the ligament. Fixation strength and stiffness and intra-articular strength and stiffness of the device and normal control should be compared at implantation and at various time intervals.

Particulate migration studies are used for comparison with clinical study results. Some animals should be kept a minimum of one year. Regional lymph nodes should be examined for migration of particles.

If the device has not been previously used for implantation in humans for a significant period of time, the carcinogenic risk to humans must be addressed. This requires that a two-year implant bioassay be performed using a maximum dose implantation in the paravertebral muscle of rats.

A typical PMA is described below for a ligament replacement device.

9.3.1 PMA application for ligament device (anterior cruciate ligament replacement)

The PMA application typically consists of the following parts:

- general information
- indications
- device description
- alternative practices
- contraindications
- potential adverse effects
- summary of pre-clinical studies
- summary of clinical studies.

General information
This section includes general information including device name, device tradename, applicant's name and address, and PMA number.

Indications
The indications of all approved ligament devices involve either reinforcement of an autogenous replacement or as a permanent replacement for the anterior cruciate ligament (ACL) in patients who have had at least one failed autogenous, intra-articular reconstruction of the ACL.

Device description
The tendon/ligament device is composed of a polymeric material that is fabricated into a multifilament device that has sufficient porosity to allow tissue ingrowth.

Alternative practices or procedures
Alternative surgical procedures to treat ACL insufficiency when previous attempts at intra-articular reconstruction of the ACL have failed include extra-articular reinforcement and further attempts at ACL replacement with other autogenous grafts including fascia lata, tendon, or semi-tendinosus muscle. In extreme cases of instability and arthritis, total knee replacement is indicated.

Contraindication
Use of a an ACL replacement is contraindicated in patients with incomplete bone growth and skeletal maturity. The device is also contraindicated in the presence of systemic or localized infection. The package insert should provide all warnings and precautions.

Potential adverse effects
The adverse effects that have been reported include inflammatory effusion, failure of the device or recurrent instability of the joint. Both of these conditions can result from improper implantation or inadequate tensioning; soft tissue irritation, deep and superficial infection, loosening of the fixation screws, fractures associated with bone tunnels or screw holes and neurovascular damage during implantation can be observed.

Summary of preclinical studies
Typically the following in vitro tests are conducted:

- cytotoxicity (agar overlay and MEM elution)
- LAL pyrogenicity
- haemolysis
- bioburden
- chemical purity
- mutagenicity
- carcinogenicity
- sterility
- mechanical testing
- animal testing.

Bioburden Results of cytotoxicity, LAL pyrogen and haemolysis tests were presented in Table 9.3 above and therefore the reader is referred there for details. The bioburden test is performed to determine the amount of aerobic and spore-forming organisms present on the non-sterile product. The sample is mixed with buffer and allowed to incubate for 40 hours. Total aerobic and spore-forming bacteria are determined following this incubation period. The results are required to show a low number of colony-forming units per unsterilized product.

Chemical purity Synthetic polymeric materials are traditionally characterized by infrared spectroscopy since each polymer has a unique fingerprint. The spectrum is compared to a standard of the material. Inorganic heavy metal contamination is evaluated by testing for mercury, lead, iron, nickel, bismuth, copper, zinc, cadmium, thallium and manganese. Trace inorganic elements can be established based on multi-element neutron activation analysis. Trace organic elements are established based on gas chromatography/mass spectroscopy.

Summary of mutagenicity/carcinogenicity testing Tests such as the Ames test, Balb/3t3 ouabain resistance mutagenesis assay and L5178Y Tk +/− mutagenesis assay are performed. Carcinogenicity is assessed based on the Balb/3T3 transformation assay.

Summary of sterilization data Some devices are furnished non-sterile and then are sterilized by either ethylene oxide exposure or steam autoclaving. The implants are evaluated after sterilization for loss of mechanical stability. Other implants are supplied in a sterilized state. In the latter case, a sterility validation is required.

Summary of mechanical testing Mechanical testing is conducted to evaluate mechanical properties for the ligament device. Tests include ultimate tensile strength, ultimate tensile load, creep, fatigue lifetime, bending fatigue, flex testing, and abrasion.

Summary of animal studies In an intra-articular location, a ligament replacement normally is rigorously tested to assess the in vivo tissue response, in vivo performance in providing knee stability and post-implantation mechanical properties. These responses in animals can be evaluated in a sheep model, using standard mechanical tests to test fixation and bone attachment strength. At least five animals are tested per time period with additional animals planned for the longest time period in case of unexpected animal losses in the earlier time periods.

Knee stability and prosthesis fixation are evaluated for periods of up to one year in sheep weighing between 50 and 75 kg. The device can be routed over the top of the bone and fixed to the bone with screws. Initial fixation strengths are measured immediately post-operative with bone screws intact. Fixation strengths in three animals are measured after about three months and six months. They are also measured without the tibial screw in place to measure biological fixation.

Gross examination of the specimens is required to evaluate intactness of the implant. Histological evaluation of ligaments is used to measure attachment and ingrowth of tissue into the prosthesis. Intra-articularly and in the bone tunnels, the amount of fibrous tissue and osseous tissue, respectively, that is deposited is evaluated. Synovial tissue and synovial fluid samples are taken for histological evaluation. Gross observations are used to assess foreign body reactions and inflammatory responses.

Clinical studies

A multi-centre study is used to evaluate the safety and effectiveness of an ACL replacement. The performance is evaluated by assessing knee stability, method of implantation, speed of rehabilitation and nature and incidence of adverse consequences of the procedure and implant. In one study 19 investigators at 27 centres and about 1000 patients were involved over a period of $3\frac{1}{2}$ years.

Controls include pre-operative status of the patient, so that post-operative results can be compared to initial baseline values for both objective and subjective measures of knee stability and knee status. Another set of controls consist of literature data on reconstruction using other techniques and implants.

Objective measures of knee stability include the anterior drawer test, the Lachman test and the pivot shift test. The anterior drawer test is evaluated by attempting to displace the patient's tibia anteriorly with the knee held in 90 degrees of flexion. The Lachman test is similar to the anterior drawer test except the knee is near full extension (20°) where the hamstring muscles, the collateral ligaments and the posterior horn of the medial meniscus are less effective at resisting anterior displacement of the tibia. The pivot test measures displacement of the joint while applying stress to the knee on the lateral aspect of the distal part of the thigh. At the same time, an internal rotation torque stress is applied at the ankle while the knee is taken from flexion to extension. The pivot shift and Lachman tests are considered most reliable for evaluating ACL insufficiency (Katz and Fingeroth, 1986).

Qualitative assessment of the success of the procedure is evaluated from a standardized series of questions asked to each patient. Pre-operatively and at follow-up exams patients are asked to respond to questions related to knee 'giving way', ability to return to activities of daily living, ability to ascend and descend stairs, episodes of locking, degree of pain and degree of swelling. At post-operative visits only, the patients were asked to evaluate the condition of their knees.

Patient selection criteria Patients admitted to the study consisted of those who exhibited disabilities caused by ACL deficiency of sufficient severity to warrant reconstructive surgery. Patients not included showed evidence of skeletal immaturity, pre-existing conditions such as infection that precluded any reconstructive procedure; and those for whom post-operative follow-up was unlikely.

Evaluation criteria Patients are grouped according to whether or not they had undergone a previous intra-articular reconstruction and the length of follow-up. Comparison of the quantitative and qualitative assessments of knee stability are statistically made to show significant differences between these groups and controls.

Safety Results of the study are evaluated by determining the number of patients with complications divided by the total number of patients (complication rate). The complication rate is also divided by the total number of months to determine the complication rate per month.

Complications to be noted include device rupture, recurrent instability, infection, effusions, bone screw associated events and other events. Histological evaluation is conducted to determine the presence of minute amounts of polymer particles in the tissues about the knee.

References

Abbas, A.K., Lichtman, A.H. and Pober, J.S. (1991) *Cellular and Molecular Immunology*, W.B. Saunders, Philadelphia, Pa., Chs 5 and 16.

Abbink, E.P. (1988) Clinical experience in correction of chronic anterior cruciate ligament deficiency with bovine xenograft: A 5-year study, in *Prosthetic Ligament Reconstruction of The Knee*, (eds M.J. Friedman and R.D. Ferkel), W.B. Saunders Co., Philadelphia, 101.

Abrahams, M., (1967) Mechanical behaviour of tendon in vitro: A preliminary report. *Med. Biol. Eng.*, **5**, 433.

Adams, J.S. (1991) Facial augmentation with solid alloplastic implants: A rational approach to material selection, in *Applications of Biomaterials in Facial Plastic Surgery*, (eds A.I. Glasgold and F.H. Silver), CRC Press, Boca Raton, Fl, Ch. 17.

Alavi, M.A. and Moore, S. (1987) Proteoglycan composition of rabbit arterial wall under conditions of experimentally induced atherosclerosis. *Atherosclerosis*, **63**, 65.

Alexander, H., Parsons, J.R., Strauchler, I.D., Corcoran, S.F., Gona, O. and Weiss, A.B. (1981) Canine patellar tendon replacement with a polylactic acid polymer-filamentous carbon degrading scaffold to form new tissues. *Orthop. Rev.*, **X**, 41.

Alho, A.M. and Underhill, C.B. (1989) The hyaluronate receptor is preferentially expressed on proliferating epithelial cells. *Cell Biol.*, **108**, 1557–65.

Alvarez, O.M. and Biozes, D.G. (1984) Cultured epidermal autografts. *Clinics in Dermatol.*, **2**, 54.

Amiel, D., Frank, C., Harwood, F., Fronek, J. and Akeson, W. (1984) Tendons and ligaments: a morphological and biochemical comparison. *J. Orthop. Res.*, **1**, 257.

Andrish, J.T. and Woods, L.D. (1984) Dacron augmentation in anterior cruciate ligament reconstruction in dogs. *Clin. Orthop.*, **183**, 298.

Angell, W.W., Angell, J.D., Woodruff, A., Sywak, A. and Kojek, J.C. (1977) The tissue valve as a superior cardiac valve replacement. *Surgery*, **82**, 875.

Annis, D., Bornat, A., Edwards, R.D., Higham, A., Loveday, B. and Wilson, J. (1978) An elastomeric vascular prosthesis. *Trans. Am. Soc. Art. Intern. Org.*, **14**, 209.

Apple, D.J., Brems, R.N., Park, R.B., Kavka-Van Norman, D., Hansen, S.O., Tetz, M.R., Richards, S.C. and Letchinger, S.D. (1987) Anterior chamber lenses, Part I: complications and pathology and a review of designs. *J. Cataract Refract. Surg.,* **13**, 157.

Apple, D.J., Mamalis, N., Loftfield, K., Googe, J.M., Novak, L.C., Kavka-Van Norman, D., Brady, S.E. and Olson, R.J. (1984) Complications of intraocular lenses: a historical and histopathological review. *Survey Ophthalmol.,* **29**, 1.

Aragona, J., Parsons, J.R., Alexander, H. and Weiss, A.B. (1981) Soft tissue attachment of a filamentous carbon-absorbable polymer tendon and ligament replacement. *Clin. Orthop.,* **160**, 268.

Arem, A.J., Rasmussen, D. and Madden, J.W. (1972) Soft tissue response to Proplast: quantitation of scar ingrowth. *Plast. Resconstr. Surg.,* **61**, 214.

Arndt, J.O., Klauske, J. and Mersch, F. (1970) The diameter of the intact carotid artery in man and its change with pulse pressure. *Pfluegers Arch. Gesamte Physiol. Menschen Tiere,* **318**, 130.

Arndt, J.D., Stegall, H.F. and Wicke, H.J. (1971) Mechanics of the aorta in vivo: A radiographic approach. *Circ. Res.,* **28**, 693.

Arnoczky, S.P. (1983) Anatomy of the anterior cruciate ligament. *Clin. Orthop. Rel. Res.,* **172**, 19.

Arnoczky, S.P., Tarvin, G.B. and Marshall, J.L. (1982) Anterior cruciate ligament replacement using patellar tendon. *J. Bone Jt. Surg.,* **64-A**, 217.

Arnoczky, S.P., Warren, R.F. and Ashlock, M.A. (1986) Replacement of the anterior cruciate ligament using a patellar tendon allograft. *J. Bone Jt. Surg.,* **68-A**, 376.

Aron-Rosa, D., Cohn, H.C., Aron, J.-J. and Bouquety, C. (1983) Methylcellulose instead of Healon® in extracapsular surgery with intraocular lens implantation. *Ophthamology,* **90**, 1235-8.

Arshinoff, S. (1989) Comparative physical properties of ophthalmic viscoelastic materials. *Ophthalmic Practice,* **7**, 16–37.

Asaga, H., Kikuchi, S. and Yoshizato, K. (1991) Collagen gel contraction by fibroblasts requires cellular fibronectin but not plasma fibronectin. *Experimental Cell Research,* **193**, 167.

Ashley, F.L. (1970) A new type of breast prosthesis, preliminary report. *Plast. Recontsr. Surg.,* **45**, 421.

Ashley, F.L. (1972) Further studies of the Natural Y breast prosthesis. *Plast. Reconstr. Surg.,* **49**, 414.

Asplund, O. (1984) Capsular contracture in silicone gel and saline-filled breast implants after reconstruction. *Plast. Reconstr. Surg.,* **73**, 270.

Bach, B.R., Warren, R.F., Flynn, W.M., Kroll, M. and Wickiewicz, T.L. (1990) Arthrometric evaluation of knees that have a torn anterior cruciate ligament. *J. Bone Jt. Surg.,* **72A**, 1299.

Bahn, C.F., Grosserode, R., Musch, D.C., Feder, J., Meyer, R.F., MacCallum, D.K., Lillie, J.H. and Rich, N.M. (1986) Effect of 1%

sodium hyaluronate (HealonR) on nonregenerating (feline) corneal endothelium. *Invest. Ophthalmol. Vis. Sci.*, **27**, 1485–94.

Baker, J., Kolin, I. and Bartlett, E. (1974) Psychosexual dynamics of patients undergoing breast augmentation. *Plast. Reconstr. Surg.*, **53**, 652.

Baker, J.L., Jr., LeVier, R. and Spielvogel, D. (1982) Positive identification of silicone in human mammary capsular tissue. *Plast. Reconstr. Surg.* **61**, 1.

Balazs, E.A. (1960) Physiology of the vitreous body, in *Importance of the Vitreous Body in Retina Surgery with Special Emphasis on Reoperations*, (ed. C. L. Schepens), Mosby, St. Louis, Mo, pp. 29–48.

Balazs, E.A. (1983) Sodium hyaluronate and viscosurgery, in *Healon: A Guide to its Use in Ophthalmic Surgery*, (eds D. Miller and R. Stegmann), John Wiley and Sons, New York, pp. 19–24.

Balazs, E. A., Freeman, M.I., Kloti, R., Meyer-Schwickerath, G., Regnault, F. and Sweeney, D.B. (1972) Hyaluronic acid and replacement of vitreous and aqueous humor. *Mod. Probl. Ophthalmol.*, **10**, 3–21.

Baldock, W.T., Hutchens, L.H., McFall, W.T. and Simpson, D.M. (1985) An evaluation of tricalcium phosphate implants in human periodontal osseous defects of two patients. *J. Periodontol.*, **56**, 1.

Baldwin, C.M. and Kaplan, E.N. (1983) Silicone-induced human adjuvant disease? *Ann. Plastic Surg.*, **10**, 270.

Barker, D. and Schultz, S. (1978) Reaction to silicone implants in the guinea pig. *Aesthetic Plast. Surg.*, **1**, 371.

Barker, D., Ritsky, M. and Schultz, S. (1978) Bleeding of silicone from bag-gel breast implants and its clinical relation to fibrous capsule reaction. *Plast. Reconstr. Surg.*, **61**, 836.

Barnett, G.O., Mallos, A.J. and Shapiro, A. (1961) Relationship of aortic pressure and diameter in the dog. *J. Appl. Physiol.*, **16**, 545.

Barrett, G. and Moore, M.B. (1988) A new method of lathing corneal lenticules for keratorefractive procedures, *J. Refr. Surg.*, **4**, 142.

Barry, D. and Ahmod, A.M. (1986) Design and performance of a modified buckle transducer for the measurement of ligament tension. *J. Biomech. Eng.*, **108**, 149.

Bartholomew, J.S. and Anderson, J.C. (1983) Distribution of proteoglycans and hyaluronic acid in transverse sections of bovine thoracic aorta. *Histochem. J.*, **15**, 941.

Batich, C. and DePalma, D. (1992) Materials used in breast implants: Silicones and polyurethanes. *J. Long-Term Effects of Medical Implants*, **1**, 253.

Batich, C., Williams, J. and King, T. (1989) Toxic hydrolysis products from biodegradable foam implant. *J. Biomed. Mater. Res.: Appl. Biomater.*, **23**, 311.

Bear, R.S. (1952) The structure of collagen fibrils. *Adv. Protein Chem.,* **7**, 69.

Beekhuis, G.J. and Colton, J.J. (1991) Mesh materials for facial augmentation, in *Applications of Biomaterials in Facial Plastic Surgery*, (eds A.I. Glasgold and F.H. Silver), CRC Press, Boca Raton, Fl, Ch. 18.

Behar, D., Juszynski, M., Ben Hur, N., Golan, J., Eldad, A., Tuchman, Y., Sterenberg, N. and Rudensky, B. (1986) Omniderm, a new synthetic wound covering: Physical properties and drug permeability studies *J. Biomed. Mat. Res.,* **20**, 731.

Bell, E., Ehrlich, H.P., Sher, S., Merrill, C., Sarber, R., Hull, B., Nakatsuji, T., Church, D. and Buttle, D.J. (1981) Development and use of a living skin, *Plastic and Reconstructive Surgery,* **67**, 386.

Bell, E., Ehrlich, P., Buttle, D.J. and Nakatsuji, T. (1981a) Living tissue formed in vitro and accepted as skin equivalent tissue of full thickness. *Science,* **211**, 1052.

Bell, E., Ivarsson, B. and Merrill, C. (1979) Production of a tissue-like structure by contraction of collagen lattices by human fibroblasts of different proliferative potential in vitro. *Proc. Natl. Acad. Sci. USA,* **76**, 1274.

Bell, E., Moore, H., Mitchie, C. Sher, S. and Coon, H. (1984) Reconstitution of a thyroid gland equivalent from cells and matrix materials. *J. Experimental Zoology,* **232**, 277.

Bell, E. Rosenberg, M., Kemp, P., Parenteau, N., Haimes, H., Chen, J., Swiderek, M., Kaplan, F., Kagan, D., Mason, V. and Boucher, L. (1989) Reconstitution of living organ equivalents from specialized cells and matrix biomolecules, *Hybrid Artificial Organs*, (eds C. Baquey and B. Dupuy), *Colloque INSERM,* **177**, 13.

Bell, E., Sher, S. and Hull, B. (1984a) The living skin equivalent as a structural and immunological model in skin grafting. *Scanning Electron Microscopy,* **4**, 1957.

Bell, E., Sher, S., Hull, B., Merrill, C., Rosen, S., Chamson, A., Asselineau, D., Dubertret, L., Coulomb, B., Lapiere, C., Nusgens, B. and Neveux, Y. (1983) The reconstitution of living skin. *J. Invest. Derm.,* **81**, 2s.

Benedetto, D. (1992) Viscoelastics, in *The Surgical Rehabilitation of Vision,* (eds L.T. Nordan, W.A. Maxwell and J.A. Davison), Gower Medical Publishing, New York, NY, Ch. 8.

Benya, P.D. and Padilla, S.R. (1986) Isolation and characterization of type VIII collagen synthesized by cultured rabbit corneal endothelial cells. *J. Biol. Chem.,* **261**, 4160.

Bergan, J.J., Veith, F., Bernhard, V.M., Yao, J.S.T., Flinn, W.R., Gupta, S.K., Scher, L.A., Samson, R.H. and Towne, J.B. (1982) Randomization of autogenous vein and polytetrafluoroethylene grafts in femoral-distal reconstruction. *Surgery,* **92**, 921.

Bergel, D.H. (1960) Arterial viscoelasticity, in *Pulsatile Blood Flow,* (ed E. Attinger) McGraw-Hill, NY, 281.
Bergel, D.H. (1961a) The static elastic properties of the arterial wall. *J. Physiol.,* **156**, 445.
Bergel, D.H. (1961b) The dynamic elastic properties of the arterial wall. *J. Physiol.,* **156**, 458.
Berghaus, A. (1985) Porous polyethylene in reconstructive head and neck surgery. *Arch. Otolaryngology,* **111**, 154.
Berkowitz, F. and Elam, M.V. (1985) Augmentation mammoplasty 20 years of clinical experience. *Am. J. Cosmetic Surg.,* **2**, 48.
Berrino, P., Galli, A., Rainero, M.L. and Santi, P.L. (1986) Long-lasting complications with the use of polyurethane-covered breast implants. *Br. J. Plastic Surg.,* **39**, 549.
Berson, F.G., Patterson, M.M. and Epstein, D.L. (1983) Obstruction of aqueous outflow by sodium hyaluronate in enucleated human eyes. *Am. J. Ophthalmol.,* **95**, 668.
Bertram, C.D. (1977) Ultrasonic transit-time system for arterial diameter measurement. *Med. Biol. Eng. Comput.,* **15**, 489.
Billingham, R.E. and Reynolds, J. (1952) Transplantation studies on sheets of pure epidermal epithelium and on epidermal cell suspensions. *Br. J. Plast. Surg.,* **5**, 25.
Binder, P.S. and Zavala, E.Y. (1987) Why do some epikeratoplasties fail? *Arch. Ophthalmol.,* **105**, 63.
Binder, W.J., Kamer, F.M. and Parker, M.L. (1981) Mentoplasty – a clinical analysis of alloplastic implants. *Laryngoscope,* **91**, 383.
Birk, D.E. and Silver, F.H. (1986) Molecular structure and physical properties of type IV collagen in solution. *Int. J. Biol. Macromol.,* **9**, 7–10.
Birk, D.E. and Trelstad, R.L. (1986) Extracellular compartments in tendon morphogenesis: collagen fibril, bundle and macroaggregate formation. *J. Cell Biology,* **103**, 231.
Birk, D.E., Fitch, J.M., Babiarz, J.P. and Linsenmayer, T.F. (1988) Collagen type I and type V are present in the same fibril in the avian corneal stroma. *Cell Biology,* **106**, 999–1008.
Birk, D.E., Silver, F.H. and Trelstad, R.L. (1991) Matrix polymerization, in *The Cell Biology of the Extracellular Matrix,* 2nd edn, (ed. E.D. Hay), Academic Press, NY, 221.
Birk, D.E., Zycband, E.I., Winkelman, D.A. and Trelstad, R.L. (1989) Collagen fibrillogenesis in situ: fibril segments are intermediates in matrix assembly. *Proc. Natl. Acad. Sci. USA,* **86**, 4549.
Black, J. (1988) *Orthopaedic Biomaterials in Research and Practice,* Churchill Livingstone, Chs 6, 7 and 13.
Black, J. (1989) Requirements for successful total knee replacement. *Orthopaedics Clinics of North America,* **20**, 1.

Blackwell, J. (1982) The macromolecular organization of cellulose and chitin, in *Cellulose and other Natural Polymer Systems*, (ed R.M. Brown Jr.) Plenum Press, NY, Ch. 20.

Bloom, W. and Fawcett, D.W. (1975) *A Textbook of Histology*, W.B. Saunders, Philadelphia, 401.

Blumenthal, N. and Steinberg, J. (1990) The use of collagen membrane barriers in conjuction with combined demineralized bone-collagen gel implants in human infrabony defects. *J. Periodontol*, **61**, 319.

Blumenthal, N., Sabet, T. and Barrington, E. (1986) Healing responses to grafting of combined collagen decalcified bone in periodontal defects in dogs. *J. Periodontol.*, **57**, 84.

Bolton, C.W. and Bruchman, W.C. (1985) The GORE-TEX expanded polytetrafluoroethylene prosthetic ligament: An in vitro and in vivo evaluation. *Clin. Orthop.*, **196**, 201.

Bonchek, L.I. and Starr, A. (1975) Ball valve prostheses: current appraisal of late results. *Am. J. Cardiol.*, **35**, 843.

Bouvier, M. (1989) The biology and composition of bone, in *Bone Mechanics*, (ed. S.C. Cowin), CRC Press, Boca Raton, Fl, Ch. 1.

Boyce, S.T. and Hansbrough, J.F. (1988) Biologic attachment, growth, and differentiation of cultured human epidermal keratinocytes on a graftable collagen and chondroitin-6-sulfate substrate. *Surgery*, **103**, 421.

Boyce, S.T., Christianson, D.J. and Hansbrough, J.F. (1988) Structure of a collagen-GAG dermal skin substitute for cultured human keratinocytes. *J. Biomed. Mat. Res.*, **22**, 939.

Boyko, G.A., Brunette, D.M. and Melcher, A.H. (1980) Cell attachment of demineralized root surface in vitro. *J. Periodont. Res.*, **15**, 297.

Braden, B.J. and Bryant, R. (1990) Innovations to prevent and treat pressure ulcers. *Geriatric Nursing*, July/August,182.

Brand, R.A. (1986) Knee ligaments: A new view. *J. Biomech. Eng.*, **108**,106.

Brandt, B., Breiting, V., Christensen, B.L., Neilsen, M. and Thomson, J.L. (1984) Five years experience of breast augmentation using silicone gel prostheses with emphasis on capsular skrinkage. *Scand. J. Plast. Reconstr. Surg.*, **18**, 311.

Broadbent, T. and Woolf, R. (1967) Augmentation mammoplasty. *Plast. Reconstr. Surg.*, **40**, 517.

Brodie, H.A. and Donald, P.J. (1991) Facial, pericranial and dural grafts in surgery of the head and neck, in *Applications of Biomaterials in Facial Plastic Surgery*, (eds A.I. Glasgold and F.H. Silver), CRC Press, Boca Raton, Fl, Ch. 12.

Brodsky, B., Eikenberry, E.F., Belbruno, C. and Sterling, K. (1982) Variations in collagen fibril structure in tendons. *Biopolymers,* **21**, 935.

Brown, D.C. and Vogel, K.G. (1989) Characteristics of the *in vitro* interaction of a small proteoglycan (PGII) of bovine tendon with type I collagen. *Matrix,* **9**, 468.

Bruck, S.D. and Silver, F.H. (1991) The safe medical devices act of 1990. *J. Long-Term Effects of Medical Implants,* **1**, 121.

Buja, L.M. (1987) The vascular system, in *Basic Pathology,* (eds S.L. Robbins and V. Kumar), W. D. Saunders, Philadelphia, Pa., Ch. 10.

Buntin, C.M. and Silver, F.H. (1988) Noninvasive measurement of rabbit aortic wall thickness using ultrasound and histological analysis. *Biomedical Sciences Instrumentation. Proc. 25th Ann. Rocky Mountain Bioeng. Symp.,* **29**, 119.

Burke, D.W. Gates, E.I. and Harris, W.H. (1984) Centrifugation as a method of improving tensile and fatigue properties of acrylic bone cement. *J. Bone Joint Surg.,* **66A**, 1265.

Burke, J.F., Yannas, I.V., Quinby, W.C. Jr., Bondoc, C.C. and Jung, W.K. (1981) Successful use of a physiologically acceptable artificial skin in the treatment of extensive burn injury. *Ann. Surg.,* **194**, 413.

Burkhardt, B.R., Dempsey, P.D., Schnur, P.L. and Tofield, J.J. (1986) Capsular contracture: a prospective study of the effect of local antibacterial agents. *Plast. Reconstr. Surg.,* **77**, 919.

Burnstein, N.L., Ding, M., and Pratt, M.V. (1988) Intraocular lens evaluation by iris abrasion in vitro: a scanning electron microscopy study. *J. Cataract Refr. Surg.,* **14**, 520.

Byron, M.A., Venning, V.A. and Mowat, A.G. (1984) Post-mammoplasty human adjuvant disease. *Br. J. Rheumatol.,* **23**, 227.

Cabaud, H.E., Feagin, J.A. and Rodkey, W.G. (1982) Acute anterior cruciate ligament injury and repair reinforced with a biodegradable intraarticular ligament. Experimental studies. *Am. J. Sports Med.,* **10**, 259.

Cabaud, H.E., Rodkey, W.G. and Feagin, J.A. (1979) Experimental studies of acute anterior cruciate ligament injury and repair. *Am. J. Sports Med.,* **7**, 18.

Cairns, T.S. and de Villiers, W. (1980) Capsular contracture after breast augmentation – A comparison between gel- and saline-filled prostheses. *S. Afr. Med. J.,* **57**, 951.

Campbell, C.D., Goldfarb, D., Detton, D.D., Roe, R., Goldsmith, K. and Diethrich, E.B. (1974) Expanded polytetrafluoroethylene as a small artery substitute, *Trans. Am. Soc. Artif. Intern. Organs,* **20**, 86.

Canton, J. and Zander, H. (1976) Osseous repair of an infrabony pocket without new attachment of connective tissue. *J. Periodontol.,* **3**, 54.

Carpentier, A., Dubost, C., Lane, E., Nashef, A., Carpentier S., Relland, J., Deloche A., Fabiani, J.N., Chauvaud, S., Perier P. and Maxwell, S. (1982) Continuing improvements in valvular bioprostheses. *J. Thorac. Cardiovasc. Surg.,* **83**, 27.

Carter, D.M., Lin, A.N., Vargese, M.C., Caldwell, D., Pratt, L.A. and Eisinger, M. (1987) Treatment of junctional epidermolysis bullosa with epidermal autografts. *J. Am. Acad. Dermatol.*, **17**, 246.

Cetta, G., Tenni, R., and Zanaboni, G. (1982) Biochemical and morphological modification in rabbit achilles tendon during maturation and aging. *Biochem. J.*, **204**, 61.

Chambers, T.J. (1980) The cellular basis of bone resorption. *Clin. Orthop. Rel. Res.*, **151**, 283.

Charnley, J. (1965) A biomechanical analysis of the use of cement to anchor the femoral head prosthesis. *J. Bone Jt. Surg.*, **47B**, 354.

Charnley, J. (1972) Post-operative infection after total hip replacement with special reference to air contamination in the operating room. *Clin. Orthop.*, **87**, 167.

Chen, E.H. and Black, J. (1990) Materials design and analysis of the prosthetic anterior cruciate ligament. *J. Biomed. Mat. Res.*, **14**, 567.

Cho, K.O. (1975) Reconstruction of the anterior cruciate ligament by semitendinosus tenodesis. *J. Bone Jt. Surg.*, **57-A**, 608.

Choi, H.U., Johnson, T.L., Pal, S., Tang, L.-H., Rosenberg, L. and Neame, P.J. (1989) Characterization of dermatan sulfate proteoglycans, DS-PGI and DS-PGII, from bovine articular cartilage and skin isolated by octyl-sepharose chromatography. *J. Biol. Chem.*, **264**, 2876.

Christiansen, D.L., Riley, D.J., Tozzi, C.A. and Silver, F.H. (1991) The mechanical properties of the extracellular matrix in *The Extracellular Matrix and the Uterus, Cervix and Foetal Membranes,* (eds P.C. Leppert and F. Woessner), Perinatology Press, Ithaca, NY, Ch. 4.

Chung, E. and Miller, E.J. (1974) Collagen polymorphism: characterization of molecules with the chain composition $[\alpha 1(III)]3$ in human tissues. *Science,* **183**, 1200.

Chung, E., Rhodes, R.K. and Miller, E.J. (1976) Isolation of three collagenous components of probable basement membrane origin from several tissues. *Biochem. Biophys. Res. Commun.*, **71**, 1167.

Churukian, M.M., Cohen, A., Kamer, F.M., Lefkoff, L., Palmer, F. R., III and Ross, C.A. (1991) Injectable collagen: A ten-year experience, in *Applications of Biomaterials In Facial Plastic Surgery*, (eds A.I. Glasgold and F.H. Silver), CRC Press, Boca Raton, Fl, Ch. 15.

Chvapil, M. (1982) Considerations on maunfacturing principles of a synthetic burn dressing: A review. *J. Biomed. Mat. Res.*, **16**, 245.

Chvapil, M., Gibeault, D. and Wang, T.-F. (1987) Use of chemically purified and cross-linked bovine pericardium as a ligament substitute. *J. Biomed. Mat. Res.*, **21**, 1383.

Ciarkowski, A.A. (1986) Preclinical testing evaluation of biomaterials: in vitro and in vivo, in *Handbook of Biomaterials Applications,* (ed. A. F. von Recum), Macmillan Publishing Co., New York, NY, Ch. 42.

Clancy, W.G., Narechania, R.G., Rosenberg, T.D., Gmeiner, J.G., Wisnefske, D.D. and Lange, T.A. (1981) Anterior and posterior cruciate ligament reconstruction in rhesus monkeys. *J. Bone Jt. Surg.*, **63**-A, 1270.

Clark, I.C. (1974) Articular cartilage: a review and electron microscopy study. II The territorial fibrillar architecture. *J. Anat.*, **118**, 261.

Clark, J.M. and Glagov, S. (1979) Structural integration of the arterial wall. I. Relationship and attachments of medial smooth muscle cells in normally distended and hyperdistended aorta. *Lab. Invest.*, **40**, 587.

Clark, J.M. and Sidles, J.A. (1990) The interrelation of fibre bundles in the anterior cruciate ligament. *J. Orthop. Res.*, **8**, 180.

Clegg, H.W., Foster, M.T., Sanders, W.E., Jr. and Baine, W.B. (1983) Infection due to organisms of the Mycobacterium fortuitum complex after augmentation mammoplasty: clinical and epidemiologic features. *J. Infect. Dis.*, **147**, 427.

Cleland, R.L. and Wang, J.L. (1970) Ionic polysaccharides, III. Dilute solution properties of hyaluronic acid fractions. *Biopolymers*, **9**, 799.

Cobanoglu, A., Grunkemeier, G.L., Aru, G.M., McKinley, C.L. and Starr, A. (1985) Mitral replacement: Clinical experience with a ball-valve prosthesis. Twenty-five years later. *Ann. Surg.*, **202**, 376.

Cocke, W., Leathers, H. and Lynch, J. (1975) Foreign body reactions to polyurethane covers of some breast prostheses. *Plast. Reconstr. Surg.*, **56**, 527.

Cohn, D. and Younes, H. (1988) Biodegradable PEO/PLA block copolymers. *J. Biomed. Mat. Res.*, **22**, 993–1009.

Cohn, L.H. (1984) The long-term results of aortic valve replacement. *Chest*, **85**, 387.

Cohney, B. C., Cohney, T.B. and Hearne, V.A. (1992) Augmentation mammoplasty – a further review of 20 years using the polyurethane-covered prosthesis. *J. Long-Term Effects of Medical Implants*, **1**, 269.

Compton, C.C., Gill, J.M., Bradford, D.A., Regauer, S., Gallico, G.G. and O'Connor, N.E. (1989) Skin regenerated from cultured epithelial autografts on full-thickness burn wounds from 6 days to 5 years after grafting. *Lab. Invest.*, **60**, 600.

Compton, C.C., Regauer, S., Seiler, G.R. and Landry, D.B. (1990) Human merkel cell regeneration in skin derived from cultured keratinocyte grafts. *Lab. Invest.*, **62**, 233.

Contri, M.B., Fornieri, C. and Ronchetti, I.P. (1985) Elastin-proteoglycan association revealed by cytochemical methods. *Connect. Tissue Res.*, **13**, 237.

Cook, S.D., Walsh, K.A. and Haddad, R.J., Jr (1985) Interface mechanics and bone growth into porous Co-Cr-Mo alloy implants. *Clin. Orthop. Rel. Res.*, **193**, 271.

Cowin, S.C. (1989) The mechanical properties of cortical bone tissue, in *Bone Mechanics*, (ed. Cowin, S.C.), CRC Press Inc., Boca Raton, Fl, Chs 6 and 7.

Cracchiolo, A., III and Revell, P. (1982) Metal concentration in synovial fluids of patients with prosthetic knee arthroplasty. *Clin. Orthop. Rel. Res.*, **170**, 169.

Cuono, C., Longdon, R. and McGuire, J. (1986) Use of cultured epidermal autografts and dermal allografts as skin replacement after burn injury. *Lancet,* **1123**.

Dagalakis, N., Flink, J., Stasikelis, P., Burke, J.F. and Yannas, I.V. (1980) Design of artificial skin. III. Control of pore structure. *J. Biomed. Mat. Res.*, **14**, 511.

Dahlstedt, L.J., Netz, P. and Dalen, N. (1989) Poor results of bovine xenograft for knee cruciate ligament repair. *Acta Orthop. Scand.*, **60**, 3.

Dandy, D.J. (1973) The safety of acrylic bone cement. *Injury*, **5**, 169.

Daniels, A.U., Chang, M.K.O., Andriano, K.P. and Heller, J. (1990) Mechanical properties of biodegradable polymers and composites proposed for internal fixation of bone. *J. Applied Biomaterials*, **1**, 57–78.

Danylchuk, K.D., Finlay, J.B. and Krcek, J.P. (1978) Microstructural organization of human and bovine cruciate ligament *Clin. Orthop.*, **131**, 294.

Dardik, D. (1986) in *Vascular Graft Update: Safety and Performance,* ASTM STP-898, (eds H.E. Kambic, A. Kantrowitz and P. Sung), American Society for Testing and Materials, Philadelphia, Pa, 50.

Dardik, H., Ibrahim, I.M. and Dardik, I. (1975a) Modified and unmodified umbilical vein; allografts and xenografts as arterial substitutes: morphological assessment. *Surg. For.,* **26**, 286.

Dardik, I. and Dardik, H. (1975) The fate of human umbilical cord vessels used as interposition arterial grafts in the baboon. *Surg. Gyn. Obstet.,* **140**, 567.

Davidson, P.F., Hong, B.S. and Cannon, D.J. (1979) Quantitative analysis of the collagens in bovine cornea. *Experimental Eye Research,* **29**, 97.

Deck, D.J. (1990) Histology and cytology of the aortic valve, in *The Aortic Valve,* (ed. M. Thubrikar), CRC Press, Boca Raton, Fl, Ch. 2.

Deck, J.D., Thubrikar, M.J., Schneider, P.J. and Nolan, S.P. (1988) Structure, stress, and tissue repair in aortic valve leaflets. *Cardiovascular Research,* **22**, 7.

Delmage, J.M., Powars, D.R., Jaynes, P.K. and Allerton, S.E. (1986) The selective suppression of immunogenicity by hyaluronic acid. *Ann. Clin. Lab. Sci.,* **16**, 303–10.

DeLustro, F., Smith, S.T., Sundsmo, J., Salem, G., Kincaid, S. and Ellingsworth, L. (1987) Reaction to injectable collagen: Results in animal models and clinical use. *Plastic and Reconstructive Surgery,* **79**, 581.

Dershaw, D.D. and Chaglassian, T.A. (1989) Mammography after prosthesis placement for augmentation or reconstructive mammoplasty. *Radiology*, **170**, 69.

DeVore, D.P. (1991) Long-term compatibility of intraocular lens implant materials. *J. Long-Term Effects of Medical Implants*, **1**, 205.

Diamant, J., Keller, A., Baer, E., Lith, N. and Arridge, R.G.C. (1972) Collagen ultrastructure and its relationship to mechanical properties as a function of aging. *Proc. Roy. Soc. Lond.*, **B180**, 293.

diFiore, M.S.H. (1981) *Atlas of Human Histology*, 5th edn, Lea & Febiger, Philadelphia, Pa.

Dingemans, K.P., Jansen, N. and Becker, A.E. (1981) Ultrastructure of the normal human aortic media. *Virchows Arch. Pathol. Anat. Physiol.*, 199.

Dingman, R.O. and Crabb, W.C. (1960) Costal cartilage homografts preserved by irradiation. *Plast. Reconstr. Surg.*, **28**, 562.

Doillon, C.J., Dunn, M.G., Berg, R.A. and Silver, F.H., (1985) Collagen deposition during wound repair. *Scanning Microscopy*, **II**, 897.

Doillon, C.J., Silver, F.H., Olson, R.M., Kamath, C.Y. and Berg, R.A. (1988) Fibroblast and epidermal cell-type I collagen interactions: cell culture and human studies. *Scanning Microscopy*, **2**, 985.

Doillon, C.J., Whyne, C.F., Berg, R.A., Olson, R.M. and Silver, F.H. (1984) Fibroblast-collagen sponge interactions and spatial deposition of newly synthesized collagen fibers in vitro and in vivo. *Scanning Microscopy*, **III**, 1313.

Donald, P.J. (1986) Collagen implants: here today and gone tomorrow? *Otolaryngol. Head and Neck Surg.*, **95**, 607.

Donald, P.J. and Brodie, H.A. (1991) Cartilage autografts, in *Applications of Biomaterials in Facial Plastic Surgery*, (eds A.I. Glasgold and F.H. Silver), CRC Press, Boca Raton, Fl, Ch. 9.

Drews, R.C. (1983) Polypropylene in the human eye. *Am. Intra-Ocular Implant Soc. J.*, **9**, 137.

Dunn, M.G. and Silver, F.H. (1983) Viscoelastic behavior of human connective tissues: Relative contribution of viscous and elastic components. *Connect Tissue Res.*, **12**, 59.

Dunn, M.G., Tria, A.J., Kato, Y.P., Bechler, J.R., Ochner, R.S., Zawadsky, J.P. and Silver, F.H. (1992) Anterior cruciate ligament replacement using a composite collagenous prosthesis: A biomechanical and histological study in rabbits. *J. Sports Med.*, **20**, 507.

Durselen, L. and Claes, L. (1990) Mechanical properties of artificial ligaments, in *Clinical Implant Materials*, (eds G. Heimke, U. Soltesz and A.J.C. Lee), *Advances in Biomaterials*, Vol. 9, Elsevier Science Publishers, Amsterdam, pp. 439–44.

Eaglstein, W.H., Mertz, P.M. and Falanga, V. (1987) Occlusive dressings. *Am. Fam. Physician*, March, 211.

Edwards, B. (1963) Teflon-silicone breast implants. *Plast. Reconstr. Surg.*, **32**, 519.

Edwards, W.S. (1959) Progress in synthetic graft development – An improved crimped graft on tendon. *Surgery*, **45**, 298.

Eisinger, M. (1985) Regeneration of epidermis by cells grown in tissue culture. *J. Am. Acad. Dermatol.*, **12**, 402.

Eisinger, M., Monden, M., Raaf, J.H. and Fortner, J.G. (1980) Wound coverage by a sheet of epidermal cells grown in vitro from dispersed single cell preparations. *Surgery*, **88**, 287.

Ellenberg, A.H. and Braun, H. (1980) A 3½ year experience with double-lumen implants in breast surgery. *Plast. Reconstr. Surg.*, **65**, 307.

Ellenberger, P., Graham, W.P. 3rd, Manders, E.K. and Basarab, R.M. (1986) Labeled leukocyte scans for detection of retained polyurethane foam. *Plast. Reconstr. Surg.*, **77**, 77.

Elliott, D.H. (1965) Structure and function of mammalian tendon. *Biol. Rev.*, **40**, 392.

Elsdale, T. and Bard, J. (1972) Collagen substrata for studies on cell behavior. *J. Cell Biol.*, **54**, 626.

Embriano, P.J. (1989) Postoperative pressures after phacoemulsification: sodium hyaluronate vs. sodium chondroitin sulfate-sodium hyaluronate. *Ann. Ophthalmol.*, **21**, 85.

Endo, L.P., Edwards, N.L., Longley, S., Corman, L.C. and Parnush, R.S. (1987) Silicone and rheumatic disease. *Semin. Arthritis Rheu.*, **17**, 112.

Ersek, R.A.(1991) Molecular impact surface textured implants (MSTI) alter beneficial breast capsule formation at 36 months. *J. Long-Term Effects of Medical Implants*, **1**, 155.

Fanning, J.C., Yates, N.G. and Cleary, E.G. (1981) Elastin-associated microfibrils in aorta: species differences in large animals. *Micron*, **12**, 339.

Faure, M., Mauduit, G., Demidem, A. and Thivolet, J. (1986) Langerhans cell free cultured epidermis used as permanent skin allografts in humans. *J. Invest. Derm.*, **86**, 474.

Faure, M., Mauduit, G., Schmitt, D., Kanitakis, J., Demidem, A. and Thivolet, J. (1987) Growth and differentiation of human epidermal cultures used as auto- and allografts in humans. *Br. J. Dermatol.*, **116**, 161.

Feagin, J.A. (1988) *The Knee: Joint of Necessity in The Cruciate Ligaments*, Churchill Livingstone, NY, 398.

Fechner, P.U. and Fechner, M.U. (1983) Methylcellulose and lens implantation. *Brit. J. Ophthalmol.* **67**, 259–63.

Feigl, E.D., Peterson, L.H. and Jones, A.W. (1963) Mechanical and chemical properties of arteries in experimental hypertension. *J. Clin. Invest.*, **42**, 1640.

Ferkel, R.D., Fox, J.M., DelPizzo, W., Freedman, M.J., Snyder, S.J., Dorey, F. and Kasimian, D. (1988) Reconstruction of the anterior cruciate ligament using a torn meniscus. *J. Bone Jt. Surg.*, **70-A**, 715.

Ferl, J.G., Goldenthal, K.L. and Mishra, N.K. (1988) FDA regulation of prosthetic ligament devices, in *Prosthetic Ligament Reconstruction of The Knee*, (eds M.J. Friedman and R.D. Ferkel), W.B. Saunders Co., Philadelphia, 202.

Fischer, G. M. and Llaurado, J.G. (1966) Collagen and elastin content in canine arteries from functionally different vascular beds. *Circ. Res.*, **19**, 3984.

Fisher, J.C. and Brody, G.S. (1992) Breast implants under siege: An historical commentary, *J. Long-Term Effects of Medical Implants*, **1**, 243.

Flaherty, J.T., Pierce, J.E., Ferrans, V.J., Patel, D.J., Tucker, W.K. and Fry, D.L. (1972) Endothelial nuclear patterns in the canine arterial tree with particular reference to hemodynamic events. *Circ. Res.* **30**, 23.

Fock, K.M., Feng, P.H. and Tey, B.H. (1984) Autoimmune disease developing after augmentation mammoplasty: report of 3 cases. *J. Rheumatol.*, **11**, 98.

Folkman, J. (1982) Angiogenesis: initiation and control. *Ann. N.Y. Acad. Sci.*, **401**, 212.

Forrester, J.V. and Lackie, J.M. (1981) Effect of hyaluronic acid on neutrophil adhesion. *J. Cell Sci.*, **48**, 315–31.

Fox, J.M., Sherman, O.H. and Markolf, K. (1985) Arthroscopic anterior cruciate ligament repair: preliminary results and instrumented testing for anterior stability. *Arthroscopy*, **1**, 175.

Frank, C., Woo, S.L-Y., Amiel, D., Harwood, F, Gomez, M. and Akeson, W.A.J. (1983) Medial collateral ligament healing: a multidisciplinary assessment in rabbits. *Am. J. Sports Med.*, **11**, 379.

Frank, C., Woo, S.L-Y., Andriacchi, T., Brand, R., Oakes, B., Dahners, L., Dehave, K., Lewis, J. and Sabiston, T. (1988) in *Injury and Repair of the Musculoskeletal Soft Tissues,* (eds S.L-Y. Woo and J. Buckwalter), American Academy of Orthopaedic Surgeons, Park Ridge, Illinois, p. 45.

Franks, W.A., Adams, G.G.W., Dart, J.K.G., and Minassian, D. (1988) The relative risks of different types of contact lenses. *Br. Med. J.*, **297**, 534.

Freeman, A.E., Igel, H.J., Waldman, N.L. and Losikoff, A. M. (1974) A new method for covering large surface area wounds with autografts, I. In vitro multiplication of rabbit-skin epithelial cells. *Arch. Surg.*, **108**, 721.

Freeman, I.L. (1982) The eye, in *Collagen in Health and Disease*, (eds J.B. Weiss and M.I.V. Jayson), Churchill Livingstone, Ch. 21.

Fried, J.A., Bergfeld, J.A., Weiker, G. and Andrish, J.T. (1985) Anterior cruciate reconstruction using the Jones-Ellison procedure. *J. Bone Jt. Surg*, **67-A**, 1029.

Friedman, M.J. and Ferkel, R.J. (1988) *Prosthetic Ligament Reconstruction of Knee*, W.B. Saunders Co., Philadelphia, Pa.

Friedman, M.J., Sherman, O.H., Fox, J.M., Del Pizzo, W., Snyder, S.J. and Ferkel, R.J. (1985) Autogeneic anterior cruciate ligament (ACL) anterior reconstruction of the knee. *Clin. Othop. Rel. Res.*, **196**, 9.

Fujikawa, K. (1988) *Prosthetic Ligament Reconstruction of the Knee*, (eds M.J. Friedman and R.D. Ferkel), W.B. Saunders Co., Philadelphia, 1329.

Fung, Y.C.B. (1967) Elasticity of soft tissues in simple elongation. *Am. J. of Physiol.*, **213**, 1532.

Fung, Y.C.B. (1972) Stress-strain history relations of soft tissues in simple elongation, in *Biomechanics: Its Foundations and Objectives*, (eds Y.C.B. Fung *et al.*), Prentice-Hall, Englewood Cliffs, New Jersey, 181.

Galin, M.A., Tuberville, A.W. and Dotson, R.S. (1982) Immunological aspects of intraocular lenses. *Int. Ophthalmol. Clin.*, **22**, 227.

Galin, M.A., Turkish, L. and Chowchuvech, E. (1977) Detection, removal, and effect of unpolymerized methylmethacrylate in intraocular lenses. *Am. J. Ophthalmol.*, **84**, 153.

Gallico, G.G., O'Connor, N.E., Compton, C.C., Kehinde, O. and Green, H. (1984) Permanent coverage of large burn wounds with autologous cultured human epithelium. *New Eng. J. Med.*, **311**, 448.

Gallico, III, G.G., O'Connor, N.E., Compton, C.C., Remensnyder, J.P., Kehinde, O. and Green, H. (1989) Cultured epithelial autografts for giant congenital nervi. *Plas. Recon. Surg.*, **84**, 1.

Galway, R.D., Beaupre, A. and MacIntosh, D.L. (1972) Pivot shift: a clinical sign of symptomatic anterior cruciate insufficiency. *J. Bone Jt. Sur.*, **54B**, 763.

Gay, S., Muller, P.K., Meigel, W.N. and Kuhn, K. (1976) Polymorphic de Kollagens neire Aspekte Fur Struktur and Funktion des Binegewebes. *Der Hautartz*, **27**, 196.

Geesin, J. C. and Berg, R.A. (1991) Biochemistry of skin, bone and cartilage, in *Applications of Biomaterials in Facial Plastic Surgery*, (eds A.I. Glasgold and F.H. Silver), CRC, Boca Raton, Florida, Ch. 2.

Gibson, T. (1977) Transplantation of cartilage, in *Reconstructive Plastic Surgery*, (eds J.M. Converse and J.G. McCarthy), Vol 1, 2nd edn, W.B. Saunders Co, Philadelphia, Pa, pp. 301.

Gibson, T. and Davis, W.B. (1959) The encapsulation of preserved cartilage grafts with prolonged survival. *Br. J. Plast. Surg.*, **12**, 22.

Gillespie, W.J., Frampton, C.M.A., Henderson, R.J. *et al.* (1983) The incidence of cancer following total hip replacement. *J. Bone Jt. Surg.*, **70B**, 539.

Glasgold, A.I. and Glasgold, M.J. (1991) Cartilage autografts, in *Applications of Biomaterials in Facial Plastic Surgery*, (eds A.I. Glasgold and F.H. Silver), CRC Press, Boca Raton, Fl, Ch. 8.

Glasgold, A.I. and Silver, F.H. (1991) *Applications of Biomaterials in Facial Plastic Surgery*, CRC Press, Boca Raton, FL.

Glasgold, M.J., Kato, Y.P., Christiansen, D., Haugue, J.A., Glasgold, A.I. and Silver, F.H. (1988) Mechanical properties of septal cartilage homografts. *Otolaryngology Head and Neck Surgery*, **99**, 374.

Goldfischer, S., Coltoff-Schiller, B., Schwartz, E. and Blumenfeld, O.O. (1983) Ultrastructure and staining properties of aortic microfibrils. *J. Histochem. Cytochem.*, **31**, 382.

Goldring, S.R., Schiller, A.L., Roelke, M. *et al.* (1983) The synovial-like membrane at the bone-cement interface in loose total hip replacements and its proposed role in bone lysis. *J. Bone Jt. Surg.*, **65A**, 575.

Good, L., Odenstein, M., Pettersson, L. and Gillquest, J. (1989) Failure of a bovine xenograft for reconstruction of the anterior cruciate ligament. *Acta Orthop. Scand.*, **60**, 8.

Goodship, A.E., Wilcock, S.A. and Shah, J.S. (1985) The development of tissue around various prosthetic implants used as replacements for ligaments and tendons. *Clin. Orthop.*, **196**, 61.

Gotoh, T. and Sugi, Y. (1985) Electron-microscopic study of the collagen fibrils of the rat tail tendon as revealed by freeze-fracture and freeze-etching techniques, *Cell Tissue Res.*, **240**, 529.

Gozna, E.R., Marble, A.F., Shaw, A.J. and Winter, D.A. (1973) Mechanical properties of the ascending thoracic aorta of man. *Circ. Res.*, **7**, 261.

Graham, L.M., Burkel, W.E., Ford, J.W., Vinter, D.W., Kahn, R. G. and Stanely, J.C. (1982) Expanded polytetrafluoroethylene vascular prostheses seeded with enzymatically derived and cultured canine endothelial cells. *Surgery*, **91**, 550.

Greenfield, J.C. and Patel, D.J. (1962) Relation between pressure and diameter in the ascending aorta of man. *Circ. Res.*, **10**, 778.

Gross, L. and Kugel, M.A. (1931) Topographic anatomy and histology of the valves in the human heart. *Am. J. Pathol.* **7**, 445.

Grossman, A. (1976) Psychological and psychosexual aspects of augmentation mammaplasty. *Clin. Plast. Surg.*, **3**, 167.

Guidry, C. and Grinnell, F. (1987) Heparin modulates the organization of hydrated collagen gels and inhibits gel contraction by fibroblasts. *J. Cell Biol.*, **104**, 1097.

Gullberg, D., Tingstrom, A., Thuresson, A.-C., Olsson, L., Terracio, L., Borg, T.G. and Rubin, K. (1990) Beta 1 integrin mediated collagen gel contraction is stimulated by PDGF. *Exp. Cell Res.*, **186**, 264.

Haimann, M.H. and Phelps, C.D. (1981) Prophylactic Timolol for the prevention of high intraocular pressure after cataract extraction. *Ophthalmol.*, **88**, 233.

Hakansson, L. and Venge, P. (1987) The molecular basis of the hyaluronic acid-mediated stimulation of granulocyte function, **138**, 4347–52.

Hall, G.W., Liotta, D., Ghidoni, J.J., DeBakey, M.E. and Dressler, D.P. (1967) Velous fabrics applied to medicine, *J. Biomed. Mater. Res.*, **1**, 179.

Hall-Craggs, E.C.B. (1990) *Anatomy as a Basis for Clinical Medicine,* 2nd edn, Urban & Schwarzenberg, Baltimore-Munich, p.167.

Hampton, S.J., Andriacchi, T.P. and Galante, J.O. (1980) Three-dimensional stress analysis of the femoral stem of a total hip prosthesis. *J. Biomech.*, **13**, 443.

Hansen, A.D. and Rand, J.A. (1988) A comparison of primary and revision total knee arthroplasty using the Kinematic stabilized prosthesis. *J. Bone Jt. Surg.*, **70 A**, 491.

Hansborough, J.F., Boyce, S.T., Cooper, M.L. and Foreman, T.J. (1989) Burn wound closure with cultured autologous keratinocytes and fibroblasts attached to a collagen-glycosaminoglycan substrate. *JAMA,* **262**, 2125.

Harkness, R.D. (1961) Biological functions of collagen. *Biol. Rev.*, **36**, 399.

Harris, W.H. (1975) A new approach to total hip repacement without osteotomy of the greater trocanter. *Clin. Orthop.*, **106**, 19.

Harrison, S.E., Soll, D.B., Shayegan, M. and Clinch, T. (1982) Chondroitin sulfate: a new and effective protective agent for intraocular lens insertion. *Amer. Acad. Ophthalmol.* **89**, 1254–60.

Hartley, J. H. and Schatten, W. E. (1971) Postoperative complication of lactation after augmentation mammoplasty. *Plast. Reconstr. Surg.*, **47**, 150.

Hartley, J.H., Jr. (1976) Specific applications of the double-lumen prosthesis. *Clin Plast. Surg.*, **3**, 247.

Hayes, H., Jr., Vandergrift, J. and Diner, W.C. (1988) Mammography and breast implants. *Plast. Reconstr. Surg.*, **82**, 1.

Heatley, F. and Scott, J.E. (1988) A water molecule participates in the secondary structure of hyaluronan. *Biochem. J.*, **254**, 489–93.

Heck, E.L., Bergstresser, P.R. and Baxter, C.R. (1985) Composite skin graft: Frozen dermal allografts support the engraftment and expansion of autologous epidermis. *J. Trauma,* **25**, 106.

Hefton, J.M., Caldwell, D., Biozes, D.G., Balin, A.K. and Carter, D.M. (1986) Grafting of skin ulcers with cultured autologous epidermal cells. *J. Am. Acad. Dermatol.*, **14**, 399.

Hefton, J.M., Madden, M.R., Finkelstein, J.L. and Shires, G.T. (1983) Grafting of burn patients with allografts of cultured epidermal cells. *Lancet,* 428.

Heimke, G. (1986) Ceramics, in *Handbook of Biomaterials Evaluation,* (ed. A.F. von Recum), Macmillan Publishing Co., NY, Ch. 3.

Heinegard, D. and Paulsson, M. (1984) Structure and metabolism of proteoglycans, in *Connective Tissue Biochemistry*, (eds K. Piez and H. Reddi), Elsevier, NY, 277.

Herman, S. (1984) The Meme implant. *Plast. Reconstr. Surg.,* **73**,.

Hertzer, N.R. (1981) Regeneration of endothelium in knitted and velour Dacron vascular grafts in dogs. *J. Cardiovasc. Surg.,* **22**, 223.

Herzog, S.R., Meyer, A., Woodley, D. and Peterson, H.D. (1988) Wound coverage with cultured autologous keratinocytes: Use after burn wound excision including biopsy follow up. *J. Trauma,* **28**, 195.

Herzog, W.R. and Peiffer, R.L., Jr. (1987) Comparison of the effect of polymethylmethacrylate and silicone intraocular lenses on rabbit corneal endothelium in vitro. *J. Cataract Refr. Surg.,* **13**, 397.

Hetter, G. (1979) Satisfactions and dissatisfactions of patients with augmentation mammoplasty. *Plast. Reconstr. Surg.,* **64**, 151.

Hipps, C.J., Raju, R. and Straith, R.E. (1978) Influence of some operative and postoperative factors on capsular contracture around breast prostheses. *Plast. Reconstr. Surg.,* **61**, 384.

Hobden, J. A., Reidy, J.J., O'Callaghan, R.J., Hill, J.M., Insler, M.S. and Rootman, D.S. (1988) Treatment of experimental pseudomonas keratitis using collagen shields containing tobramycin. *Arch. Ophthalmol.,* **106**, 1605.

Hobson, R.W., II, O'Donnell, J.A., Jamil, Z. and Mehta, K. (1980) Below knee bypass for limb salvage. *Arch. Surg.,* **115**, 833.

Holly, F.J. and Lemp, M.A. (1977) Tear physiology and dry eyes. *Surv. Ophthalmol.,* **21**, 69.

Hughes, D.J., Babbs, C.F., Geddes, L.A. and Bourland, J.D. (1979) Measurements of Young's modulus of elasticity of the canine aorta with ultrasound. *Ultrasonic Imag.,* **1**, 356.

Hughes, D.J., Fearnot, N.E., Babb, C.F., Bourland, J.D., Geddes, L.A. and Eggelgton, R. (1985) Continuous measurement of aortic radius change in vivo with an intra-aortic ultrasonic catheter. *Med. Biol. Eng. Comput.,* **23**, 197.

Hughes, D.J., Geddes, L.A., Bourland, J.D. and Babbs, C.F. (1979a) *Dynamic Imaging of the Aorta In Vivo ith 10 MHz Ultrasound, Acoustical Imaging.* (ed. A. Metherell) Plenum Press, New York.

Hughston, J.C., Andrews, J.R., Cross, M.J. and Moschi, A. (1976) Classification of knee ligament instabilities Part I. *J. Bone Jt. Surg.,* **58A**, 159.

Hull, B.E., Finley, R.K. and Miller, S.F. (1990) Coverage of full-thickness burns with bi-layered skin equivalents: A preliminary clinical trial. *Surgery,* **107**, 496.

Hulmes, D.J.S., Jesior, J.-C, Miller, A., Berthet-Colominas, C. and Wolff, C. (1981) Electron microscopy shows periodic structure in collagen fibril cross-sections. *Proc. Natl. Acad. Sci. USA,* **78**, 3567.

Hunderford, D.S. and Kenna, R.V. (1983) Preliminary experience with a total knee prosthesis with porous coating used without cement. *Clin. Orthop. Rel. Res.*, **176**, 95.

Hurley, F.L. (1986) Clinical trials of biomaterials and medical devices, in, *Handbook of Biomaterials Evaluation*, (ed. A.F. von Recum), Macmillan, NY, Ch. 43.

Hutchinson, J.J. and McGuckin, M. (1990) Occlusive dressings: A microbiologic and clinical review. *Am. J. Infect. Control,* **18**, 257.

Hynes, R.O. (1987) Integrins: A family of cell surface receptors. *Cell,* **48**, 549.

Igel, H.J., Freeman, A.E., Boeckman, C.R. and Kleinfeld, K.L. (1974) A new method for covering large surface area wounds with autografts. *Arch. Surg.*, **108**, 724.

Ingber, D.E. (1990) Fibronectin controls capillary endothelial cell growth by modulating cell shape. *Proc. Natl. Acad. Sci. USA,* **87**, 3579.

Jackson, D.W., Grood, E.S., Arnoczky, S.P., Butler, D.L. and Simon, T.M. (1987) Freeze-dried anterior cruciate ligament allografts. Preliminary studies in a goat model. *Am. J. Sports Med.,* **15**, 295.

Jackson, D.W., Windler, G.E. and Simon, T.M. (1990) Intraarticular reaction associated with the use of freeze-dried, ethylene oxide-sterilized bone-patellar tendon-bone allografts in the reconstruction of the anterior cruciate ligament. *Am. J. Sports Med.,* **18**, 1.

Jacobsen, K. (1977) Stress radiographical measurements of post-traumatic knee instability: a clinical study. *Acta Orthop. Scand.,* **48**, 301.

James, J.H. and Watson, A.C.H. (1975) The use of Opsite, a vapour permeable dressing, on skin graft donor sites. *Brit. J. Plast. Surg.,* **28**, 107.

Jenkins, D.H.R., Forster, I.W., McKibbin, B. and Ralis, Z.A. (1977) Induction of tendon and ligament formation by carbon implants. *J. Bone Jt. Surg.* **59-B**, 53.

Jerusalem, C., Hess, F. and Werner, H. (1987) The formation of a neo-intima in textile prostheses implanted in the aorta of rats and dogs *Cell Tissue Res.,* **248**, 505.

Jimenez, S.A., Yankowski, R. and Bashey, R. (1978) Identification of two new collagen α chains in extracts of lathyritic chick embryo tendon. *Biochem. Biophys. Res. Commun.,* **81**, 1298.

Johnson, R.J., Eriksson, E., Haggmark, T. and Pope, M.H. (1984) Five to ten-year follow-up evaluation after reconstruction of the anterior cruciate ligament. *Clin. Orthop.*, **183**, 122.

Jolley, W.B., Sharma, B., Charmi, R., Ng, C. and Bullington, R. (1988) Long-term skin allograft survival by combined therapy with suboptimal dose of cyclosporine and ribavarin. *Transplantation Proceedings XX,* 703.

Jones, K.G. (1980) Results of use of the central one-third of the patellar ligament to compensate for anterior cruciate ligament deficiency. *Clin. Orthop.*, **147**, 39.

Jonkman, M. F., Bruin, P., Hoeksma, E. A., Nieuwenhuis, P., Klasen, H. J., Pennings, A.J. and Molennar, I. (1988) A clot-inducing wound covering with high vapor permeability: Enhancing effects on epidermal healing in partial-thickness wounds in guinea pigs. *Surgery,* **104**, 537.

Kalath, S., Tsipouras, P. and Silver, F.H. (1986) Non-invasive assessment of aortic mechanical properties. *Ann. Biomed. Eng.,* **14**, 513.

Kalath, S., Tsipouras, P. and Silver, F.H. (1987) Increased aortic root stiffness associated with osteogenesis imperfecta. *Ann. Biomed. Eng.,* **15**, 91.

Kamer, F.M. and Churukian, M.M. (1984) Clinical use of injectable collagen: A three-year retrospective review. *Archives Otolaryngology,* **110**, 93.

Kanitakis, J., Maudoit, G., Faure, M., Schmitt, D. and Thivolet, J. (1987) Ultrastructural studies of cultured epithelial sheets used as skin allografts. *Virchows Archiv. A,* **410**, 523.

Kaplan N., Wickiewicz, T.L. and Warren, R.F. (1990) Primary surgical treatment of anterior cruciate ligament ruptures. *Am. J. Sports Med.,* **18**, 354.

Karasek, M.A. and Charlton, M.E. (1971) Growth of post-embryonic skin epithelial cells on collagen gels. *J. Invest. Dermatol.,* **56**, 205.

Kastelic, J., Galeski, A. and Baer, E. (1978) The multicomposite structure of tendon. *Connec. Tissue Res.,* **6**, 11.

Kato, Y.P., Dunn, M.G., Zawadsky, J.P., Tria, A.J. and Silver, F.H. (1991) Regeneration of Achilles tendon using a collagen tendon prosthesis: results of a one year implantation study. *J. Bone Jt. Surg.,* **73-A**, 561.

Katz, J.L., Yoon, H.B., Lipson, S., Maharidge, R., Meunier, A. and Christel, P. (1984) The effects of bone remodeling on the elastic properties of bone. *Calcif. Tissue Int.*, **36**, S31.

Katz, J.S. and Fingeroth, J. (1986) The diagnostic accuracy of ruptures of the anterior cruciate ligament comparing the Lachman test, the anterior draw sign, and the pivot shift test in acute and chronic knee injuries. *Am. J. Sports Med.,* **14**, 88.

Keene, D.R., Sakai, L.Y., Bachinger, H.P. and Burgeson, R.E. (1987) Type III collagen can be present on banded collagen fibrils regardless of fibril diameter. *J. Cell Biol.,* **105**, 2393.

Kennedy, J.C., Hawkins, R.J., Willis, R.B. and Danylchuk, K.D. (1976) Tension studies of human knee ligaments. *J. Bone Jt. Surg.,* **58-A**, 350.

Kennedy, J.C., Weinberg H.W. and Wilson, A.S. (1974) The anatomy and function of the anterior cruciate ligament. *J. Bone Jt. Surg.,* **54A**, 223.

King, A.L. (1950) Circulatory system: arterial pulse; wave velocity, in *Medical Physiology,* Vol. 2, (ed. O. Glasser), Year Book Publishers, Chicago, 188.

Klebe, R.J., Caldwell, H. and Milan, S. (1989) Cells transmit spatial information by orienting collagen fibers. *Matrix,* **91**, 451.

Kleiner, J.B., Amiel, D., Harwood, F.L. and Akeson, W.H. (1989) Early histologic, metabolic, and vascular assessment of anterior cruciate ligament autografts. *J. Orthop. Res.,* **7**, 235.

Knapp, T.R., Kaplan, E.N. and Daniels, J.R. (1977) Injectable collagen for soft tissue augmentation. *Plast. Reconstr. Surg.,* **60**, 398.

Knudson, C.B. and Toole, B.P. (1987) Hyauronate-cell interactions during differentiation of chick embryo limb mesoderm. *Dev. Biol.,* **124**, 82–90.

Knutson, K.A.J., Linstrand, A. and Lidgren L. (1986) Survival of knee arthroplasties. A nation-wide multicentre investigation of 8000 cases. *J. Bone Jt. Surg.,* **68 B**, 795.

Krause, W.R., Miller, J. and Ng, P. (1982) The viscosity of acrylic bone cements. *J. Biomed. Mat. Res.,* **16**, 219.

Kronenthal, R.L. (1981) Nylon in the anterior chamber. *Ophthalmology,* **88**, 965.

Ksander, G.A., Pratt, B.M., Desilets-Avis, P., Gerhardt, C.O. and McPherson, J.M. (1990) Inhibition of connective tissue formation in dermal wounds covered with synthetic, moisture vapor-permeable dressings and its reversal by transforming growth factor-beta. *J. Investigative Dermatology,* **95**, 195.

Labat-Robert, J., Szendroi, M., Godeaiu, G. and Robert, L. (1985) Comparative distribution patterns of type I and III collagen and fibronectin in human arteriosclerotic aorta. *Pathol. Biol.,* **33**, 261.

Langdon, R.C., Cuono, C.B., Birchall, N., Madri, J. A., Kuklinska, E., McGuire, J. and Moellmann, G.E. (1988) Reconstitution of structure and cell function in human skin grafts derived from cryopreserved allogeneic dermis and autologous cultured keratinocytes. *J. Investigative Dermatology,* **91**, 479.

Larson, R.L. (1983) Physical examination in the diagnosis of rotary instability. *Clin. Orthop.,* **172**, 38.

Laurent, T.C., Ryan. M. and Pietruszkiewicz, A. (1960) Fractionation of hyaluronic acid. The polydispersity of hyaluronic acid from the bovine vitreous body. *Biochim. Biophys. Acta,* **12**, 416.

Lean, J.S., Leaver, P.K., Cooling, R.J. and McLeod, D. (1982) Management of complex retinal detachments by vitrectomy and fluid/silicone exchange. *Trans. Ophthalmol. Soc. UK,* **102**, 203.

Leenslag, J.W., Pennings, A.J., Bos, R.R.M., Rozema, F.R. and Boering, G. (1987) Resorbable materials of poly (L-lactide). VI. Plates and screws for internal fracture fixation. *Biomaterials,* **8**, 70–73.

Leenslag, J.W., Pennings, A.J., Bos, R.R.M., Rozema, F.R. and Boering, G. (1987a) Resorbable materials of poly (L-lactide). VII. In vivo and in vitro degradation. *Biomaterials,* **8**, 311–314.

Lelah, M.D. and Cooper, S.L. (1986) *Polyrethanes in Medicine,* CRC Press Inc., Boca Raton, Fl, Ch. 11.

Lemp, M.A. (1973) Artificial tear solutions. *Int. Ophthalmol. Clin.,* **13**, 221.

Lemp, M.A., Goldberg, M. and Reddy, M.R. (1975) The effect of tear substitutes on tear break-up time. *Invest. Ophthalmol. Vis. Sci.,* **14**, 1255.

Leushner, J.R.A. and Haust, M.D. (1985) Glycoproteins on the surface of smooth muscle cells involved in their interaction with type I collagen. *Can. J. Biochem. Cell Biol.,* **63**, 1176.

Levine, N.S., Lindberg, R.A., Salsbury, R.E., Mason, A.D. Jr. and Pruitt, B.A. Jr. (1976) Comparison of coarse mesh gauze with biologic dressings on granulating wounds. *Am. J. Surg.,* **131**, 727.

Levy, J.H. and Piscano, A.M. (1988) Clinical cell loss following phacoemulsification and silicone or polymethylmethacrylate lens implantation. *J. Cataract Refract. Surg.,* **14**, 299.

Levy, M., Torzilli, P.A., Gould, J.D. and Warren, R.F. (1989) The effect of lateral meniscectomy on motion of the knee, *J. Bone Jt. Surg.,* **71A**, 40–6.

Lewis, J.L. and Lew, W.D. (1987) Bioengineering of total joint replacement, in *Handbook of Bioengineering,* (eds R. Skalak and S. Chien), McGraw-Hill Book Co., NY, Ch. 40.

Liesegang, T.J. (1990) Viscoelastic substances in ophthalmolgy. *Survey of Ophthalmology,* **34**, 268–293.

Liesegang, T.J., Bourne, W.M. and Ilstrup, D.M. (1986) The use of hydroxypropyl methylcellulose in extracapsular cataract extraction with intraocular lens implantation. *Amer. J. Ophth.,* **102**, 723–26.

Limberg, M.B., McCaa, C., Kissling, G.E. and Kaufman, H.E. (1987) Topical application of hyaluronic acid and chondroitin sulfate in the treatment of dry eyes. *Amer. J. Ophth.,* **103**, 194.

Linsenmayer, T.F., Bruns, R.R., Mentzer, A. and Mayne, R. (1986) Type VI collagen: immunohistochemical identification as a filamentous component of the extracellular matrix of the developing avian corneal stroma. *Dev. Biol.,* **118**, 425–31.

Liotta, D., Bracco, D., Ferrari, H., Bertolozzi, E., Pisanu, A. and Donato, O. (1977) Low profile bioprosthesis for cardiac valve replacement: early clinical results. *Cardiovascular Diseases,* Bulletin of the Texas Heart Institute, **4**, 371.

Lippman, J.I. (1990) Contact lens materials: A critical review. *Contact Lens Association of Ophthalmologists Journal,* **16**, 287.

Lipscomb, A.B. and Anderson, A.F. (1986) Tears of the anterior cruciate ligament in adolescents, *J. Bone Jt. Surg.,* **68A**, 19.

Losee, R.E., Johnson, T.R. and Southwick, W.O. (1978) Anterior subluxation of the lateral tibial plateau. *J. Bone Jt. Surg.,* **60A**, 1015.

Lyman, D.J., Albo, D., Jr., Jackson, R. and Knutson, K. (1977) Development of small diameter vascular protheses. *Trans. Am. Soc. Artif. Intern. Org.,* **23**, 253.

MacMillan, B.G. (1984) Present status of bioadherent materials, barrier dressings, and biosynthetics as skin substitutes, in *Burn Wound Coverings,* Vol. 1, (ed. D.L. Wise), CRC Press, Inc, Boca Raton, Fl, 115.

MacRae, S.M., Edelhauser, H.F., Hyndick, R.A., Burd, E.M. and Schultz, R.O. (1983) The effects of sodium hyaluronate, chondroitin sulfate, and methylcellulose on the corneal endothelium and intraocular pressure. *Amer. J. Ophthal.,* **95**, 332–41.

Madden, M.R., Finkelstein, J.L., Staiano-Coico, L., Goodwin, C.W., Shires, G.T., Nolan, E.E. and Hefton, J.M. (1986) Grafting of cultured allogenic epidermis on second and third degree burn wounds on 26 patients. *J. Trauma,* **26**, 955.

Madsen, K., Stenevi, U., Apple, D.J. and Harfstrand, A. (1989) Histochemical and receptor binding studies of hyaluronic acid binding sites on corneal endothelium. *Ophthalmic Practice,* **7**, 2–8.

Maguire, J.K., Jr., Coscia, M.F. and Lynch, M.H. (1987) Foreign body reaction to polymeric debris following total hip arthroplasty. *Clin. Orthop. Rel. Res.,* **216**, 213.

Marble, A.E., McGonald, A.S., Hilliard, W.G., Holland, J.G., Miller, C.H. and Winter, D.A. (1973) Measurement of aortic wall thickness in living dogs. *Med. Biol. Eng.,* **11**, 39.

Marentette, L.J. (1991) Bone grafts in facial reconstruction, in *Applications of Biomaterials in Facial Plastic Surgery,* (eds A.I. Glasgold and F.H. Silver), CRC Press, Boca Raton, Fl., Ch. 10.

Marshall, J.L., Warren, R.F. and Wickiewicz, T.L. (1982) Primary surgical treatment of anterior cruciate ligament lesions. *Am. J. Sports Med.,* **10**, 103.

Matsuda, K., Suzuki, S., Isshiki, N., Yoshioka, K., Okada, T. and Ikada, Y (1990) Influence of glycosaminoglycans on the collagen sponge component of a bilayer artificial skin. *Biomaterials,* **11**, 351.

Maurice, D.M. (1969) *The Eye,* (ed. H. Davson), Academic Press, New York and London, pp. 489–600.

Mayne, R. and Irwin, M.H. (1986) Collagen types in cartilage, in *Articular Cartilage Biochemistry,* (eds K.E. Kuettner, R. Schleyer, and V. Hascall), Raven Press, NY, 23.

Mayne, R. and von der Mark, K. (1983) Collagens of cartilage, in *Cartilage: Structure, Function and Biochemistry,* Vol. 1, (ed. B.K. Hall) Academic Press, NY, 181.

McBride, D.J., Jr., Hahn, R.A. and Silver, F.H. (1985) Morphological characterization of tendon development during chick embryogenesis: measurement of birefringence retardation. *Int. J. Biol. Macromol.*, **7**, 71.

McBride, D.J., Jr., Trelstad, R.L. and Silver, F.H. (1988) Structural and mechanical assessment of developing chick tendon. *Int. J. Biol. Macromol.*, **10**, 194.

McDermott, M.L. and Chandler, J.W. (1989) Therapeutic uses of contact lenses. *Surv. Ophthalmology*, **33**, 381.

McDonald, D.A. (1960) *Blood Flow in Arteries*, 2nd edn, Williams and Wilkins, Baltimore.

McDonald, D.A. (1968) Regional pulse-wave velocity in the arterial tree. *J. Appl. Physiol.*, **24**, 73.

McDonald, M.B. (1988) The future direction of refractive surgery. *Refract. Corneal Surg.*, **3**, 158.

McDonald, M.B., Kaufman, H.E., Aquavella, J. V., Durrie, D.S., Hiles, D.A., Hunkeler, J.D., Keates, R.H., Morgan, K.S. and Sanders, D.R. (1987) The nationwide study of epikeratophakia for myopia. *Amer. J. Ophthal.*, **103**, 375.

McDonald, M. B., Kaufman, H.E., Durrie, D.S., Keates, R.H. and Sanders, D.R. (1986) Epikeratophakia for keratoconus. *Arch. Ophthalmol.*, **104**, 1294.

McDonald, M.B., Klyce, S.D., Suarez, H., Kandarakis, A., Friedlander, M. H. and Kaufman, H. E. (1985) Epikeratophakia for myopia correction. *Ophthalmology*, **92**, 1417.

McGrath, M. H. and Burkhardt, B. R. (1984) The safety and efficacy of breast implants for augmentation mammoplasty. *Plast. Reconstr. Surg.*, **74**, 550.

McKinney, P. and Tresley, G. (1983) Long-term comparison of patients with gel and saline mammary implants. *Plast. Reconstr. Surg.*, **50**, 220.

McMaster, W.C. (1985) A histologic assessment of canine anterior cruciate substitution with bovine xenograft. *Clin. Orthop.*, **196**, 196.

McPherson, G.K., Mendenhall, H.V., Gibbons, D.F., Plenk, H., Rottmann, W., Sanford, J.B., Kennedy, J.C. and Roth, J.H. (1985) Experimental mechanical and histological evaluation of the Kennedy ligament augmentation device. *Clin. Orthop. Rel. Res.*, **196**, 186.

Meek, K.M., Elliott, G.F. and Nave, C. (1986) A synchrotron X-Ray diffraction of bovine cornea stained with cupromeronic blue. *Collagen and Related Research*, **6**, 203–18.

Meffert, R.M., Thomas, J.R., Hamilton, K.M. and Brownstein, C.N. (1985) Hydroxylapatite as an alloplastic graft in the treatment of human periodontal osseous defects. *J. Periodontol.*, **56**, 63.

Melcher, A.H. (1976) On the repair potential of periodontal tissues. *J. Periodontol.*, **47**, 256.

Melmed, E.P. (1988) Polyurethane implants: a 6-year review of 416 patients. *Plast. Reconstr. Surg.*, **82**, 285.

Mendler, M., Eich-Bender, S.G., Vaughan, L., Winterhalter, K.H. and Bruchkner, P. (1989) Cartilage contains mixed fibrils of collagen types II, IX and XI. *J. Cell Biol.*, **108**, 191.

Merillon, J.P., Motte, G., Fruchaud, J. and Gourgon, R. (1978) Evaluation of the elasticity and characteristic impedance of the ascending aorta in man. *Cardiovasc. Res.*, **12**, 401.

Merrilees, M.J., Tiang, K.M. and Scott, L. (1987) Changes in collagen fibril diameters across artery walls including a correlation with glycosaminoglycan content. *Connect. Tissue Res.*, **16**, 237.

Meyer, L. and Ringberg, A. (1987) Augmentation mammoplasty-psychiatric and psychosocial chracteristics and outcome in a group of Swedish women. *Scand. J. Plast. Reconstr. Surg. Hand Surg.*, **21**, 199.

Michna, H. (1984) Morphometric analysis of loading-induced changes in collagen-fibril populations in young tendons. *Cell Tissue Res.*, **236**, 465.

Miller, E.J. and Gay, S. (1987) The collagens: an overview and update. *Methods Enzymol.*, **144**, 3.

Miller, T.A., Switzer, W.E., Foley, F.D. and Moncrief, J.A. (1967) Early homografting of second degree burns. *Plast. Reconstr. Surg.*, **40**, 117.

Milnor, W.R. (1975) Arterial impedance as ventricular afterload. *Circ. Res.*, **36**, 565.

Minabe, M., Kogou, T., Kodama, T., Sugaya, A., Tamura, T., Hori, T. and Watanabe, Y. (1988) Effect of collagen solution application on healing following surgical treatment in colony-bred monkeys. *J. Periodont. Res.*, **23**, 313.

Minabe, M., Takeuchi, K., Tamura, T., Hori, T. and Umemoto, T. (1989) Subgingival administration of tetracycline on a collagen film. *J. Periodontol.*, **60**, 552.

Minabe, M., Uemutsu, Nishhijima, K., Tomomatsu, E., Tamura, T., Hori, T., Umemoto, T. and Hino, T. (1989a) Application of a local drug delivery system to periodontal therapy. I. Development of the collagen preparations with immobilized tetracycline. *J. Periodontol.*, **60**, 113.

Mitchell, R. (1983) A new biological dressing for areas denuded of mucous membrane. *Br. Dent. J.*, **155**, 346.

Miyauchi, S. and Iwata, S. (1986) Evaluations on the usefulness of viscous agents in anterior segment surgery. I. The ability to maintain the deepness of the anterior chamber. *J. Ocular Pharm.*, **2**, 267–74.

Mobray, S.L., Chang, S.-H. and Casella, J.F. (1983) Estimation of the useful lifetime of polypropylene fiber in the anterior chamber. *Am. Intra-Ocular Implant Soc., J.*, **9**, 143.

Mochitate, K., Pawele, R.P. and Grinnell, F. (1991) Stress relaxation of contracted collagen gels: disruption of actin filament bundles, release of cell surface fibronectin, and down-regulation of DNA and protein synthesis. *Experimental Cell Research,* **193**, 198.

Moore, J.W. (1989) The Allergan Advent™-flexible fluoropolymer for daily or extended wear. *Contact Lens Forum,* August, 27.

Morris, I.R. (1988) Functional anatomy of the upper airway. *Airway Management Anesth.,* **6**, 639.

Morton, L.F. and Barnes, M.J. (1982) Collagen polymorphism in the normal and diseased blood vessel wall. *Atherosclerosis,* **42**, 41.

Mosler, E., Folkhard, W., Knorzer, E., Nemetschke-Gansler, H., Nemetschek, Th. and Koch, M.H.J. (1985) Stress-induced molecular rearrangement in tendon collagen. *J. Mol. Biol.,* **182**, 589.

Mukai, N., Lee, P.F. and Schepens, C.L. (1972) Intravitreous injection of silicone: An experimental study. II. Histochemistry and electron microscopy. *Ann. Ophthalmol.,* **4**, 273.

Muller, W. (1983) Kinematics of the Rolling-Gliding Principle, in *The Knee,* Springer-Verlag, New York, NY, p.8.

Murata, K., Motayama, T. and Kotake, C. (1986) Collagen types in various layers of the human aorta and their changes with the atherosclerotic process. *Atherosclerosis.* **60**, 251.

Nanchahal, J., Otto, W.R., Dover, R. and Dhital, S.K. (1989) Cultured composite skin grafts: Biological skin equivalents permitting massive expansion. *Lancet,* 191.

Neame, P.J., Choi, H.U. and Rosenberg, L.C. (1989) The primary structure of the core protein of the small, leucine-rich proteoglycan (PG I) from bovine articular cartilage. *J. Biol. Chem.,* **264**, 8653.

Nelson, J.D. and Farris, R. L. (1988) Sodium hyaluronate and polyvinyl alcohol artificial tear preparations. A comparison in patients with keratoconjunctivitis. *Archives Ophthalmology,* **106**, 484.

Nestler, F.H., Hvidt, S., Ferry, J.D. and Veis, A. (1983) Flexibility of collagen determined from dilute solution viscoelastic measurements. *Biopolymers,* **22**, 1747.

Newton, P.O., Horibe, S. and Woo, S.L-Y., (1990) Experimental studies of anterior cruciate ligament autografts and allografts: mechanical studies, in *Knee Ligaments, Structure, Function, Injury and Repair,* (eds D. Daniel, W. Akeson and J. O'Connor), Raven Press, NY, 389.

Nichols, W.W. and McDonald. D.A. (1972) Wave velocity in the proximal aorta. *Med. Biol. Eng.,* **10**, 327.

Nicosia, J.E. and Petro, J.A. (1983) *Manual of Burn Care,* Raven Press, NY, vii.

Nikolaou, P.K., Seaber, A.V., Glesson, R.R., Ribbeck, B.M. and Bassett, F.H. (1986) Anterior cruciate ligament allograft transplantation: long-term function, history revascularization and operative technique. *Amer. J. Sports Med.,* **14**, 348.

Niven, H., Baer, E. and Hiltner, A. (1982) Organization of collagen fibres in rat tail tendon at the optical microscope level. *Collagen Rel. Res.*, **2**, 131.

Nokagawa, Y., Totsuka, M., Soto, T., Fukuda, Y. and Kirota, K. (1989) Effect of disease on the ultrastructure of the achilles tendons in rats. *Eur. J. Appl. Physiol.*, **59**, 239.

Norn, M.S. and Opauski, A. (1977) Effects of ophthalmic vehicles on stability of the precorneal film. *Acta Ophthalmol.*, **55**, 23.

Noyes, F.R. and Grood, E.S. (1976) The strength of the anterior cruciate ligament in humans and rhesus monkeys. *J. Bone Jt. Surg*, **58-A**, 1074.

Noyes, F.R., Butler, D.L., Grood, E.S., Bassett, R.W. and Hosea, T.M. (1978) Clinical paradoxes of anterior cruciate instability and a new test to detect its instability. *Orthop. Trans.*, **2**, 36.

Noyes, F.R., Butler, D.L., Paulos, L.E. and Grood, E.S. (1983) Intraarticular cruciate reconstruction. *Clin. Orthop.*, **172**, 71.

O'Connor, N.E., Gallico, G., Compton, C., Kehinde, O. and Green, H. (1984) Grafting of burns with cultured epithelium prepared from autologous epidermal cells: Intermediate term results on three paediatric patients, in *Soft and Hard Tissue Repair, Biological and Clinical Aspects*, Vol. 11, (eds Hunt, T.K., Heppenstal, K.B., Pines, E. and Rovee, D.), Praeger Scientific, New York.

O'Connor, N.E., Mulliken, J.B., Banks-Schledels, S., Kehinde, O. and Green, H. (1981) Grafting of burns with cultured epithelium prepared from autologous epidermal cells. *Lancet*, Jan. 10, 75.

O'Donoghue, D.H., Frank, G.R., Jeter, G.L., Johnson, W., Zeiders, J.W. and Kenyon, R. (1971) Repair and reconstruction of the anterior cruciate ligament in dogs. *J. Bone Jt. Surg.*, **53-A**, 710.

O'Donoghue, D.H., Rockwood, C.A., Jr., Jack, S.C. and Kenyon, R. (1966) Repair of the anterior cruciate ligament in dogs. *J. Bone Jt. Surg.*, **48-A**, 503.

O'Neill, D.A. and Harris, W.H. (1984) Failed total hip replacement assessment by plain radiographs, athrograms, and aspiration of the hip joint. *J. Bone Jt. Surg.*, **66A**, 540.

Oakes, B.W. and Bialkower, B. (1977) Biomechanical and ultrastructural studies on the elastic wing tendon from the domestic fowl. *J. Anat.*, **123**, 369.

Oh I. and Harris, W.H. (1978) Proximal strain distribution in the loaded femur: An in-vitro comparison of the distributions in the intact femur and after insertion of different hip replacement femoral components. *J. Bone Jt. Surg.*, **60-A**, 75.

Oliver, R.F., Grant, R.A., Hulme, M.J. and Mudie, A. (1977) Incorporation of stored cell-free dermal collagen allografts into skin wounds: A short term study. *Brit. J. Plast. Surg*, **30**, 88.

Oliver, R.F., Grant, R.A. and Kent, C.M. (1972) The fate of cutaneously and subcutaneously implanted trypsin purified dermal collagen in the pig. *Br. J. Exp. Path.*, **53**, 540.

Olson, L.J., Subramanian, R. and Edwards, W.D. (1984) Surgical pathology of pure aortic insufficiency: a study of 225 cases, *Mayo Clin. Proc.*, **59**, 835.

Olson, R.M., Shelton, O. and Olson, D.B. (1971) Ultrasonic measurement of aortic diameter versus time, position, and pressure. *Proc. 24th Annu. Conf. Engineering in Medicine and Biology*, Las Vagas, Nevada, **13**, 264.

Oppenheimer, B.S. (1952) Sarcomas induced in rodents by imbedding various plastic films. *Proc. Soc. Exp. Biol. Med.*, **79**, 366.

Orentreich, D.S. and Orentreich, N. (1991) Injectable fluid silicone for soft-tissue augmentation, in *Applications of Biomaterials in Facial Plastic Surgery*, (eds A.I. Glasgold and F.H. Silver), CRC Press, Boca Raton, Fl, Ch. 14.

Orlandi, G.E., Ruggiero, C. and Orlandini, S.Z. (1986) The corrected circumference of human pulmonary trunk and arteries in relation to the size of the aorta and principal bronchi. *Anat. Anz. Jena.*, **162**, 251.

Oyer, P.E., Stinson, E.B., Miller, D.C., Jamieson, S.W., Mitchell, R.S. and Shumway, N.E. (1984) Thromboembolic risk and durability of the Hancock bioprosthetic cardiac valve, *Eur. Heart J.*, **5**, 81.

Pachence, J., Berg, R.A. and Silver, F.H. (1987) Collagen: Its place in the medical device industry. *Medical Device and Diagnostic Industry*, **9**, 49.

Packer, A.J., McCuen, B.W., II, Hutton, W.L. and Ramsay, R.C. (1989) Procoagulation effects of intraocular sodium hyaluronate (healon) after phakic diabetic vitrectomy. *Ophthalmol.*, **96**, 1491.

Parish, L.C., Witkowski, J.A. and Crissey, J.T. (1983) *The Decubitus Ulcer*, Masson Publishing USA, Inc., NY, p. 11.

Park, J.B. (1984) *Biomaterials,* Plenum Press, NY, Ch. 5.

Park, J.P., Grana, W.A. and Chitwood, J.S. (1975) A high strength dacron augmentation for cruciate ligament reconstruction. *Clin. Orthop.*, **196**, 175.

Parry, D.A.D. and Craig, A.S. (1977) Quantitative electron microscope observations of the collagen fibrils in rat tail tendon. *Biopolymers*, **16**, 1015.

Parry, D.A.D., Craig, A.S. and Barnes, G.R.G. (1978) Tendon and ligament from the horse: An ultrastructural study of collagen fibres as a function of age. *Proc. Ro. Soc. Lond.*, **B203**, 293.

Parsons, J.R., Rosario, A., Weiss, A. and Alexander, H. (1984) Achilles tendon repair with an absorbable polymer-carbon fiber composite. *Foot and Ankle,* **5**, 49.

Passik, C.S., Ackermann, D.M., Pluth, J.R. and Edwards, W.D. (1987) Temporal changes in the causes of aortic stenosis: a surgical pathologic study of 646 cases. *Mayo Clin. Proc.*, **62**, 119.

Passo, M.S., Ernest, J.T. and Goldstick, T.K. (1985) Hyaluronate increases intraocular pressure when used in cataract extraction. *Br. J. Ophthalmol.*, **69**, 572.

Patel, D.I. and Fry, D.L. (1964) In situ pressure-radius-length measurements in ascending aorta of anesthetized dogs. *J. Appl. Physiol.*, **19**, 413.

Patel, D.J., Schilder, D.P. and Mallos, A.J. (1960) Mechanical properties and dimensions of the major pulmonary arteries. *J. Appl. Physiol.*, **15**, 92.

Pattee, G.A. and Friedman, M.J. (1988) in *Prosthetic Ligament Reconstruction of the Knee,* (eds M.J. Friedman and R.D. Ferkel), W.B. Saunders Co., Philadelphia, 22.

Paulos, L.E., Butler, D.L., Noyes, F. and Grood, E.S. (1983) Intraarticular cruciate reconstruction, II: replacement with vascularized patellar tendon. *Clin. Orthop.*, **172**, 78.

Pellet, S., Menesi, L., Novak, J. and Temesi, A. (1984) Freeze-dried irradiated porcine skin as a burn wound covering, in *Burn Wound Coverings,* Vol I, CRC Press, Inc, Boca Raton, Fl, p. 85.

Percival, P. (1987) Capsular bag implantation of the hydrogel lens. *J. Cataract Refract. Surg.*, **13**, 627.

Pessac, B and Defendi, V. (1972) Cell aggregation: Role of acid mucopolysaccharides. *Science,* **175**, 898–900.

Peterson, L.M., Jensen, R.E. and Parnell, J. (1960) Mechanical properties of arteries in vivo. *Circ. Res.*, **8**, 622.

Petersen, M.J., Lessane, B. and Woodley, D.T. (1990) Characterization of cellular elements in healed cultured keratinocyte autografts used to cover burn wounds. *Arch. Dermatol.*, **126**, 175.

Petro, J.A. (1983) Emergency room evaluation and triage of burns, in *Manual of Burn Care,* (eds Nicosia, J.E. and Petro, J.A.), Raven Press, NY, 5.

Phelps, J.R. and Dormer, R.A. (1986) Legal aspects of biomaterials in medical treatment in *Handbook of Biomaterials Evaluation*, (ed. A.F. von Recum), Macmillan Publishing Corporation, New York, NY, 503.

Phillips, R.W. (1991) *Skinner's Science of Dental Materials*, 9th edn, W.B. Saunders Co., Philadelphia, Pa.

Phillips, T.J., Bhawan, J., Leigh, I.M., Baum, H.J. and Gilchrest, B.A. (1990) Cultured epidermal autografts and allografts: A study of differentiation and allograft survival. *J. Am. Acad. Dermatol.*, **23**, 189.

Phillips, T.J., Kehinde, O., Green, H. and Gilchrest, B.A. (1989) Treatment of skin ulcers with cultured epidermal allografts. *J. Am. Acad. Dermatol.*, **21**, 191.

Pitaru, S., Tal, H., Soldinger, M., Grosskopf, A. and Noff, M. (1988) Partial regeneration of periodontal tissues using collagen barriers. Initial observations in the canine. *J. Clin. Periodontol.*, **59**, 380.

Pittelkow, M.R. and Scott, R.E. (1986) New techniques for the in vitro culture of skin keratinocytes and perspectives on their use for grafting of patients with extensive burns *Mayo Clin. Proc.*, **61**, 771.

Pizzoferato, A. (1979) Evaluation of the tissue response to the wear products of the hip joint endo-arthroprosthesis. *Biomat. Med. Dev. Art. Org.*, **7**, 257.

Poggio, E.C., Glynn, R.J., Schein, O.D., Seddon, J. M., Shannon, M.J., Scardino, U.A. and Kenyon, K.R. (1989) The incidence of ulcerative keratitis among users of daily-wear and extended-wear soft contact lenses. *N. Engl. J. Med.*, **321**, 779.

Polack, F.M., Demong, T. and Santella, H. (1981) Sodium-hyaluronate (Healon) in keratoplasty and IOL implantation. *Ophthalmol.*, **88**, 425.

Polson, A.M. and Heijl, L.C. (1978) Osseous repair in infrabony periodontal defects. *J. Clin. Periodontol.*, **5**, 13.

Polson, A.M. and Proye, M.P. (1983) Fibrin linkage: A precursor for new attachment. *J. Periodontol.*, **54**, 141.

Poss, R., Brick, G.W., Wright, R.J., Roberts, D.W. and Sedge, C.B. (1988) The effects of modern cementing techniques on the longevity of total hip arthroplasty. *Orthop. Clin. N. Am.*, **19**, 591.

Postlethwaite, A.E., Seyer, J.M. and Kang, A.H. (1978) Chemotactic attraction of human fibroblasts to type I, II, and III collagen and collagen-derived peptides. *Proc. Natl. Acad. Sci. USA*, **75**, 871–5.

Pratt, R.M., Larsen, M.A. and Johnson, M.C. (1975) Migration of cranial neural crest cells in a cell-free hyaluronate rich matrix. *Dev. Biol.*, **44**, 298–305.

Praus, R., Brettschneider, I. and Adam, M. (1979) Heterogeneity of bovine corneal collagen. *Experimental Eye Research*, **29**, 409.

Pruett, R.C., Schepens, C.L., Constable, I.J. and Swann, D.A. (1977) Hyaluronic acid vitreous substitute, in *Vitreous Surgery and Advances in Fundus Diagnosis and Treatment*, (eds H.M. Freeman, T. Hirose and C.L. Schepens), Appleton-Century-Crofts, New York, p. 433.

Pruett, R.C., Schepens, C.L. and Swann, D.A. (1979) Hyaluronic acid vitreous substitute: A six-year clinical evaluation. *Arch. Ophthalmol*, **97**, 2325.

Pruitt, B.A. and Levine, N.S. (1984) Characteristics and uses of biologic dressings and skin substitutes. *Arch. Surg.*, **119**, 312.

Pulapura, S., Li, C., Engelberg, I. and Kohn, J. (1990) Structure-property relationships for the design of poly(iminocarbonates). *Biomaterials*, **11**, 666.

Ransj'o, U., Asplund, O.A., Gylbert, L. and Jurell, G. (1985) Bacteria in the female breast. *Scand. J. Plast. Reconstr.*, **19**, 87.

Redfern, A.B., Ryan, J.J. and Su, T.C. (1977) Calcification of the fibrous capsule about mammary implants. *Plast. Reconstr. Surg.,* **59**, 249.

Rees, T.D., Guy, C.L. and Colburn, R.J. (1973) The use of inflatable breast implants. *Plast. Reconstr. Surg.,* **52**, 609.

Refojo, M.F. (1982) Current status of biomaterials in ophthalmology. *Surv. Ophthalmol.,* **26**, 257.

Refojo, M.F. (1986) Biomedical materials to repair retinal detachments. *Mat. Res. Soc. Symp. Proc.,* **55**, 55.

Reis, R.L., Hancock, W.D., Yarbrough, J.W., Glancy, D.L. and Morrow, A.G. (1971) The flexible stent: a new concept in the fabrication of tissue valve prostheses, *J. Thorac. Cardiovasc. Surg.,* **62**, 683.

Rheinwald, J.G. and Green, H. (1975) Serial cultivation of strains of human epidermal keratinocytes: the formation of keratinizing colonies from single cells. *Cell,* **6**, 331.

Ritter, M.A., Gioe, T.J. and Sieber, J.M. (1984) Systemic effects of polymethylmethacrylate. Increased serum levels of gamma-glutamyl-transpeptidase following arthroplasty. *Acta Orthop. Scand.,* **55**, 411.

Roach, M.R. (1983) The pattern of elastin in the aorta and large arteries of mammals, in *Development of the Vascular System,* Ciba Foundation Symposium 100, Pitman Books, London, 37.

Roberts, B. and Peiffer, R. L., Jr. (1989) Experimental evaluation of a synthetic viscoelastic material on intraocular pressure and corneal endothelium. *J. Cataract. Refract. Surg.,* **15**, 321–6.

Rodriguez, F. (1982) *Principles of Polymer Systems,* McGraw-Hill Book Co., NY.

Rogers, G.J., Milthrope, B.K., Muratore, A. and Schindhelm, K. (1990) Measurement of the mechanical properties of the ovine ACL bone-ligament-bone complex: a basis for prosthetic evaluation. *Biomaterials,* **11**, 89.

Rosenberg, A.S., Katz, S.I. and Singer, A. (1989) Rejection of skin allografts by CD4+ T cells is antigen-specific and requires expression of target alloantigen on Ia- epidermal cells. *J. Immunology* **143**, 2452.

Rosenberg, L.C. and Buckwalter, J.A. (1986) Cartilage proteoglycans, in *Dynamics of Connective Tissue Macromolecules,* (eds P.M.C. Burleigh and A.R. Poole), North-Holland, Amsterdam, Ch. 5.

Rosenthal, P. (1985) Daily and extended wear performance of the Boston IV contact lens. *Current Canadian Ophthalmology Practice,* **3**, 94.

Ross, R. (1986) The pathogenesis of atherosclerosis-an update. *N. Engl. J. Med.,* **314**, 488.

Rovee, D.T. (1991) Evolution of wound dressings and their effects on the healing process. *Clinical Materials,* **8**, 183.

Rowe, R.W.D. (1985) The structure of rat tail tendon. *Connective Tissue Res,* **14**, 9.

Royer, J. and Montard, M. (1981) Modification in vivo du matériel de suture intra-oculaire: étude comparative au microscope electronique. *J. Fr. Ophthalmol.*, **4**, 375.

Rubin, L.R., Bromberg, B.E. and Walden, R.H. (1981) Long-term human reaction to synthetic plastics. *Surg. Gynecol. Obstet.*, **132**, 603.

Rummelt, V., Lang., G.K., Yanoff, M. and Naumann, O.H. (1990) A 32-year follow-up of a rigid Schreck anterior chamber lens: A clinicopathological correlation. *Arch. Ophthalmol.*, **108**, 401.

Ruoslahti, E. (1991) Integrins *J. Clin. Invest.*, **87**, 1.

Ruoslahti, E. and Pierschbacher M.D. (1987) New perspectives in cell adhesion: RGD and integrins. *Science*, **238**, 491.

Rusch, R.M., Nelson, E.F. and Noel, D. (1988) Integraft anterior cruciate ligament reconstruction: Arthroscopic technique, in *Prosthetic Ligament Reconstruction of the Knee*, (eds M.J. Friedman and R.D. Ferkel), W.B. Saunders Co., Philadelphia, 59.

Sailer, H.F. (1983) *Transplantation of lyophilized cartilage in maxillofacial surgery: experimental foundations in clinical success*, S. Kargev, NY, 42.

Sathyanarayana, B.K. and Rao, V.S.R. (1971) Conformational studies of β-glucans. *Biopolymers*, **10**, 1605.

Sauvage, L.R., Berger, K., Wood, S.J., Nakagawa, Y. and Manfield, P.B. (1971) An external velour surface for porous arterial prostheses. *Surgery*, **70**, 940.

Sauvage, L.R., Smith, J.C., Davis, C.C., Rittenhouse, E.A., Hall, D.G. and Mansfield, P.B. (1986) Dacron® arterial grafts; Comparative structures and basis for successful use of current prostheses, in *Vascular Graft Update: Safety and Performance*, ASTM STP 898, (eds H. E. Kambic, A. Kantrowitz and P. Sung), American Society For Testing Materials, Philadelphia, p. 16.

Sawada, H., Konomi, H. and Hirosawa, K. (1990) Characterization of the collagen in the hexagonal lattice of Descemet's membrane: Its relation to type VIII collagen. *Cell Biology*, 219–27.

Schein, O.D., Glynn, R.J., Poggio, E.C. Seddon, J.M. and Kenyon, K.R. (1989) The relative risk of ulcerative keratitis among users of daily-wear and extended-wear soft contact lenses: A case-control study. *N. Engl. J. Med.*, **321**, 773.

Schmidt, S.P., Hunter, T. J., Sharp, W. V., Malindzak, G.S. and Evancho, M. M. (1984) Endothelial cell-seeded four-millimeter Dacron vascular grafts: effects of blood flow manipulation through the grafts. *J, Vas. Surg.*, **1**, 434.

Schoen, F.J. (1987) Cardiac valve prostheses: pathological and bioengineering considerations. *J. Cardiac Surg.*, **2**, 65.

Schoen, F.J. (1987a) Cardiac valve prostheses: Review of clinical status and contemporary issues. *J. Biomed. Mat. Res.*, **21**, 91.

Schoen, F.J. and Sutton, M.S.T. (1987) Contemporary issues in the pathology of valvular heart disease. *Human Pathology,* **18**, 568.

Schuller, D.E., Bardach, J., and Krause, C.J. (1977) Irradiated homologous costal cartilage for facial contour restoration. *Arch Otolaryngology Head Neck Surg.,* **103**, 12.

Schwartz, S.D., Harrison, S.A., Engstrom, R.E., Bawdon, R.E., Lee, D.A. and Mondino, B. J. (1990) Collagen Shield Delivery of Amphotericin B. *Am. J. Ophthalmol.,* **109**, 701.

Scott, J.D. (1981) Use of liquid silicone in vitrectomised eyes. *Dev. Ophthalmol.,* **2**, 185.

Scott, J.E. (1992) Supramolecular organization of extracellular matrix glycosaminoglycans, in vitro and in the tissues. *FASEB Journal,* **6**, 2639.

Scott, J.E. and Orford, C.R. (1981) Dermatan sulphate proteoglycan associated with rat tail tendon collagen and the d band in the gap region. *Biochem. J.,* **197**, 213.

Scott, J.E., Cummings, C., Brass, A. and Chen, Y. (1991) Secondary and tertiary structures of hyaluronan in aqueous solution, investigated by rotary shadowing-electron microscopy and computer simulation. *Biochem. J.,* **274**, 699–705.

Scott, J.E., Orford, C.R. and Hughes, E.W. (1981) Proteoglycan-collagen interactions in developing rat tail tendon. *Biochem. J.,* **195**, 573.

Scott, W.N., Ferriter, P. and Marino, M. (1985) Intra-articular transfer of the iliotibial tract: two- to seven-year follow-up results. *J. Bone Jt. Surg.,* **67**, 532.

Sears, D., and Sears, X. (1974) Blood-aqueous barrier and alpha-chymotrypsin glaucoma in rabbits, *Am. J. Ophthalmol.,* **77**, 378.

Sell, S. and Scully, R.E. (1965) Aging changes in the aortic and mitral valves. *Am. J. Pathol.,* **46**, 345.

Sergott, T. J., Limoli, J.P., Baldwin, C.M., Jr. and Laub, D.R. (1986) Human adjuvant disease after silicone implantation. *Plast. Reconstr. Surg.,* **78**, 104.

Sheldon, H. (1983) Transmission electron microscopy of cartilage, in *Cartilage, Structure, Function and Biochemistry,* Vol. I, (ed. B.K. Hall), Academic Press, NY, 87.

Shepard, A. D., Eldrup-Jorgensen, J., Keough, E.M., Foxall, T. F., Ramberg, K., Connolly, R.J., Mackey, W. C., Garvis, V., Auger, K.R., Libby, P., O'Donnel, T. F. and Callow, A.D. (1986) Endothelial cell seeding of small-caliber synthetic grafts in the baboon. *Surgery,* **90**, 318.

Sher, S.E., Hull, B.E., Rosen, S., Church, D., Friedman, L. and Bell, E. (1983) Acceptance of allogeneic fibroblasts in skin equivalent transplants. *Transplantation,* **36**, 552.

Shieh, S-J., Zimmerman, M.C. and Parsons, J.R. (1990) Preliminary characterization of bioresorbable and nonresorbable synthetic fibers for the repair of soft tissue injuries. *J. Biomed. Mat. Res.*, **24**, 789.

Shipley, R., O'Donnell, J. and Bader, K. (1977) Personality characteristics of women seeking breast augmentation. Result: they are as stable psychologically as other women. *Plast. Reconstr. Surg.*, **60**, 369.

Sievers, H. and Von Domarus, D. (1984) Foreign-body reaction against intraocular lenses. *Am. J. Ophthalmol.*, **97**, 743.

Silver, F.H. (1987) *Biological Materials: Structure, Mechanical properties, and Modeling of Soft Tissues*, NYU Press, NY.

Silver, F.H. and Birk, D.E. (1984) Molecular structure of collagen in solution: Comparison of types I, II, III and V. *Int. J. Biol. Macromol.*, **6**, 125–32.

Silver, F. and Doillon, C. (1989) *Biocompatibility: Interactions of Biological and Implantable Materials*, Vol. 1, Polymers, VCH Publishers, New York, NY, Ch. 4.

Silver, F. and Doillon, C. (1989) Organ and tissue structure, in *Biocompatibility*, VCH Publishers, New York, NY, 27.

Silver, F.H. and Parsons, J.R. (1991) Repair of skin, cartilage and bone, in *Applications of Biomaterials in Facial Plastic Surgery*, (eds A.I. Glasgold and F.H. Silver), CRC Press, Boca Raton, Fl.

Silver, F.H. and Pins, G. (1992) Cell culture on collagen: A review of tissue engineering using scaffolds containing extracellular matrix. *J. Long-Term Effects of Medical Implants*, **2**, 67.

Silver, F.H. and Swann, D.A. (1982) Laser light scattering measurements on vitreous and rooster comb hyaluronic acids. *Int. J. Biol. Macromol.*, **4**, 425–9.

Silver, F.H., Christiansen, D. L. and Buntin, C.M. (1989) Mechanical properties of the aorta: a review. *Critical Reviews in Biomedical Engineering*, **17**, 323.

Silver, F.H., Doillon, C.J., Rojo, B., Olson, R.M., Kamath, C.Y. and Berg, R.A. (1989a) Collagenous materials enhance healing of chronic skin ulcers. *Mat. Res. Soc. Symp. Proc.*, **110**, 371.

Silver, F.H., Kato, Y.P., Ohno, M. and Wasserman, A.J. (1992) Analysis of mammalian soft tissues: Relationship between hierarchical structures and mechanical properties, in *Biomedical Applications of Composites*, (eds C. Migliaresi and J. Kardos), CRC Press Inc., Boca Raton, Fl, in press.

Silver, F.H., Librizzi, J. and Benedetto, D. (1992a) Use of viscoelastic solutions in ophthalmology: A review of physical properties and long-term effects. *J. Long-Term Effects Of Medical Implants*, in press.

Silver, F.H., Tria, A.J., Zawadsky, J.P. and Dunn, M.G. (1991) Anterior cruciate ligament replacement: structures, healing and repair. *J. Long-Term Effects of Medical Implants*, **1**, 135.

Silverstein, M.J., Handel, N., Gamagami, P. et al. (1985) Breast cancer in women after augmentation mammoplasty. *Arch. Surg.*, **123**, 681.

Slade, C. and Peterson, H. (1982) Disappearance of the polyurethane cover of the Ashley Natural-Y prosthesis. *Plast. Reconstr. Surg.*, **70**, 379.

Slatter, D.H., Costa, N.D. and Edwards, M.E. (1982) Ocular inserts for application of drugs to bovine eyes-in vivo and in vitro studies on the release of gentamicin from collagen inserts. *Australian Veterinary J.*, **59**, 4.

Smahel, J. (1978) Tissue reactions to breast implants coated with polyurethane. *Plast. Reconstr. Surg.*, **61**, 1.

Snowden, J.M. and Swann, D.A. (1980) Vitreous structure V. The morphology and thermal stability of vitreous collagen fibres and comparison to articular cartilage (type II) collagen. *Invest. Ophthalmol. Vis. Sci.*, **19**, 610.

Speer, D.P., Chvapil, M., Eskelson, C.D. and Ulreich, J. (1980) Biological effects of residual glutaraldehyde in glutaraldehyde-tanned collagen biomaterials. *J. Biomat. Res.*, **14**, 753.

Spiera, H. (1988) Sceroderma after silicone augmentation mammoplasty. *J. Amer. Med. Assoc.*, **260**, 236.

Sprague Zones, J. (1992) The political and social context of silicone breast implant use in the United States. *J. Long-term Effects of Medical Implants*, **1**, 225.

Starr, A. (1960) Total mitral valve replacement fixation and thrombosis. *Surg. Forum*, **11**, 258.

Stegman, S.J., Chu, S., Bensch, K. and Armstrong, R. (1987) A light and electron microscopic evaluation of Zyderm collagen and Zyplast implants in aging human facial skin. *Archives Dermatology*, **123**, 1644.

Stein, M.D., Salkin, L.M., Freedman, A.L. and Glushko, V. (1984) Collagen sponge as a topical hemostatic agent in mucogingival surgery. *J. Periodontol.*, **55**, 35.

Steiner, M.E., Brown, C., Zarins, B., Brownstein, B., Koval, P.S. and Stone, P. (1990) Measurement of anterior-posterior displacement of the knee. *J. Bone Jt. Surg.*, **72A**, 1307.

Stonebrook, S.N., Berman, A.B., Bruchman, W.C. and Bain, J.R. (1988) Functional biomechanics of the GORE-TEX cruciate ligament prosthesis: effects of implant tensioning, in *Prosthetic Ligament Reconstruction of the Knee*, (eds M.J. Friedman and R.D. Ferkel), W.B. Saunders Co., Philadelphia, 140.

Subramanian, R., Olson, L.J. and Edwards, W.D. (1984) Surgical pathology of pure aortic stenosis: a study of 374 cases. *Mayo Clin. Proc.*, **59**, 683.

Swanson, W.M. and Clark, R.E. (1974) Dimensions and geometric relationships of human aortic valve as a function of pressure. *Cir. Res.*, **35**, 871.

Szilagyi, D.E., Smith, R.F., Elliott, J.P. and Vrandecic, M.P. (1972) Infection in arterial reconstruction with synthetic grafts. *Ann. Surg.*, **176**, 321.

Tardieu, A. and Delaye, M. (1988) Eye lens proteins and transparency: From light transmission theory to solution X-ray structural analysis. *Ann. Rev. Biophys. Chem.*, **17**, 47–70.

Tavis, M.J., Thorton, J., Danet, R. and Bartlett, R.H. (1978) Current status of skin substitutes. *Surg. Clin. North Am.*, **58**, 1233.

Teijeira, F.J., Lamoureux, G., Tetreault, J.-P., Bauset, R., Guidoin, R., Marois, Y., Paynter, R. and Assayed, F. (1989) Hydrophilic polyurethane versus autogenous femoral vein as substitutes in the femoral arteries of dogs: quantification of platelets and fibrin deposits. *Biomaterials*, **10**, 80.

Thiele, H. (1964) Sols while rebuilding biological materials. *Chem. Eng. News*, **42**, 40.

Thivolet, J., Faure, M., Demidem, A. and Mauduit, G. (1986) Long-term survival and immunological tolerance of human epidermal allografts produced in culture. *Transplantation*, **42**, 274.

Thompson, K.P., Hanna, K., Waring, G.O., Gipson, I., Liu, Y., Gailitis, R.P., Johnson-Wint, B. and Green, K. (1991) Current status of synthetic epikeratoplasty. *Refractive and Corneal Surgery*, **7**, 240.

Thomson, P.D. and Parks, D.H. (1984) Amnion as a burn dressing, in *Burn Wound Coverings*, Vol I, (ed. D.L. Wise), CRC Press, Boca Raton, Fl, 47.

Thubrikar, M. (1990) Replacement cardiac valves, in *The Aortic Valve*, (ed. M. Thubrikar), CRC Press, Boca Raton, Fl, Chs. 1, 2, 5, and 9.

Thubrikar, M., Piepgrass, W.C., Bosher, L.P. and Nolan, S.P. (1980) The elastic modulus of canine aortic valve leaflets in vivo and in vitro. *Cir. Res.*, **47**, 792.

Thubrikar, M.J., Aouak, J. and Nolan, S.P. (1986) Comparison of the in vivo and in vitro mechanical properties of aortic valve leaflets. *J. Thorac. Cardioivascular Surg.*, **92**, 29.

Tillberg, B. (1977) The late repair of torn cruciate ligaments using menisci. *J. Bone Jt. Surg.*, **59-B**, 15.

Toole, B.P. and Trelstad, R. (1971) Hyaluronic acid production and removal during corneal development in the chick. *Dev. Biol.*, **26**, 28–35.

Topol, B., Haimos, H., Dubertret, L. and Bell, E. (1986) Transfer of melanosomes in a skin equivalent model in vitro. *Invest. Dermatol.*, **87**, 642.

Torg, J.S., Conrad, W. and Kalen, V. (1976) Clinical diagnosis of anterior cruciate ligament instability in the athlete. *Am. J. Sports Med.*, **4**, 84.

Toriumi, D.M. and Larrabee, W.F. (1991) Induced osteogenesis for craniofacial reconstruction, in *Applications of Biomaterials in Facial*

Plastic Surgery, (eds A.I. Glasgold and F.H. Silver), CRC Press, Boca Raton, FL, Ch. 11.

Trelstad, R.L. and Kang, A.H. (1974) Collagen heterogeneity in the avian eye: lens, vitreous body, cornea and sclera. *Experimental Eye Research,* **18**, 395.

Tuberville, A.W., Galin, M.A., Perez, H.D., Banda, D., Ong, R. and Goldstein, I.M. (1982) Complement activation by nylon- and polypropylene-looped prosthetic intraocular lenses. *Invest. Ophthalmol. Vis. Sci.*, **22**, 727.

Turner, F.C. (1941) Sarcomas at the site of subcutaneously implanted Bakelite discs in rats. *J. Natl. Cancer Found.*, **2**, 181.

Unterman, S.R., Rootman, D.S., Hill, J.M., Parelman, J.J., Thompson, H.W. and Kaufman, H.E. (1988) Collagen shield drug delivery: Therapeutic concentrations of tobramycin in the rabbit cornea and aqueous humor. *J. Cataract Refract. Surg.*, **14**, 500.

Vainionpaa, S., Kilpikari, J., Laiho, J., Kelevirta, P., Rokkanen, P. and Tormala, P. (1987) Strength and strength retention in vitro, of absorbable, self-reinforced polyglycolide (PGA) rods for fracture fixation. *Biomaterials,* **8**, 46048.

Van der Rest, M. and Garrone, R. (1991) Collagen family of proteins, *FASEB,* **5**, 2814.

Varga, J. (1989) Systemic sclerosis after augmentation mammoplasty with silicone implants. *Ann. Intern. Med.*, **111**, 377.

Vasseur, P.B., Rodrigo, J.J., Stevenson, S., Clark, G. and Sharkey, N. (1987) Replacement of the anterior cruciate ligament with a bone-ligament-bone anterior cruciate ligament allograft in dogs. *Clin. Orthop.*, **219**, 268.

Vasseur, P.B., Pool, R.R. and Arnoczky, S.P. (1985) Correlative biomechanical and histologic study of the cranial cruciate ligament in dogs. *Am. J. Vet. Res.*, **46**, 1842.

Vert, M., Christel, P., Chabat, F. and Leray, J. (1984) Bioresorbable plastic materials for bone surgery. in *Macromolecular Biomaterials,* (eds G.W. Hastings and P. Ducheyne), CRC Press, Boca Raton, Fl, pp. 120–42.

Verzar, F. (1957) The ageing of connective tissue. *Gerontologie,* **X**, 363.

Viidik, A. (1987) Properties of tendons and ligaments, in *Handbook of Bioengineering,* (eds R. Skalak, and S. Chien) McGraw-Hill Book Co., New York, Ch. 6.

Viidik, A. (1990) Structure and function of normal and healing tendons and ligaments, in *Biomechanics of Diarthrodial Joints,* (eds V.C. Mow, A. Ratcliffe and S.L-Y. Woo), Springer-Verlag, NY, 3.

Vinard, E., Eloy, R., Descotes, J., Brudon, J.R., Guidicelli, H., Patra, P., Streichenberger, R. and David, M. (1991) Human vascular graft failure and frequency of infection. *J. Biomed. Mat. Res.*, **25**, 499.

Volker, W., Schmidt, A. and Buddecke, E. (1986) Compartmentation and characterization of different proteoglycans in bovine arterial wall. *J. Histochem. Cytochem.*, **34**, 1293.

von Recum, A.F. (ed.) (1986) *Handbook of Biomaterials Evaluation,* Macmillan Publishing Co., NY, Chs 14–21.

Wagner, W.D. (1985) Proteoglycan structure and function as related to atherosclerosis. *Ann. N.Y. Acad. Sci.,* **454**, 52.

Walker, A.B. (1984) Use of amniotic membranes for burn wound coverage, in *Burn Wound Coverings,* Vol I, CRC Press, Inc, Boca Raton, Fl, 55.

Walker, P.S. (1989) Requirements for successful total knee replacements: Design considerations. *Orthop. Clin. N. Am.* **20**, 15.

Walsh, J.J. (1972) Meniscal reconstruction of the anterior cruciate ligament. *Clin. Orthop.,* **89**, 171.

Warton, G., Seifert, L. and Sherwood, R. (1980) Late leakage of inflatable silicone breast protheses. *Plast. Reconstr. Surg.,* **65**, 302.

Wasserman, A.J. and Dunn, M. G. (1991) Morphology and mechanics of skin, cartilage and bone, in *Applications of Biomaterials in Facial Plastic Surgery,* (eds A.I. Glasgold and F.H. Silver), CRC Press, Boca Raton Fl.

Waterman, A.H. and Schrik, J.J. (1985) Allergy in hip arthroplasty. *Contact Dermatitis,* **13**, 294.

Weisman, M.H., Vecchione, T.R., Albert, D., Moore, L.T. and Mueller, M.R. (1988) Connective-tissue disease following breast augmentation: a preliminary test of the human adjuvant disease hypothesis. *Plast. Reconstr. Surg.,* **82**, 626.

Weissman, B.A. and Lee, D.A. (1988) Oxygen transmissibility, thickness, and water content of three types of collagen shields. *Archives of Ophthalmology,* **106**, 1706.

Werblin, T.P. and Klyce, S.D. (1981) Epikeratophakia: The surgical correction of aphakia: I. Lathing of corneal tissue. *Curr. Eye Res.,* **1**, 123.

Whipple, T.L. (1988) Arthroscopic anterior cruciate ligament reconstruction with Procol xenograft bioprosthesis, in *Prosthetic Ligament Reconstruction of the Knee,* (eds M.J. Friedman and R.D. Ferkel), W.B. Saunders Co., Philadelphia, 112.

White, R.A. (1987) Vascular prostheses: Present status and future development, in *Blood Compatibility,* Vol II, (ed. D.F. Williams), CRC Press, Boca Raton, Fl, Ch. 3.

Whitley, J.E. and Whitley, N.O. (1971) *Angiography: Techniques and Procedures,* W.H. Green, St. Louis, 10.

Willert, H.-G. and Semlitsch, M. (1977) Reactions of the articular capsule to wear products of artificial joint prostheses. *J. Biomed. Mat. Res.,* **11**, 157.

Willey, D. E., Williams, I., Faucett, C. and Openshaw, H. (1991) Ocular acyclovir delivery by collagen discs: a mouse model to screen anti-viral agents. *Current Eye Research*, **10**, 167.

Williams, D.F. (1987a) Blood physiology and biochemistry: Hemostasis and thrombosis, in *Blood Compatibility*, Vol. I, (ed. D.F. Williams) CRC Press, Inc., Boca Raton, Fl, Chs 2,6.

Williams, I.F., McCullagh, K.G. and Silver, I.A. (1984) The distribution of Types I and III collagen and fibronectin in the healing equine tendon. *Connec. Tissue Res.*, **12**, 211.

Williams, J.E. (1972) Experiences with a large series of Silastic breast implants. *Plast. Reconstr. Surg.*, **49**, 253.

Winter, G.D. (1962) Formation of the scab and rate of epithelialization of superficial wounds in the skin of the young domestic pig. *Nature*, **193**, 293.

Wixon, R.L., Lautenschlager, E.P. and Novak, M. (1985) Vacuum mixing of methylmethacrylate bone cement. *Trans. Orthop. Res. Soc.*, 31st Annual Meeting, Las Vegas, 325.

Wong, E., Christiansen, D., Rizvi, A., Geller, H. and Silver, F.H. (1990) A method for preparation of etched collagen fibers that support neurite outgrowth. *J. Applied Biomaterials*, **1**, 225.

Woo, S.L.-Y. and Adams, D.J. (1990) Tensile properties of human ACL and ACL graft tissues, in *Knee Ligaments, Structure, Function, Injury and Repair*, (eds D. Daniel, W. Akeson and J. O'Connor), Raven Press, NY, pp. 279–89.

Woo, S.L.-Y., Inoue, M., McGurk-Burleson, E. and Gomez, M.A. (1987) Treatment of medial collateral ligament injury; II: structure and function of canine knees in response to differing treatment regimens. *Am. J. Sports Med.*, **115**, 22.

Woo, S.L.-Y., Orlando, C.A., Camp, J.F. and Akeson, W.H. (1986) Effects of postmortem storage by freezing on ligament tensile behavior. *J. Biomechanics*, **19**, 399.

Woodley, D.T., Peterson, H.D., Herzog, S.R., Stricklin, G.P., Burgeson, R.E., Briggaman, R.A., Cronce, D.J. and O'Keefe, E.J. (1988) Burn wounds resurfaced by cultured epidermal autografts show abnormal reconstitution of anchoring fibrils. *JAMA*, **258**, 2566.

Worst, P.K.M., Valentine, E.A. and Fusenig, N.E. (1974) Formation of epidermis after reimplantation of pure primary epidermal cell cultures from perinatal mouse skin. *J. Nat. Cancer Institute*, **53**, 1061.

Wroble, R.R., Grood, E.S., Noyes, F.R. and Schmitt, D.J. (1990) Reproducibility of Genucom knee analysis system testing. *Am. J. Sports Med.*, **18**, 387.

Wroble, R.R., Van Ginkel, L.A., Grood, E.S., Noyes, F.R. and Shaffer, B.L. (1990a) Repeatability of the KT-1000 arthrometer in a normal population, *Am. J. Sports Med.*, **18**, 396.

Yaffee, A., Ehrlich, J. and Shoshan, S. (1982) One-year follow up for the use of collagen for biological anchoring of acrylic dental roots in the dog. *Archs Oral Biol.*, **27**, 999.

Yahia, L.-H. and Drouin, G. (1989) Microscopical investigation of canine anterior cruciate ligament and patellar tendon: Collagen fascicle morphology and architecture. *J. Orthop. Res.*, **7**, 243.

Yamada, H. (1970) in *Strength of Biological Materials,* (ed. F.G. Evans), Williams and Wilkins, Baltimore, 239.

Yamaguchi, T. and Katake, K. (1960) Study on strength of auricular cartilages of men and animals. *J. Kyoto Pref. Med. Univ.*, **67**, 420.

Yanachi, T. and Yamaguchi, T. (1990) Temporary network formation of hyaluronate under a physiological condition. 1. Molecular-weight dependence. *Biopolymers,* **30**, 415–25.

Yannas, I.V. (1981) Use of artificial skin in wound management, in *The Surgical Wound,* (eds P. Dineen and G. Hildick-Smith), Lea & Febiger, Philadelphia, Pa., 171.

Yannas, I.V. and Burke, J.F. (1980) Design of an artificial skin. I. Basic design principles. *J. Biomed. Mat. Res.*, **14**, 65.

Yannas, I.V., and Orgill, D.P. (1986) Artificial skin: A fifth route to organ repair and replacement in *Polymeric Biomaterials,* (eds E. Piskin and A.S. Hoffman), Martinus Nijhoff Publishers: Dordrecht.

Yannas, I.V., Burke, J.F., Gordon, P.L., Huang, C. and Rubenstein, R.H. (1980) Design of an artificial skin. II. Control of chemical composition. *J. Biomed. Mat. Res.*, **14**, 65.

Yannas, I.V., Burke, J.F., Orgill, D.P. and Skrabut, E.M. (1981) Wound tissue can utilize a polymeric template to synthesize a functional extension of skin. *Science,* **215**, 174.

Zarins, B. and Adams, M. (1988) Medical progress: knee injuries in sports. *New England J. Medicine,* **318**, 950.

Zarins, C.K. and Glagov, S. (1987) Pathophysiology of human atherosclerosis, in *Vascular Surgery,* (eds S.E. Wilson, F.J. Veith, R.W. Hobson and R.A. Williams) McGraw-Hill, NY.

Index

A
Annealing (heat treatment)   16
Anodization   17
Aorta
   aneurysm   181
   aortic valves   154
   mechanical properties   168–170
   replacement   183–187
   structure   153, 154
Artificial skin   80, 90
Atherosclerosis   153, 181

B
Biological grafts
   bone   211, 212
   cartilage   207
Blood compatibility   28
Blood coagulation   64
Bone structure   93, 198
   mechanical properties   5
Brazing   16
Breast implants   240
   complications   247
Burn injury   2, 66, 70, 84, 87

C
Carbons   22, 24
Carburization   18
Carcinogenicity   28
Cartilage structure   195
   mechanical properties   202
Cell culture   80
Cell cytoxicity   27
Cellulose acetate   146
Ceramics   5, 22

Chondroitin sulphate   128, 132, 150
Class I device   1
Class II device   1
Class III device   1
Cobalt-like alloys   12, 20
Collagen   136
   dental implants   232
   eye shields   148
   fibers   51
   tendon   96
   viscoelastic   128, 136
   wound dressings   79
Composites   24
Contact lens   145

D
Dental implants   12
   cements   229
   denture base resins   225
   impression materials   222
   restorative resins   225
Device   1
Drawing   16

E
Elastin   51, 55
Electroplating   17
Eye   120
   cornea   124
   lens   125
   sclera   124
   structure   121–122
   vitreous body   125

F
Facial implants   194, 213

302 Index

Facial implants *contd*
  injectable 214
  mesh 219
  solid 27
FDA
  Federal Food, Drug and Cosmetic Act 38
  good manufacturing practices 41
  510(k) 40, 252
  investigational device exemption 42
  Medical Device Amendments 1, 39
  medical device reporting 42
  performance standards 44
  PMA 41, 257
  Safe Medical Device Act 43

G
Graft
  allo- 31
  auto- 31
  rejection 34–36
  xeno- 31
Grinding 18

H
Hard tissue 4
Heart valves 12
Hemolysis 28
Hyaluronan (hydaluronate or hyaluronic acid) 57, 130, 150
Hydroxyapatite 5, 22, 23
Hydroxypropylmethylcellulose 128, 131

I
Immune response
  cell mediated 32
  humoral 32
  mixed leukocyte reaction 32
  suppression 37
Implantation 127
Inflammation 64
Intracutaneous injection 28
Intraocular lens 143

J
Joint, components 12
  biological response 117
  degenerative joint disease 113
  replacement 113
    total hip 114
    total knee 115

L
Ligament 93
  anterior cruciate 95
  clinical evaluation 105
  posterior cruciate 95
  replacements 107–111
  rupture 107
Long-term implantation 28

M
Machining 16
Major histocompatibility complex 29
  alpha chain 29
  beta chain 30
  class I products 29
  class II products 29
  human leukocyte antigens 30
Markets 2
Mechanical properties
  ligaments 100
  ocular tissues 125
  skin 57–62
Medical Device Amendments 1, 39
Menisci 93
Mucous membrane irritation 28
Mutagenicity 28

N
Nylon 143

P
Passivation 18
Plasticizers 10
Polishing 18
Polyacrylamide 128, 136
Poly(dimethyl siloxane) 8
  (see silicone)
Polydispersity index 10
Poly(ethylene) 8, 143, 150
  facial implants 218
Poly(ethylene terephthalate) 8, 184
Poly(hydroxyethylacrylate) 143
Polymerization 6

Polymers 5, 6, 8
   sterilization 11
Poly(methyl methacrylate) 8, 143, 145
Poly(propylene) 145
Poly(tetrafluoroethylene) 184
   facial implants 218
Poly(urethane) 8
   breast implants 243
Precipitation hardening 17
Pre-clinical testing 25
   safety testing 26
Proteoglycans 54, 56, 99
Pyrogenicity 29

Q
Quenching 16, 17

R
Rejection
   cellular 31
   first set 31
   graft 34, 36
   second set 32
Rheology 137

S
Sand blasting 18
Sensitization 28
Silicone 143, 146, 150
   breast implants 242
   facial implants 217
   injectable 213, 214
Skin 46
   basement membrane 53
   dermis 46, 54
   epidermis 46
   extracellular components 52
   intracellular components 52
   keratinocytes 52
   keratins 52
   mechanical properties 57, 60, 61
   papillary layer 48
   repair 62–66
   reticular dermis 48
   ulcers 66, 68–70, 73, 79, 84
Skin irritation 27
   excision 66
Soft tissue 4
Steel 12
   austenitic 18
   ferritic 18
   martensitic 18
Surface alloying 18
Systemic injection 28

T
Tempering 17
Tendon 92
Tissue engineering 82
Titanium 12

V
Vessel wall structure 158
   mechanical properties 170
   replacement 187
Viscoelastics 126, 137
   long-term effects 140
   optimum properties 127

W
Welding 16
Wound dressings 73
   barrier dressings 74
   biodegradable dermal
      substitutes 78
   biological dressings 76
Wound healing 64
   cardiovascular 179
   corneal 126
   facial 204
   granulation 64
   ligament 103
   remodelling 64

Printed in the United States
1289800001BC/12